# Gastrointestinal system

Series Editor

**Daniel Horton-Szar**
BSc (Hons), MBBS (Hons)
Northgate Medical Practice
Canterbury
Kent, UK

Faculty Advisor

**Martin Lombard**
Consultant Gastroenterologist
Royal Liverpool University
Hospital
Liverpool, UK

**Rusheng Chew** BMedSci (Hons)
School of Clinical Medicine
University of Cambridge
Cambridge
UK

MOSBY

Edinburgh • London • New York • Oxford • Philadelphia • St Louis • Sydney • Toronto 2008 ELSEVIER

# MOSBY
## ELSEVIER

| | |
|---|---|
| Commissioning Editor: | Fiona Conn, Alison Taylor |
| Development Editor: | Lulu Stader |
| Project Manager: | Andrew Palfreyman |
| Design Direction: | Sarah Russell |
| Illustrations Manager: | Merlyn Harvey |
| Illustrator: | Cactus |

First edition 1998
Second edition 2002
Reprinted 2003 (twice), 2005
Third edition 2008
Reprinted 2009

ISBN: 9780723434207

**British Library Cataloguing in Publication Data**
A catalogue record for this book is available from the British Library

**Library of Congress Cataloging in Publication Data**
A catalog record for this book is available from the Library of Congress

**Note**
Neither the publisher nor the authors assume any responsibility for any loss or injury and/or damage to persons or property arising out of or related to any use of the material contained in this book. It is the responsibility of the treating practitioner, relying on independent expertise and knowledge of the patient, to determine the best treatment and method of application for the patient.
The Publisher

Printed in China

Medical education is changing. As medical science develops by leaps and bounds there is less emphasis on acquisition of knowledge for its own sake, and more on building a strong conceptual foundation on which to base further study of the subject.

In line with this, many medical curricula are now clinically focussed even from the early stages, with the basic science subject matter closely related with clinical applications. Nevertheless, this does not necessitate the 'dumbing-down' of the scientific knowledge base, as a firm grasp of basic science facilitates a proper understanding of mechanisms of disease and thus clinical study. This is especially true of the gastrointestinal system, given the anatomical and physiological variation along its length and its susceptibility to many different disease processes.

This book, therefore, was written with the goal of being a concise, easy-to-read text which yet provides a comprehensive coverage of gastrointestinal anatomy, physiology, biochemistry and pathology heavily integrated with clinically relevant material. It is not intended for use as a textbook of clinical gastroenterology. Like its predecessors, it is targeted towards the overburdened medical student, hence the continued emphasis on the essentials while still maintaining the level of detail required for those who aim for distinction.

Opinions of students and teachers alike have been taken into account when planning this edition. There is increased emphasis on pre-clinical knowledge central to practice in later years, such as clinical pharmacology, and a vigorous subscription to the clinician's adage that "common things occur commonly" when considering clinical information for inclusion. While maintaining the structure from its successful previous editions, a number of chapters have been reorganized, adding and omitting material where needed, to ensure a more streamlined and focussed presentation of information, and there is an all-new self-assessment section testing core material.

To the reader, I hope that this book will be a useful resource, whether for primary learning or revision, whatever type of medical course you are on. More importantly, I hope that it helps in your understanding of the biomedical and clinical scientific principles pertinent to this important organ system.

**Rusheng Chew**

More than a decade has now passed since work began on the first editions of the Crash Course series, and over four years since the publication of the second editions. Medicine never stands still, and the work of keeping this series relevant for today's students is an ongoing process. These third editions build upon the success of the preceding books and incorporate a great deal of new and revised material, keeping the series up to date with the latest medical research and developments in pharmacology and current best practice.

As always, we listen to feedback from the thousands of students who use Crash Course and have made further improvements to the layout and structure of the books. Each chapter now starts with a set of learning objectives, and the self-assessment sections have been enhanced and brought up to date with modern exam formats. We have also worked to integrate points of clinical relevance into the basic medical science material, which will not only add to the interest of the text but will reinforce the principles being described.

In this age of information technology, a series of revision books would not be complete without extensive web-based resources to support students as they learn. With the third editions of Crash Course, that is exactly what we have created: all titles will be enhanced with valuable online material and self-assessment questions.

But still, we hold fast to the principles on which we first developed the series: Crash Course will always bring you all the information you need to revise in compact, manageable volumes that integrate basic medical science and clinical practice. The books still maintain the balance between clarity and conciseness, and providing sufficient depth for those aiming at distinction. The authors are medical students and junior doctors who have recent experience of the exams you are now facing, and the accuracy of the material is checked by senior faculty members from across the UK.

I wish you all the best for your future careers!

**Dr Dan Horton-Szar**
**Series Editor (Basic Medical Sciences)**

Two people deserve exceptional mention for their role in bringing the 3rd edition of this book to fruition. The first is Martin Lombard, faculty advisor, whose knowledge of the gastrointestinal system and general medicine has helped maintain the goal of a textbook with a close relationship between basic and clinical sciences sharply in focus.

Secondly, Lulu Stader, development editor, who managed to keep the production process running smoothly with her dedication and attention to detail, and without whose guidance the early stages would have been much more difficult.

To Martin and Lulu, thank you for all your help and for making the writing of this book a fun and worthwhile undertaking.

My thanks also to Andrew Miller, former commissioning editor, who considered me capable enough for the privilege of authorship.

## Figure acknowledgements

Figs 3.6, 3.13, 3.14 and 5.6 adapted with permission from L Johnson. Gastrointestinal Physiology, 6th edition. Mosby, 2000

Fig. 3.15 redrawn with permission from General and Systematic Pathology, edited by JCE Underwood. Churchill Livingstone, 1992

Fig 4.4 redrawn with permission from J O'Grady, J Lake and P Howdle. Comprehensive Clinical Hepatology. Mosby, 2000

Fig. 4.12 redrawn with permission from A Gaw, R Cowan, D O'Reilly, M Stewart and J Sheperd. Clinical Biochemistry, 2nd edition. Churchill Livingstone, 1999

Fig. 4.15 adapted with permission from HP Rang, M Dale and JM Ritter. Pharmacology, 4th edition. Churchill Livingstone, 1999

Fig. 4.20 redrawn with permission from General and Systematic Pathology, 2nd edition, edited by JCE Underwood. Churchill Livingstone, 1996

Fig. 4.25 redrawn with permission from PJ Kumar and ML Clarke. Clinical Medicine, 3rd edition. Bailliere Tindall, 1994

Figs 4.30 and 4.31 reproduced with permission from L Friedman and EB Keefe. Handbook of Liver Disease. Churchill Livingstone, 1997

Fig 5.5 reproduced with permission from A Stevens and J Lowe. Human Histology, 2nd edition. Mosby, 1997

Figs 5.11, 7.16, 8.3, 8.14, 10.4 and 10.5 redrawn and reproduced with permission from Davidson's Principles and Practice of Medicine, 18th edition, edited by C Haslett. Churchill Livingstone, 1999

Fig. 6.18 redrawn with permission from RM Berne and MN Levy. Principles of Physiology, 3rd edition. Mosby, 2000

Fig 9.2 reproduced with permission from AD Cameron. Crash Course: Psychiatry, 2nd edition. Mosby, 2004

Fig 10.3 reproduced with permission from C Fox and M Lombard. Crash Course: Gastroenterology, 2nd edition. Mosby, 2004

Figs 10.7 and 10.8 reproduced courtesy of Dr A Grundy

Fig. 10.9 reproduced courtesy of Dr J Pilcher

*To my family, for all their love and support.*

## Contents

# BASIC MEDICAL SCIENCE OF THE GASTROINTESTINAL SYSTEM

# Introduction to the gastrointestinal system

## Learning objectives

After reading this chapter, you should be able to:

- Outline and reproduce the basic structure of the gastrointestinal system.
- Describe the functions of the gastrointestinal system.
- Name the major food groups and their roles.
- Describe the embryological development of the gastrointestinal tract.

## ANATOMICAL OVERVIEW

The gastrointestinal (GI) system (Fig. 1.1) develops entirely from the endoderm in the embryo. Anatomically, it is essentially a muscular tube which maintains the same basic structure throughout its length (Fig. 1.2). From the innermost to the outermost, the layers which comprise the basic structure are the mucosa (which comprises the epithelial layer, lamina propria and muscularis mucosae), submucosa, two smooth muscle layers (the outer being longitudinal and the inner circular) and the adventitia or serosa. There are also intrinsic submucosal (Meissner's) and

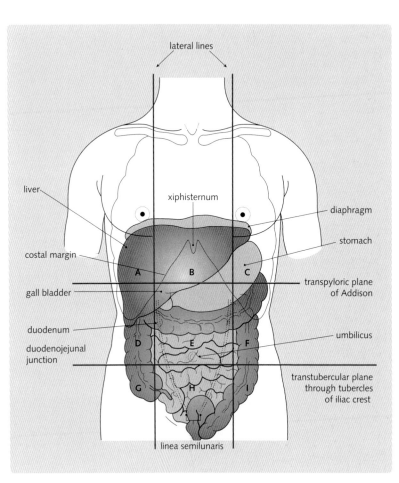

Fig. 1.1 Anatomy of the gastrointestinal tract, showing its surface markings. The transpyloric plane (of Addison) passes midway between the jugular notch and the symphysis pubis, and midway between the xiphisternum and the umbilicus. It passes through the pylorus, the neck of the pancreas, the duodenojejunal flexure and the hila of the kidneys. Surface regions: A = right hypochondriac; B = epigastric; C = left hypochondriac; D = right lumbar; E = umbilical; F = left lumbar; G = right iliac fossa; H = hypogastric; I = left iliac fossa.

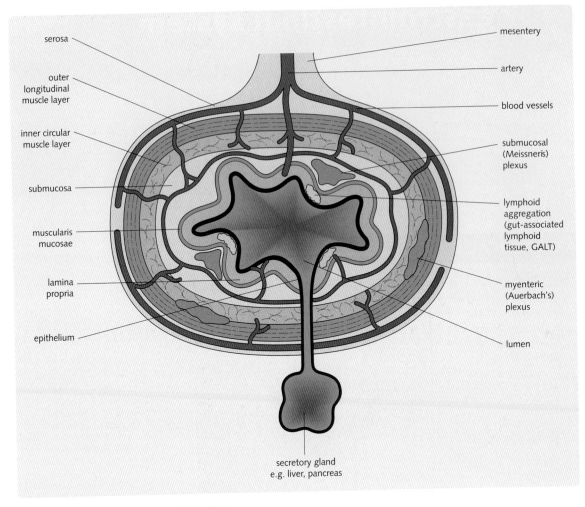

**Fig. 1.2** The basic structure of the gastrointestinal tract.

mucosal (Auerbach's) nerve plexuses, the activity of which is moderated by extrinsic innervation and hormones.

It is essential to know the basic structure of the GI tract and the order of the layers; MCQs often test this.

Food is moved through the tract by gravity, voluntary muscular action (in the oral cavity to the upper third of the oesophagus) and peristalsis (a wavelike movement involving the coordinated contraction of muscle in one area and relaxation in the next; see Chapter 6). A series of sphincters prevent any reflux, or backflow of food (Fig. 1.3).

Among other factors, the integrity of the lower oesophageal sphincter protects against reflux of acid contents from the stomach (gastro-oesophageal reflux disease, or GORD). If reflux is extensive, oesophagitis, Barrett's oesophagus (a condition which predisposes to carcinoma) or oesophageal stricture may result.

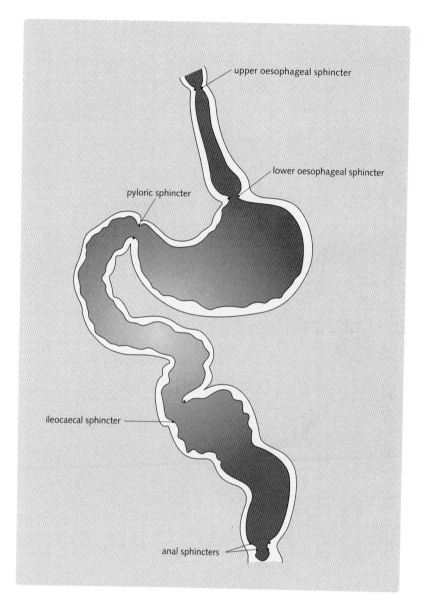

**Fig. 1.3** Sphincters of the gastrointestinal tract.

upper oesophageal sphincter

lower oesophageal sphincter

pyloric sphincter

ileocaecal sphincter

anal sphincters

# FUNCTIONS OF THE GASTROINTESTINAL TRACT

The main functions of the alimentary tract can be summarized as motility, secretion, digestion and absorption. For a complete list of its functions see Fig. 1.4.

Motility refers to the muscular contractions which cause the propulsion and mixing of gut contents. There is a constant pressure maintained on the contents of the GI tract by the tone of the smooth muscle layers and, superimposed on that, propulsive movements (peristalsis) as well as the mixing movements occur. In addition, sympathetic and parasympathetic reflexes occurring in different parts of the tract act through hormonal and neuronal mechanisms to modify the speed of food movement through the tract. The contents move through the tract at a rate at which they can be processed.

The other three principal functions are closely related. Secretory glands release digestive juices into the gut lumen. These juices contain enzymes which break up complex food structures into smaller absorbable units by hydrolysis, i.e. digestion. Following this, the products of digestion are absorbed into

**Fig. 1.4** A summary of the functions of the gastrointestinal tract. (UOS = upper oesophageal sphincter.)

| Function | Mechanism/process involved | Where it occurs |
|---|---|---|
| Digestion of food | i) Mastication | Mouth: with teeth and tongue |
| | ii) Swallowing | Oropharynx: relaxation of UOS |
| | iii) Mixing | Stomach and small intestine |
| | iv) Enzymatic digestion | Stomach and small intestine |
| | v) Absorption | Stomach, small intestine and large intestine |
| Motility | i) Peristalsis | Throughout gut |
| | ii) Mass movement | Throughout gut |
| Storage of food waste | | Stomach, sigmoid colon and rectum |
| Excretion | Defecation | Rectum and anus |
| Exocrine secretions | i) Mucus/saliva secretion | Salivary gland |
| | ii) HCl/pepsin/mucus secretion | Gastric glands of stomach |
| | iii) $HCO_3$/amylase/lipase secretion | Pancreas |
| | iv) Bile salt secretion | Liver |
| Endocrine secretions | i) Gastrin secretion | Stomach |
| | ii) Secretin secretion | Duodenal mucosa |
| | iii) Insulin secretion | Pancreas |
| Paracrine secretions | Somatostatin secretion | Mucosa |
| Defence | i) Smell, sight, taste | Oral cavity, cephalic region |
| | ii) Gastric acid secretion | Stomach |
| | iii) Vomit reflex | Stomach up to mouth |
| | iv) Gut flora | Throughout gut |
| | v) Mucus secretion | Throughout gut |
| | vi) Immune response | Peyer's patches, macrophages in mucosa |
| | vii) Secretion of IgA | Mucosal secretions |

the blood or lymph from the gut lumen. Absorption happens mainly in the small intestine.

Other functions related to the digestive process include:

- Storage of waste material in the sigmoid colon and rectum.
- Exocrine, endocrine and paracrine secretions are all involved in active digestion and the control of digestion and motility in the gut.
- Some GI peptide hormones have local and systemic effects.
- Excretion of waste products.

Although it is an internal structure, the GI tract is not sterile as it is open to the external environment. It is thus presented with a number of challenges on a daily basis, from harmful bacteria to toxic substances and so requires good defence mechanisms:

- *Sight, smell and taste* often alert us to the fact that food is contaminated. The vomit reflex exists to eject harmful material.
- *The acid in the stomach* kills most of the bacteria ingested with food.
- *The natural bacterial flora* of the gut prevent colonization by potentially harmful bacteria and can also aid digestion of food.
- *Aggregations of lymphoid tissue* (part of the immune system) are present in the walls of the gut, known as Peyer's patches. These can mount an immune response to antigens found in the diet.

# FOOD GROUPS

Food is a source of energy, minerals and vitamins. The body requires these for growth, maintenance and repair. The key food groups are carbohydrates, fat and protein, which are oxidized to generate high-energy bonds in adenosine triphosphate (ATP) and to provide materials for building new tissues.

Nevertheless, overeating is a major cause of morbidity. This is because excess food, which is stored as fat, leads to obesity and associated diseases such as ischaemic heart disease and type 2 diabetes.

Conversely, an average 70 kg man may survive for 5–6 weeks on body fat stores when deprived of food, provided he is able to drink water. Blood glucose levels drop during the initial few days, then rise and stabilize. During prolonged fasting, the body will also break down muscle, including heart muscle, to provide energy. This may lead to death from cardiac failure. However, most food-deprived people do not die from starvation directly, but from the inability to fight off infectious diseases.

A description of the major food groups follows, and Fig. 1.5 provides a summary. For a more comprehensive account of the food groups and the metabolic processes involved in starvation and overeating, see *Crash Course: Metabolism and Nutrition*.

## Carbohydrate

Carbohydrates are the main energy source in, and therefore the main constituent of, most diets. They provide 17 kJ (4 kCal) of energy per gram. Most dietary carbohydrate is in the form of polysaccharides, which consist of chains of glucose molecules. The principal ingested polysaccharides are starch, which is derived from plant sources, and glycogen from animal sources.

Other sources of carbohydrate are monosaccharides (glucose, fructose and galactose) and disaccharides (sucrose and lactose). Cellulose is an indigestible polysaccharide and is considered in the section on dietary fibre.

Carbohydrates are a cheap form of food, and so are easily taken in excess, often limiting the intake of other food constituents.

## Protein

Protein is composed of amino acids linked by peptide bonds. Nine amino acids are essential for protein synthesis and nitrogen balance; the other necessary amino acids can be manufactured *de novo* in the body. Protein is required for tissue growth and repair. Meat is the principal source of protein, especially in the developed world.

We need 0.75 g of protein per kilogram of body weight per day, but in developed countries most people exceed this. In developing countries, however, where protein from animal sources is less readily available, combinations of certain foods can provide enough of the essential amino acids even though those foods, on their own, are low in some amino acids. A good example of a non-animal

**Fig. 1.5** A summary of the dietary food groups.

| Food group | | Source | Site of digestion | Function |
|---|---|---|---|---|
| Carbohydrates | | Sugary foods, potatoes, pasta etc. | Mouth and small intestine | Energy source |
| Fats | | Meats, oil, butter etc. | Small intestine | Energy source |
| Protein | | Meat, pulses etc. | Stomach and small intestine | Synthesis and repair of tissues |
| Vitamins | Fat-soluble (A, D, E, K) | Meat, fish and vegetable oils | Not digested | Maintenance of general health |
| | Water-soluble (B, C) | Milk, meat, fruit and vegetables | Not digested | |
| Minerals | | Meat, milk, vegetables, cereals | Not digested | Maintenance of general health |
| Fibre | | Plant foods | Not digested | Bulking agent, aids gut motility |

protein source which is high in essential amino acids is soybeans.

Proteins provide about the same amount of energy per gram as carbohydrates, but are not as easily utilized under normal circumstances.

## Fat

Dietary fat is chiefly composed of triglycerides (esters of free fatty acids and glycerol, which may be saturated, monounsaturated or polyunsaturated). The essential fatty acids are linoleic acid and α-linoleic acid, which cannot be manufactured and so must be obtained from our diet.

The body is efficient at manufacturing fats (triglycerides, sterols and phospholipids) and will lay down subcutaneous fat stores even on low-fat diets.

Dietary fat provides 37 kJ (9 kcal) of energy per gram. Nevertheless, due to its ill-effects when taken in excess, fats should comprise less than 35% of the total energy intake.

## Water

Fluid intake and oxidation of food provides water for the body. About 1 L of water is needed per day to balance insensible losses such as sweating, metabolism and exhalation of water vapour (more water is required in hot climates). Excess water is excreted in the urine by the kidneys; inadequate intake leads to dehydration.

Water is also needed for digestion, as digestion involves enzymatic hydrolysis of the bonds linking the smaller units which make up complex food structures.

## Minerals

These are chemicals that must be present in the diet to maintain good health; over 20 have so far been identified, e.g. iron and calcium.

Trace elements (e.g. zinc, copper and iodine) are substances that, by definition, are present in the body in low concentrations (less than 100 parts per million) and include some minerals. It is not yet known whether all trace elements are essential for health.

## Vitamins

Vitamins are classified as fat soluble or water soluble; vitamins A, D, E and K are fat soluble, the other vitamins are water soluble.

Fat-soluble vitamins are stored in fatty tissue in the body (mainly in the liver) and are not usually excreted in the urine. It is thus possible to have an excess of these vitamins, which may be toxic, e.g. vitamin A poisoning. On the other hand, absorption of fat-soluble vitamins is dependent upon the absorption of dietary fat: deficiency can occur in cases of fat malabsorption (see Chapter 6).

Body stores of water-soluble vitamins (other than vitamin $B_{12}$) are smaller than stores of fat-soluble vitamins. They are excreted in the urine and deficiencies of water-soluble vitamins are more common.

## Dietary fibre

Dietary fibre consists of indigestible carbohydrates, primarily cellulose but also lignin and pectin. Cellulose cannot be digested as we do not have the enzymes necessary to hydrolyse the β-glycosidic bonds linking its glucose molecules, unlike starch where the glucose residues are linked by α-glycosidic bonds.

Although it does not provide energy, fibre adds bulk to the bowel contents and increases gut motility, thus preventing constipation. It also decreases absorption of toxic compounds, e.g. some carcinogens, due to its binding properties.

## DEVELOPMENT OF THE GASTROINTESTINAL TRACT

The gastrointestinal tract is the main organ system derived from the endodermal germ layer. The formation of the tube is largely passive; it depends on the cephalocaudal and lateral folding of the embryo.

The yolk sac produces blood cells and vessels, and is the site of haematopoiesis for the first 2 months from conception. Later, it becomes inverted and incorporated into the body cavity. The folding of the embryo constricts the initial communication between the embryo and the yolk sac.

The remnant of this communication is the vitelline duct, which normally disappears in utero. Where it persists, it is known as a Meckel's diverticulum.

The gut tube divides into foregut, midgut and hindgut. Their blood supply is from the coeliac trunk, superior mesenteric artery and inferior mesenteric artery respectively (Fig. 1.6). All derivatives from each division of the gut tube will thus have the

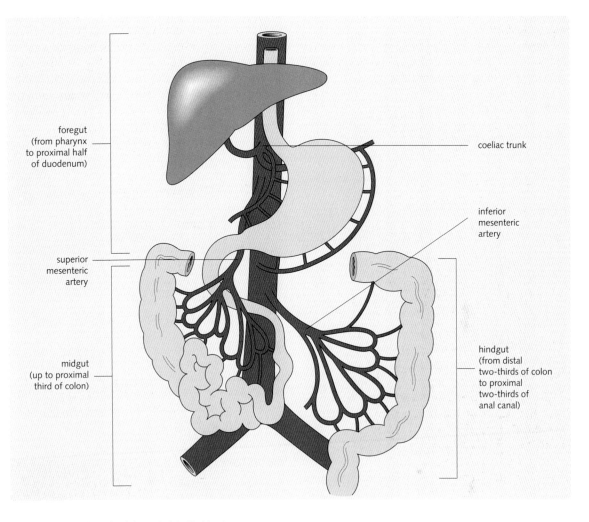

foregut
(from pharynx
to proximal half
of duodenum)

coeliac trunk

inferior
mesenteric
artery

superior
mesenteric
artery

midgut
(up to proximal
third of colon)

hindgut
(from distal
two-thirds of colon
to proximal
two-thirds of
anal canal)

**Fig. 1.6** The arterial supply of the gastrointestinal tract.

same principal blood supply. The superior mesenteric artery is in the umbilicus.

The nerve supply of the foregut and midgut is from the vagus nerve (Xth cranial nerve), while the hindgut gets its nerve supply from the pelvic splanchnic nerves.

The gut tube starts straight but twists during development and the midgut grows rapidly, with the developing liver occupying most of the space. As development progresses, there is not enough room in the fetal abdomen to accommodate the rapidly developing gut because of the large size of the liver and the two sets of kidneys. The midgut therefore herniates into the umbilical cord between weeks 7 and 11 of gestation, continuing its development outside the abdominal cavity.

In the umbilical cord, the midgut undergoes a clockwise rotation of 180° around the axis of the superior mesenteric artery and what was the inferior limb becomes the superior limb (and vice versa). At the same time, it elongates to form the loops of the jejunum and ileum.

During the 11th week, the midgut returns into the abdomen, the process being known as the reduction of the physiological midgut hernia. The reason for this is not well-explained, but is possibly due to the reduction in size of the liver and kidneys as well as the enlargement of the abdomen. The part forming the small intestine returns first to occupy the central part of the abdomen. The part forming the large intestine undergoes a 270° anticlockwise rotation as it returns so that the caecum lies under the liver. The tube then elongates again so that the caecum points downwards.

The falciform ligament lies in front of the liver and the lesser omentum lies behind the liver. The liver and pancreas develop from endodermal diverticula that bud off the duodenum in weeks 4–6 (see Fig. 4.5).

Much of the mouth (including the muscles of mastication and tongue) and the oesophagus develop from the branchial arches, of which there are six, the first four being well-defined while the fifth and sixth are rudimentary.

The muscles of mastication, mylohyoid and anterior belly of digastric develop from the first (mandibular) arch, supplied by the trigeminal nerve (Vth cranial nerve).

The anterior two thirds of the tongue develop from three mesenchymal buds from the first pair of branchial arches. The posterior belly of digastric develops from the second arch, supplied by the facial nerve (VIIth cranial nerve).

Stylopharyngeus develops from the third arch, supplied by the glossopharyngeal nerve (IXth cranial nerve).

Cricothyroid, the constrictors of the pharynx and the striated muscles of oesophagus develop from the fourth and sixth arches, supplied by branches of the vagus nerve. The fifth arch is often absent. These developmental stages are shown in Fig. 1.7.

> The embryological development of the GI tract is a common essay question in exams – make sure you know the key stages, as well as the blood supply to the gut divisions and the developments during the herniation of the midgut.

A summary of the major congenital abnormalities affecting the gastrointestinal tract is given in Fig. 1.8. These will be discussed in more depth in the relevant chapters.

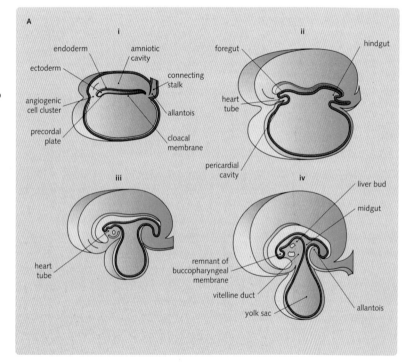

**Fig. 1.7** Stages of embryonic development of the gastrointestinal tract. (A) Schematic drawings of sagittal sections through embryos at various stages of development, showing the development of the foregut, midgut and hindgut. i. Presomite embryo. ii. 7-somite embryo. iii. 14-somite embryo. iv. Embryo at 1 month.

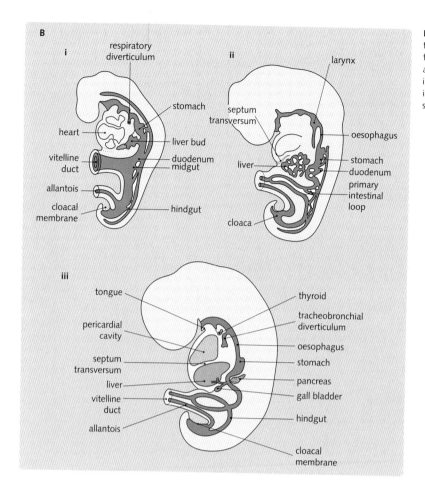

**Fig. 1.7** (B) Schematic drawings showing the primitive gastrointestinal tract and formation of the liver. i. Diagram showing a 3 mm embryo (approx 25 days). ii. Embryo at 32 days (5 mm). iii. Diagram of a 9 mm embryo (36 days) showing caudal expansion of the liver.

**Fig. 1.8** Major developmental abnormalities of the gastrointestinal system.

| Organ | Abnormality | Description |
|---|---|---|
| Mouth and oropharynx | Cleft lip | Incomplete fusion of maxillary and medial nasal prominences |
| | Cleft palate | Incomplete fusion of palatine shelves |
| Oesophagus | Oesophageal atresia | Failure of growth of oesophageal endoderm |
| Stomach | Hypertrophic pyloric stenosis | Hypertrophy of pyloric circular smooth muscle |
| Pancreas | Annular pancreas | Abnormal migration of pancreatic buds |
| | Pancreas divisum | Failure of fusion of pancreatic buds |
| Intestine | Meckel's diverticulum | Remnant of vitelline duct |
| | Exomphalos | Failure of intestine to return after herniation |
| | Gastroschisis | Herniation of bowel through abdominal wall |

# gastrointestinal tract

## Learning objectives

After reading this chapter, you should be able to:

- List the components of the upper gastrointestinal tract.
- Outline the embryological development of the structures making up the upper gastrointestinal tract.
- Describe the anatomy and histological structure of the tongue.
- Describe the anatomy and histological structure of the salivary glands.
- Outline and reproduce the structure of a salivon.
- Describe the anatomy of the pharynx.
- Describe the anatomy and histological structure of the oesophagus, and relate structure to function.
- List the factors which affect appetite.
- List the functions of saliva, and understand the factors which control the rate of salivation.
- Describe the mechanism of swallowing.
- Outline the factors which cause vomiting.
- Outline the following types of disorders of the upper gastrointestinal tract: congenital abnormalities, infections and inflammatory disease, vascular disease and neoplastic disease.

## OVERVIEW

The upper gastrointestinal tract starts at the mouth and ends at the termination of the oesophagus. Associated structures include the tongue and salivary glands. Ingestion and the initial breaking up of food occurs in the mouth, following which the resulting food boluses are swallowed and enter the oesophagus. This is helped by the action of the tongue and pharyngeal muscles, as well as saliva secreted by the salivary glands.

## FUNCTIONS AND PHYSIOLOGY

### Food intake and its control

The control of food intake is complex and the hypothalamus plays an important role.

Young people burn off excess intake as heat and through physical activity. They maintain a relatively constant weight, but this ability reduces with age, leading to middle-aged spread.

Our genetics have a huge influence on feeding and can account for up to 70% of the difference in body mass index in later life.

### Signals which affect appetite

There are a number of factors that regulate appetite:

- *Blood glucose concentration* activates glucoreceptors in the hypothalamus, either acting to upregulate hunger when blood glucose levels fall, or upregulate satiety when blood glucose concentrations rise.
- *Amino acids* in food raise body temperature, resulting in starving people feeling cold, even in hot surroundings.
- *Fat ingestion* releases cholecystokinin (CCK), which slows stomach emptying, making us feel full. Injection of CCK into the hypothalamus inhibits appetite, suggesting a central as well as peripheral role.
- *Calcitonin*, a peptide hormone secreted by the thyroid gland, acts to reduce appetite.

13

- *Insulin* acts to upregulate appetite, but *glucagon* downregulates it.
- Deposition of fat may lead to control of appetite by neuronal and hormonal signals. *Leptin*, a protein secreted by white fat cells, acts on the leptin receptors in the hypothalamus. This is thought to be part of the main satiety centre in the brain. Leptin produces a feedback mechanism between adipose tissue and the brain, acting as a 'lipostat', thus controlling fat stores. Leptin inhibits neuropeptide Y, which is the most potent peptide to stimulate feeding.
- *Cold environments stimulate appetite*, whereas hot environments inhibit it.
- *Distension of a full stomach inhibits appetite, but contraction of an empty stomach stimulates it.* However, denervation of the stomach and intestines seems to have no effect on food intake.

## Central controls

The satiety centre is found in the ventromedial wall and the paraventricular nucleus of the hypothalamus. Stimulation of this inhibits food intake (aphagia), but lesions in this area may result in hyperphagia.

Glucostats in the brain measure the utilization of glucose. Diabetic patients feel hungry despite high blood glucose concentrations, because they lack insulin and, therefore, the cellular ability to take up glucose.

A feeding centre (not specific for hunger) is found in the lateral hypothalamus. Stimulation of this area increases eating and lesions here result in aphagia.

Other important central nervous system controls include opioids, somatostatin and growth hormone releasing hormone, all of which increase appetite. 5-hydroxytryptamine (5-HT, serotonin), dopamine and γ-aminobutyric acid (GABA) all decrease appetite.

## Cortical and limbic centres

Habit and conditioning play a role in controlling appetite.

## Diurnal variation

We principally metabolize carbohydrates during the day and fats at night. The hypothalamus is responsible for the switch between the two.

## Mastication

Mastication breaks up large food particles, mixing them with salivary secretions and aiding subsequent digestion. Molecules dissolve in salivary secretions and stimulate taste buds. Odours are released that activate the olfactory system, leading to the initiation of reflex salivation and gastric acid secretions.

The muscles of mastication (see later) cause movement of the mandible at the temporomandibular joint.

The digastric and mylohyoid muscles open the mouth, while the infrahyoid muscles stabilize the hyoid bone during mastication.

The teeth, gums, palate and tongue also play an important role, manipulating food and immobilizing it between the crushing surfaces of the teeth. The tongue then propels the bolus of food along the palate towards the pharynx, initiating the swallowing reflex.

## Salivation

The average rate of salivary secretion is 1–2 L per day. Saliva composition varies according to the rate and site of production, but the main components are water, proteins and electrolytes. Primary secretion from the acini produces an isotonic fluid that is modified in the ducts (Fig. 2.1).

### Control of salivary secretion

Secretion of saliva is under the control of the salivary centre in the medulla. Both the parasympathetic and sympathetic pathways are involved. Parasympathetic innervation causes an upregulation in secretion and sympathetic innervation causes a down regulation. Parasympathetic cholinergic stimulation produces a watery secretion, which is blocked by atropine. This is given before surgery to reduce the risk of aspiration of saliva.

Sympathetic adrenergic and noradrenergic stimulation produce thick mucoid secretions, which add to the dry mouth sensation during the fright–fight–flight response.

There is a baseline level of salivary secretion, which is about 0.5 mL/min and is due to ongoing low-level parasympathetic stimulation. This baseline secretion prevents the mouth and pharynx from drying out.

On top of the baseline, increases in salivary secretion occur reflexively. There are two types of salivary reflex: the simple reflex and the conditioned,

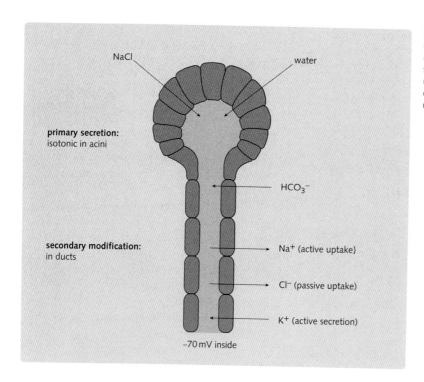

**Fig. 2.1** Secretion of saliva. The primary secretion is released into the blind-ending acini and the fluid then flows through a series of converging ducts for secondary modification, before entering the oral cavity. The parotid glands produce the most serous secretions.

or acquired, reflex. In the simple reflex, chemoreceptors in the mouth and oropharynx are activated by the presence and taste of food; for example, amyl nitrate and citric acid produce copious secretion, hence sucking on a lemon wedge increases the rate of secretion about tenfold.

In the conditioned reflex, no oral stimulation is needed. Thinking, smelling and seeing food causes salivation by activating the salivary centre via the cerebral cortex. The conditioned reflex is acquired in response to previous experience.

However salivation is initiated, the impulses to the salivary glands travel via the autonomic nerves (Fig. 2.2).

Denervation causes dribbling. This is known as Canon's law of denervation hypersensitivity. Normally receptors are localized at neuroeffector junctions, but, if nerves are cut, receptors spread all over the gland and it becomes excessively sensitive to circulating acetylcholine, producing copious amounts of saliva.

Chewing produces saliva secretion by stimulating receptors in the masticatory muscles and joints. Paradontal mechanoreceptors around the teeth can also stimulate saliva.

There are four main sites at which the sympathetic and parasympathetic nerves can act to modify saliva secretion:

- The acini producing the primary secretion.
- The ducts, which modify the secretions.

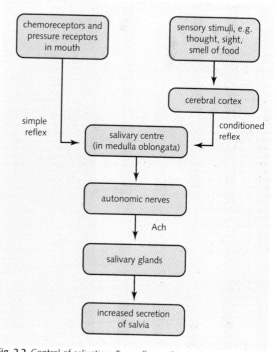

**Fig. 2.2** Control of salivation. Two reflexes, the simple reflex and the conditioned (acquired) reflex, increase salivation above the baseline level of around 0.5 mL/min.

- The blood vessels providing substances required for secretion and energy-containing nutrients, and removal of waste.
- The myoepithelial cells surrounding the ducts and acini.

## Salivary electrolytes

The major electrolytes found in saliva are $Na^+$, $K^+$, $Cl^-$ and $HCO_3^-$. The concentrations vary according to the rate of flow (Fig. 2.3). Levels of $Na^+$ and $Cl^-$ in saliva are hypotonic, but levels of $HCO_3^-$ and $K^+$ are hypertonic at higher rates of flow. Saliva is hypotonic overall (about 200 mmol/L) and alkaline, although the exact pH varies with flow.

## Salivary proteins

Salivary proteins include amylase, ribonuclease, R protein (which protects vitamin $B_{12}$ as it passes through the duodenum, jejunum and ileum), lipase (important in cystic fibrosis when pancreatic lipase is lost), lysozyme, secretory IgA (immunoglobulin A), IgG and IgM.

Epidermal growth factor (EGF) is also secreted in saliva. This has a protective role at the gastro-duodenal mucosa, by preventing the development of ulcers and promoting healing. Blood group antigens A, B, O (H) and $Le^a$ have also been identified in saliva.

## Functions of saliva and the salivary glands

The functions of saliva and the salivary glands include:

- General cleansing and protection of the buccal cavity, by washing away food particles which attract bacteria.
- Moistening of the buccal cavity for speech (by aiding movements of the lips and tongue) and breastfeeding (saliva forms a seal around the mother's nipple).
- Secretion of digestive enzymes, especially salivary amylase, which hydrolyses α-1,4 linkages in starch.
- Dissolving many food components, thus contributing to the taste of food.
- Lubrication of the buccal cavity by mucus-secreting units of glands (under sympathetic and parasympathetic control), which helps swallowing.
- Secretion of the antibacterial enzyme lysozyme, which protects teeth.

**Fig. 2.3** Salivary composition against flow rate. (Redrawn with permission from Thaysen JH et al. Secretion control in salivation. Am J Physiol 1954 178:155.)

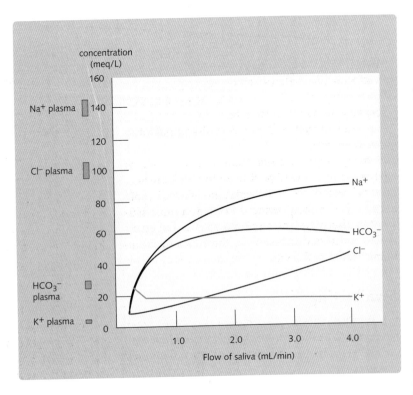

- Secretion of IgA by plasma cells in connective tissue, which act to protect the body from invasion of microorganisms. The secretory component of IgA is synthesized by striated duct cells.
- Neutralizing acid produced by bacteria as well as acids in food by the presence of bicarbonate; this helps to prevent dental caries.

## Oral absorption

Most drugs are administered orally. Although this is the most convenient method for patients, it results in the most complicated pathway to the tissues and exposes drugs to first-pass metabolism in the liver.

Drugs given orally must dissolve in the gastro-intestinal fluids and penetrate the epithelial cells lining the gastrointestinal tract by passive diffusion or active transport. Some drugs are poorly absorbed orally or are unstable in the tract. Most drugs require an un-ionized state to move passively through the gut mucosa, which may be difficult to achieve because of the pH of the gastric acid.

Sublingual administration allows diffusion into the systemic circulation through the capillary network of the oral cavity, bypassing the liver and avoiding first-pass metabolism. Lower doses can, therefore, be given. Glyceryl trinitrate used in angina treatment is commonly given this way.

## Oral defences

The alkaline pH of saliva neutralizes acid in food or in gastric contents following vomiting. Calcium and phosphate in saliva protect teeth by mineralizing newly erupted teeth and repairing pre-carious white spots in enamel.

Salivary proteins cover teeth with a protective coat called an acquired pedicle. Antibodies and anti-bacterial agents retard bacterial growth and tooth decay. The mucosa-associated lymphoid tissue (MALT) also plays an important role in protecting against microbial invasion at the mucosal membranes of the oral cavity.

## Swallowing

We swallow about 600 times a day: 200 times while eating and drinking, 350 times while awake (when not eating or drinking) and 50 times while asleep.

Swallowing is the controlled transport of a food bolus from mouth to stomach, involving a sequential swallowing motor programme, which is generated in the medullary swallowing centre and consists of three phases: buccal, pharyngeal and oesophageal (Fig. 2.4). It is an 'all-or-nothing' reflex; it is initiated voluntarily, but once it is started, it cannot be stopped.

### The buccal phase

The voluntary buccal phase occurs when the mouth is closed. The bolus of food is pushed upwards and backwards against the hard palate, forcing it into the pharynx. This phase initiates the subsequent phases, which are involuntary.

### The pharyngeal phase

The pharyngeal phase, which lasts about 1 s, is initiated by the bolus stimulating mechanoreceptors in the pharynx and firing impulses in the trigeminal (Vth cranial nerve), glossopharyngeal (IXth cranial nerve) and vagus (Xth cranial nerve) nerves. Efferent fibres pass to the tongue and the pharyngeal muscles through the trigeminal, facial and hypoglossal nerves.

This results in:

- The tongue being positioned against the hard palate, thus preventing the bolus re-entering the oral cavity.
- The nasopharynx being closed off by the soft palate, in particular the uvula.
- The larynx is elevated and its opening sealed off by the vocal folds.
- The epiglottis closing the larynx.
- The relaxation and opening of the upper oesophageal sphincter (UOS) for 0.5–1 s (once the bolus has passed through the upper oesophageal sphincter, it contracts tightly).

Note also that respiration, which would be futile as the airway is closed, is temporarily stopped because the swallowing centre inhibits the respiratory centre, which is also located in the medulla.

### The oesophageal phase

The oesophageal phase involves transport of the bolus along the oesophagus and takes between 6 and 10 s. Both primary and secondary peristaltic contractions are required.

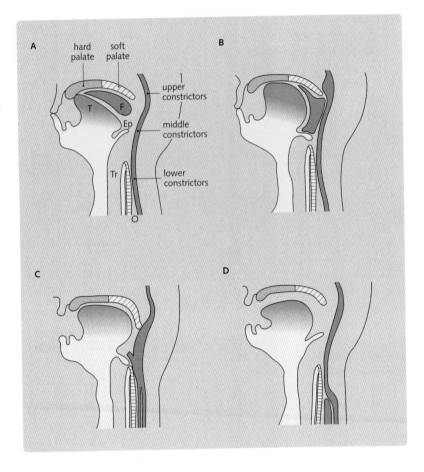

**Fig. 2.4** The stages of swallowing.
(A) The bolus of food, F is pushed into the pharynx by the tongue, T. (B) The bolus is propelled further back and the soft palate shuts off the nasopharynx. (C) The epiglottis, Ep, closes the opening to the trachea, Tr, and the bolus moves through the upper oesophageal sphincter. (D) Peristalsis now propels the bolus towards the lower oesophageal sphincter and stomach. (O = oesophagus.)

The primary peristaltic wave is initiated by swallowing and sweeps down the entire length of the oesophagus. It involves sequential activation of the vagal efferents, which supply the striated muscle in the upper oesophagus directly. The smooth muscle is supplied by the enteric nerve plexus.

The bolus of food begins to move towards the stomach with the aid of gravity. The secondary peristaltic wave is triggered in response to local distension of the oesophagus and begins on the orad (mouth) side of the bolus and runs to the lower oesophageal sphincter (LOS). This occurs by an enteric reflex and helps clear food residues. Tertiary waves are common in the elderly, but they are not peristaltic or propulsive.

The LOS relaxes when the peristaltic wave meets it. It opens for 5–10 s, allowing the bolus to pass into the stomach. Precision of tone is given by the vagal excitatory fibres (cholinergic) and the vagal inhibitory fibres (non-adrenergic non-cholinergic; NANC). These act reciprocally.

To tighten the LOS, an upregulation in vagal excitatory fibre stimulation is required, coupled with a downregulation in vagal inhibitory fibre stimulation. The opposite is true in relaxing or opening the LOS.

## Vomiting

Vomiting (emesis) is one of the most common symptoms of illness, especially in children (where it is associated with almost any physical or emotional illness), pregnancy, alcohol dependency and some metabolic disorders, e.g. uraemia.

The vomiting centre (Fig. 2.5) in the lateral reticular formation of the medulla 'coordinates' the process of vomiting. It is stimulated by:

- The chemoreceptor zone (CTZ) in the area postrema, which may itself be stimulated by circulating chemicals, drugs, motion sickness (induced by prolonged stimulation of the vestibular apparatus) and metabolic causes.

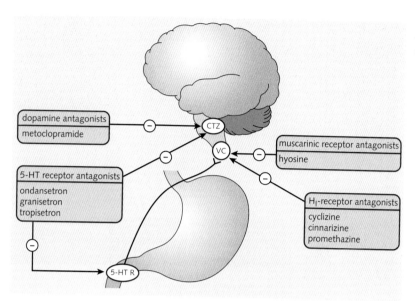

**Fig. 2.5** The mechanisms controlling vomiting and the sites of action of anti-emetic drugs.

- Vagal and sympathetic afferent neurons from the gut, which are stimulated by mucosal irritation.
- The limbic system—less is known about these circuits, but sights, smells and emotional circumstances can induce vomiting.

Lesions of the chemoreceptor zones abolish vomiting induced by some emetic drugs, uraemia and radiation sickness, but not by gastrointestinal irritation. Vomiting involves a retrograde giant contraction from the intestines, which expels some intestinal contents, e.g. bile, as well as gastric contents.

## Stages of vomiting

- A feeling of nausea is often accompanied by autonomic symptoms of sweating, pallor and hypersalivation (which protects the mucosa of the mouth from the acid contents of the stomach).
- A deep breath is taken and the epiglottis closes, protecting the trachea and lungs.
- At the same time, the retrograde giant contraction moves the contents of the upper intestine into the stomach.
- The breath is held, fixing the chest. The muscles of the abdominal wall contract, increasing intra-abdominal pressure.
- The oesophageal sphincters relax allowing expulsion of gastric contents through the mouth by reverse peristalsis.

# Pharmacology of vomiting

From a pharmacological viewpoint, it is important to understand the neural control of vomiting as most of the relevant drugs act on the receptors of the neurotransmitters involved, i.e. 5-HT, dopamine, histamine and acetylcholine. Anti-emetic drugs are by far more important than drugs which induce vomiting.

## Emetic drugs

Stimulation of vomiting may be needed in certain circumstances, for example if a toxic substance has been ingested and gastric lavage is difficult. However, stimulation of emesis should not be tried if the substance is corrosive or if the patient is not fully conscious.

Ipecacuanha, or syrup of ipecac, is a gastric irritant and the most common drug used to induce vomiting. The active ingredients of this drug are emetine and cephaeline, which are alkaloids.

Remember, however, that nausea and vomiting are common side-effects of many drugs, from anti-depressants to cytotoxic drugs.

## Anti-emetic drugs

Anti-emetic drugs are used to prevent motion sickness, as well as to prevent vomiting caused by other pharmacological agents, like the cytotoxic drugs used in the treatment of cancer. Other indications for anti-emetics are vomiting due to radiation, viral gastroenteritis and uraemia. Anti-emetics should only be given when the cause is certain, otherwise their prescription may delay the diagnosis. Also, as prevention of vomiting is easier than stopping it once it has started, anti-emetics should be given before an emetic stimulus. A description of the major classes of anti-emetics and how they work (Fig. 2.5) follows.

### 5-HT receptor antagonists

5-HT is an important neurotransmitter in the vomiting reflex. As such, selective 5-HT receptor antagonists, for example ondansetron which blocks 5-HT$_3$ receptors, are used to treat and prevent vomiting caused by cytotoxic drugs. Other drugs with a similar mechanism of action are granisetron and tropisetron. These drugs act on the CTZ and visceral afferent nerves, as 5-HT$_3$ receptors are found there.

### Metoclopramide

Metoclopramide acts by blocking dopamine receptors in the CTZ. Dopamine, like 5-HT, is a neurotransmitter in the vomiting pathway. Metoclopramide also has a stimulant effect on gastrointestinal motility, which adds to its anti-emetic function. Note, however, that metoclopramide may cause side-effects, chief of which are movement disorders due to the blockade of dopamine receptors.

### H$_1$-receptor antagonists

H$_1$-receptor antagonists are effective against motion sickness, as these receptors are found in the vestibular nuclei, and against vomiting caused by substances acting in the stomach. However, they are of no use against vomiting produced by substances acting on the CTZ. Examples of this class of drug are cyclizine, cinnarizine and promethazine.

### Muscarinic-receptor antagonists

Acetylcholine receptors are found in the vomiting centre and in the nucleus tractus solitarius. Muscarinic-receptor antagonists, such as hyoscine, are therefore effective in preventing motion sickness and vomiting caused by gastric stimuli but not against vomiting caused by substances acting on the CTZ.

The main side-effects, drowsiness and dry mouth, are predictable autonomic effects of muscarinic-receptor blockade. For a comprehensive account of the autonomic nervous system see the relevant chapter in *Crash Course: Physiology*.

The drug of choice for motion sickness is hyoscine (a muscarinic receptor antagonist); for control of vomiting induced by cytotoxic drugs it is ondansetron (a 5-HT$_3$-receptor antagonist). This is related to the presence of receptors for the relevant neurotransmitter in the sites stimulated by the emetic stimuli concerned — hence the need to know this information!

# THE MOUTH, ORAL CAVITY AND OROPHARYNX

## Anatomy

The oral cavity extends from the lips to the pillars of the fauces, which is the opening to the pharynx. It contains the tongue, alveolar arches (which anchor the teeth), gums, teeth and the openings of the salivary ducts (Fig. 2.6).

The oral cavity is divided into the vestibule (anterior to the teeth) and the oral cavity proper (posterior to the incisors).

The blood supply of the oral cavity (as well as the oropharynx) comes from branches of the external carotid artery, such as the facial artery and lingual artery. Innervation comes from branches of the cranial nerves.

The oral cavity is lined with stratifed squamous epithelium with an underlying submucosa containing collagen, elastin and salivary glands.

## Embryology and development

The head and neck derive primarily from the pharyngeal (branchial) arches, which are bars of mesenchymal tissue with an outer covering of ectoderm and inner covering of endoderm, separated by pharyngeal clefts and outpocketings called pharyngeal pouches.

Each pharyngeal arch contains neural crest cells, which contribute to skeletal components. Each also contains an arterial, cranial nerve and muscular component. Initially there are six arches, but the fifth disappears (Fig. 2.7).

At about four and a half weeks of embryological development, the 1st and 2nd arches form the mesenchymal prominences. The 1st pharyngeal

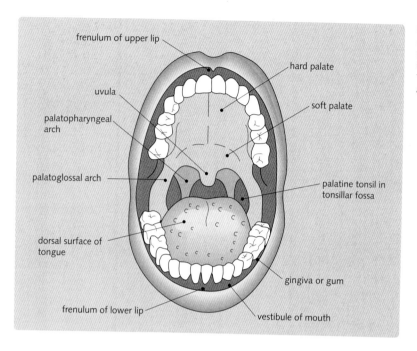

**Fig. 2.6** The oral cavity. The lateral walls of the pillars of the fauces are composed of the palatoglossal arches (anterior) and the palatopharyngeal arches (posterior). The palatine tonsils lie between the two arches, covered with mucous membrane.

arch consists of a dorsal and ventral portion called the maxillary and mandibular prominences, respectively. These fuse and develop with the frontonasal prominence to give rise to the mandible, upper lip, palate and nose. Failure to fuse results in abnormalities, such as cleft palate and cleft lip.

## The lips

These mark the boundaries of the mouth. The outer surface of the lips is covered with skin containing hairs, sebaceous glands and sweat glands, while the inner surface is lined with non-keratinizing stratified squamous epithelium.

In between the inner and outer surfaces is the vermilion border. This is the transition zone. The epithelium resembles that of the inner surface, but has a prominent rete ridge system with prominent blood vessels. It is these vessels which give the lips their red colour.

Deep to the epithelium, striated muscle is found arranged in a concentric fashion around the mouth. This is the orbicularis oris muscle which opens and closes the mouth.

The lips are supplied by the labial arteries, which come off the facial arteries. These form an arterial ring around the lips. Lightly pinching the lips with two fingers will allow their pulse to be felt.

## The teeth

The primary teeth first erupt at around age 6–8 months and number 20 in total. By age 18, however, eruption of the permanent teeth is normally complete and by then there are 32 teeth, 16 on each jaw (Fig. 2.8A). The third molars ('wisdom teeth') may or may not have erupted by that age.

Each tooth has three parts: the crown, the neck and the root (Fig. 2.8B). Histologically, most of the tooth is comprised of dentine. This is covered by enamel over the crown and cementum over the root. The root canal is the channel by which vessels and nerves enter the pulp cavity.

## The palate

The hard and soft palates form the roof of the mouth and separate it from the nasal cavity. The former is formed by the palatine processes of the maxillae and the palatine bones.

The soft palate is posterior to the hard palate. Its oral surface contains many mucous glands. The soft palate is a mobile, muscular aponeurosis attached to the posterior border of the bony hard palate. It is covered with mucous membrane and is continuous laterally with the wall of the pharynx. Between the pillars of the fauces is the palatine tonsil (Fig. 2.6).

**Fig. 2.7** Development of the mouth and pharynx (A) and the tongue (B).

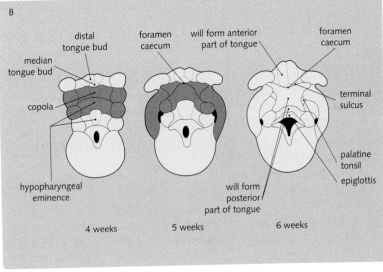

The palatoglossal and palatopharyngeal arches join the tongue and the pharynx, respectively, to the soft palate. The curved free border of the soft palate lies between the oropharynx and the nasopharynx. From this hangs the uvula, in the midline, which is seen to move when a patient says 'aahh'.

The muscles of the soft palate are:

- Levator veli palatini.
- Tensor veli palatini.
- Palatoglossus.
- Palatopharyngeus.
- Musculus uvulae.

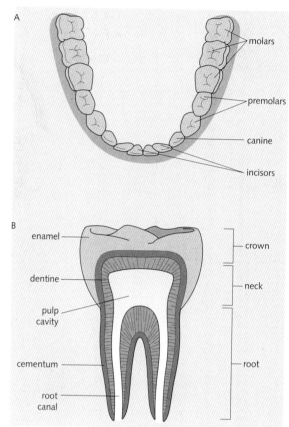

A

molars

premolars

canine

incisors

B

enamel

crown

dentine

neck

pulp
cavity

cementum

root

root
canal

**Fig. 2.8** (A) Adult human dentition. (B) The structure of a tooth.

The extrinsic muscles originate outside the tongue and attach to it. They act to control movement of the tongue.

The extrinsic muscles are:

- Genioglossus—a fan-shaped muscle that attaches to the mandible in the midline.
- Hyoglossus—attaches to the hyoid bone.
- Styloglossus—attaches to the styloid process and its fibres interdigitate with the hyoglossus.
- Palatoglossus—originates in the soft palate and enters the lateral part of the tongue.

The palatoglossus muscle is innervated by the fibres from the cranial root of the accessory nerve (XIth cranial nerve), through the pharyngeal branch of the vagus nerve. The other lingual muscles are innervated by the hypoglossal nerve (XIIth cranial nerve). The nerve supply of the tongue is summarized in Fig. 2.9.

The arterial supply to the tongue is from the lingual artery (a branch of the external carotid). The lingual vein drains the tongue. Lymph drains to the deep cervical, submandibular and submental nodes.

All are supplied by the pharyngeal motor fibres of the vagus nerve via the pharyngeal plexus, except the tensor veli palatini, which is supplied by the mandibular nerve, a branch of the trigeminal nerve.

## The tongue

### Anatomy

The tongue is a muscular structure and its dorsum (upper surface) is divided into anterior (two thirds) and posterior (one third) by a V-shaped borderline—the sulcus terminalis. At the apex of the sulcus terminalis is the foramen caecum, which is the remnant of the embryonic thyroglossal duct opening.

The tongue consists of four pairs of intrinsic muscles (superior and inferior longitudinal, transverse and vertical), which have no attachments outside the tongue itself. These muscles are involved with changing the shape of the tongue.

### Histology

The dorsal surface is covered with small papillae, especially the anterior two-thirds. Filiform papillae, which look like short bristles, are the most numerous and are found mainly in the middle of the tongue. Fungiform papillae, which are red and globular, are found among the filiform papillae and on the tip of the tongue.

**Fig. 2.9** The tongue, showing its innervation, the arrangement of the taste receptors and the areas most sensitive to the different types of taste.

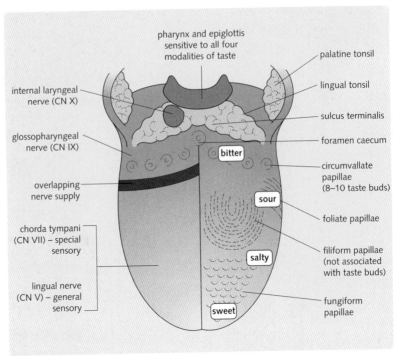

Circumvallate papillae are found just anterior to the sulcus terminalis and most of the taste buds are located in the circular trenches surrounding these papillae (Fig. 2.9). The posterior third contains the lingual tonsil. Very rudimentary foliate papillae may also be found, although these are more numerous and developed in some animals.

The four basic tastes detected by taste buds are sweet, sour, salty and bitter. Taste receptors (also called taste buds) sensitive to a particular taste are found in different areas of the tongue (Fig. 2.9). They can provide early warning that food may be bad.

### Embryology and development

Development of the tongue begins at the end of the 4th week of gestation. The tongue mucosa develops from the endoderm of the pharyngeal floor. The anterior two thirds of the tongue develop primarily from the lateral lingual swellings and the median tongue bud (or tuberculum impar), all of which are derived from the 1st pharyngeal arch.

The posterior third is formed by the growth of the hypopharyngeal eminence (a structure formed from the 3rd and 4th pharyngeal arches) over the copula, a midline structure formed by mesoderm of the 2nd, 3rd and part of the 4th arches.

The muscles of the tongue, except palatoglossus, are formed from mesoderm derived from the myotomes of the occipital somites. The muscles (except palatoglossus) are supplied by the hypoglossal nerve, which is consistent with their origin.

### Muscles of mastication

The muscles of mastication are the:

- Masseter.
- Temporalis.
- Lateral pterygoids.
- Medial pterygoids.

These develop from the mesoderm of the 1st pharyngeal (branchial) arch. Their motor nerve supply is from the mandibular branch of the trigeminal nerve. They all arise from the skull and insert into the mandible, causing movement of the mandible and the temporomandibular joint (Fig. 2.10). The muscles are summarized in Fig. 2.11.

### Salivary glands

There are three pairs of large salivary glands (the parotid, submandibular and sublingual glands) and numerous smaller glands, scattered throughout the mouth (Fig. 2.12).

The parotid gland is formed from a tubular ectodermal outgrowth at the inner surface of the cheek. The submandibular and sublingual glands

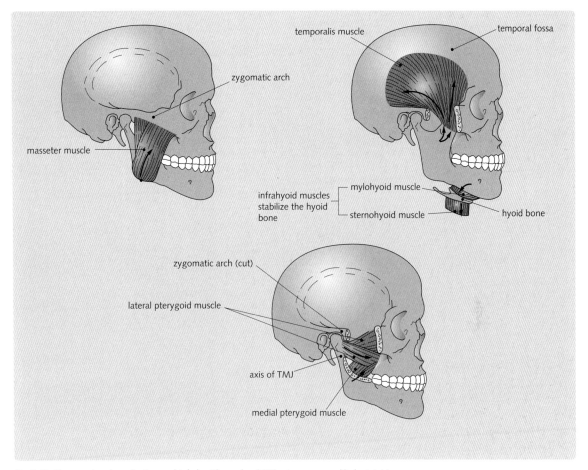

**Fig. 2.10** The muscles of mastication and infrahyoid muscles. (TMJ = temporomandibular joint.)

are formed in a similar fashion from invaginations of the endoderm of the floor of the mouth.

The salivary glands consist of parenchymal (functional) and stromal (support) components. Each parenchymal unit is called a salivon, which consists of an acinus (from the Latin word for grape) and a duct (Fig. 2.13). The duct of the salivon modifies the secretions of the acinus. The striated segment of the duct is continuous with the excretory part of the duct.

Acini consist of serous or mucous cells. The parotid gland has only serous acini, the sublingual gland contains mostly mucous acini and the submandibular gland contains predominantly serous acini. The minor salivary glands are mucous, except for von Ebner's glands and those in the tip of the tongue, which are serous. The structure of the salivary glands is very similar to that of the pancreatic exocrine glands, which secrete a wide range of digestive enzyme precursors.

## The parotid gland

This is the largest salivary gland and it produces serous saliva. It lies between the ramus of the mandible and the mastoid and coronoid processes, and its anterior border overlies the masseter. An accessory lobe may be found above this muscle. The parotid gland is covered with a fibrous capsule that is continuous with the deep investing fascia of the neck. The facial nerve (VIIth cranial nerve) passes through the parotid gland.

The parotid duct is about 5 cm long. It pierces the buccinator muscle and opens into the mouth opposite the second upper molar tooth. This opening can be felt with the tongue.

The parotid gland is supplied by branches of the external carotid artery; venous blood drains to the retromandibular vein. It is innervated by both the sympathetic and parasympathetic systems. Parasympathetic innervation is secretomotor (causing

**Fig. 2.11** A summary of the muscles of mastication.

| Muscle (Nerve supply) | Origin | Insertion | Action |
|---|---|---|---|
| Masseter ($V^3$) | Inferior border + medial surface of zygomatic arch | Lateral surface of ramus of mandible | Elevates and protrudes jaw, closing it. Retrusion of chin |
| Temporalis ($V^3$) | Temporal fossa, overlying temporal fascia | Tip and medial surface of coronoid plexus | Elevates mandible (closes jaw) retrudes mandible after protrusion |
| Lateral pterygoid ($V^3$) | **Superior head** | **Superior and inferior heads** | **Together** |
| | Infratemporal surface and crest of greater wing of sphenoid | Neck of mandible + capsule + articular disc of temporomandibular joint | Protrude mandible |
| | **Inferior head** | | **Alone** |
| | Lateral surface of lateral pterygoid plate | | Acting alternatively, they produce side to side movement |
| Medial pterygoid ($V^3$) | **Deep head** | **Superficial and deep heads** | **Together** |
| | Medial surface of lateral pterygoid plate | Medial surface of ramus of mandible, inferior to mandibular foramen | Help elevate mandible, closing jaw. Also help protrude mandible |
| | **Superficial head** | | **Alone** |
| | Tuberosity of maxilla | | Acting alternate, they produce a grinding motion |

production of saliva); sympathetic innervation is vasoconstrictor (causing a dry mouth).

Parasympathetic fibres are carried from the glossopharyngeal nerve through the otic ganglion and auriculotemporal nerve.

Sympathetic fibres from the superior cervical ganglion pass along the external carotid artery.

Lymph from the superficial part of the gland drains to the parotid nodes and from the deep part to the retropharyngeal nodes.

## The submandibular gland

The submandibular gland lies in the floor of the mouth covered by a fibrous capsule, and produces mixed serous and mucous secretions. Both its superficial and deep parts communicate around the posterior border of the mylohyoid muscle.

Its duct passes forwards between the mylohyoid and hyoglossus muscles to open onto sublingual papillae at the base of the frenulum. The lingual nerve crosses the duct.

The gland is supplied by the facial and lingual arteries (branches of the external carotid arteries); venous drainage is by the facial and lingual veins.

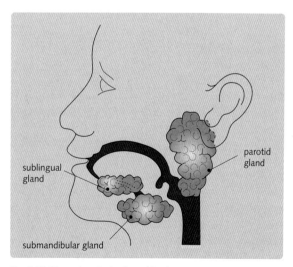

**Fig. 2.12** The main paired salivary glands.

sublingual gland

parotid gland

submandibular gland

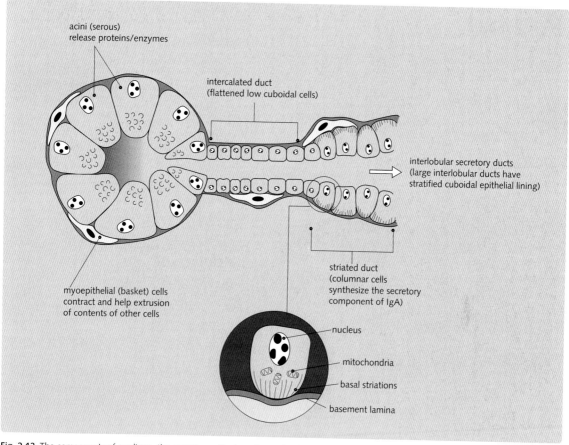

acini (serous)
release proteins/enzymes

intercalated duct
(flattened low cuboidal cells)

interlobular secretory ducts
(large interlobular ducts have
stratified cuboidal epithelial lining)

myoepithelial (basket) cells
contract and help extrusion
of contents of other cells

striated duct
(columnar cells
synthesize the secretory
component of IgA)

nucleus

mitochondria

basal striations

basement lamina

**Fig. 2.13** The components of a salivon, the secreting unit of a salivary gland.

It is innervated by both the parasympathetic and sympathetic systems.

Parasympathetic fibres are conveyed from the facial nerve through the chorda tympani and submandibular ganglion.

Sympathetic innervation is from the superior cervical ganglion, with fibres passing along the arteries of the gland.

Lymphatic drainage is to the submandibular lymph nodes, which are partly embedded in the gland and partly lie between it and the mandible.

## The sublingual gland

This is the smallest and also the most deeply situated of the paired salivary glands. It is almond-shaped and found below the mucous membrane of the floor of the mouth. It produces mainly mucous secretions, which either pass into numerous small ducts (10–20) that open into the floor of the mouth, or they pass into the submandibular duct. The inner-

vation, blood supply and venous and lymphatic drainage are similar to the submandibular gland.

## Pharynx

The pharynx is a fibromuscular tube, approximately 15 cm long, that extends from the base of the skull to the inferior border of the cricoid cartilage anteriorly, and to the inferior border of C6 vertebra posteriorly. It communicates with the nose, middle ear (by the auditory tube), mouth and larynx.

It conducts food and fluids to the oesophagus and air to the larynx and lungs (however, some air is swallowed with food).

The pharynx can be split into three functional parts: the nasopharynx, the oropharynx and laryngopharynx. Its walls have mucous, submucous and muscular layers.

The muscular layer of the pharynx consists of:

- Superior, middle and inferior constrictors.
- Salpingopharyngeus.

- Stylopharyngeus.
- Palatopharyngeus.

The cricopharyngeus muscle forms the upper oesophageal sphincter (Fig. 2.14). Stylopharyngeus is supplied by the glossopharyngeal nerve, but all the other muscles of the pharynx (Fig. 2.15) are supplied by the vagus nerve through the pharyngeal plexus on the outer surface of the middle constrictor.

> The superior, middle and inferior pharyngeal constrictor muscles are arranged so that the superior one is innermost and the inferior one is outermost – like three flowerpots stacked inside each other.

Superior to the superior constrictor muscle, the submucosa thickens to form the pharyngobasilar membrane, which blends with the buccopharyngeal fascia to form the pharyngeal recess.

The pharyngeal tonsils, or adenoids, lie submucosally in the nasopharynx. The epiglottis, a flap of cartilage covered with mucous membrane, lies posterior to the tongue in the laryngopharynx and closes the entrance to the larynx during swallowing. On either side of the epiglottis lie the piriform fossae – a common site for fish bones to lodge!

The pharynx is supplied by branches of the ascending pharyngeal, superior thyroid, maxillary, lingual and facial arteries. Venous drainage is to the internal jugular vein, via the pharyngeal venous plexus. Lymph from the nasopharynx drains to the retropharyngeal lymph nodes. The rest of the pharyngeal lymph drains to the deep cervical nodes.

Together with the lingual tonsils, the palatine tonsils and other smaller aggregations, the pharyngeal tonsils form a protective ring around the oro- and nasopharynx, called Waldeyer's ring. These lymphoid tissues are also described as mucosa-associated lymphoid tissue (MALT).

Histologically, the pharyngeal mucosa is continuous with that of the nose, oral cavity, auditory tube, larynx and oesophagus. The nasopharynx is lined with respiratory epithelium (ciliated mucous membrane with goblet cells).

The oropharynx and laryngopharynx are lined with stratified squamous epithelium to withstand abrasion from the passage of food.

# DISORDERS OF THE MOUTH AND OROPHARYNX

## Congenital abnormalities

Cleft lip and cleft palate are common defects, which present with abnormal facial appearance and defective speech. Overall, cleft lip is more common than cleft palate (1/1000 births compared with 1/2500 births). Cleft lip is more common in male babies than in female babies. A lateral cleft lip (hare lip) may result from incomplete fusion of the maxillary and medial nasal prominences, and a cleft palate from failure of fusion of the palatine shelves. Cleft lip and palate may also occur together (Fig. 2.16).

The palatine shelves in the female fetus fuse about 1 week later than they do in the male; hence cleft palate on its own is more common in female babies. Of every nine affected babies, two have a

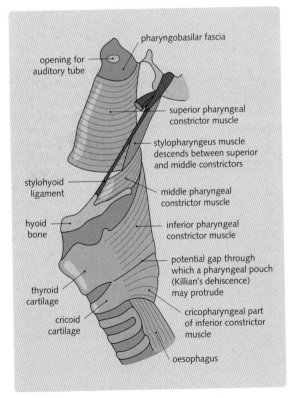

opening for auditory tube

pharyngobasilar fascia

superior pharyngeal constrictor muscle

stylopharyngeus muscle descends between superior and middle constrictors

stylohyoid ligament

middle pharyngeal constrictor muscle

hyoid bone

inferior pharyngeal constrictor muscle

potential gap through which a pharyngeal pouch (Killian's dehiscence) may protrude

thyroid cartilage

cricoid cartilage

cricopharyngeal part of inferior constrictor muscle

oesophagus

Fig. 2.14 The muscles of the pharynx.

**Fig. 2.15** A summary of the pharyngeal muscles.

| Name of muscle (nerve supply) | Origin | Insertion | Action |
|---|---|---|---|
| Superior constrictor (pharyngeal plexus) | Medial pterygoid plate, pterygoid hamulus, pterygomandibular ligament, mylohyoid line of mandible | Pharyngeal tubercle of occipital bone, midline raphe | Assists in separating oro- and nasopharynx and propels food bolus downward |
| Middle constrictor (pharyngeal plexus) | Stylohyoid ligament, lesser and greater horns of hyoid bone | Pharyngeal raphe | Propels food bolus downward |
| Inferior constrictor (pharyngeal plexus) | Lamina of thyroid cartilage, cricoid cartilage | Pharyngeal raphe | Propels food bolus downward |
| Cricopharyngeus (pharyngeal plexus) | Fibres of inferior constrictor muscle attached to cricoid cartilage | Pharyngeal raphe | Sphincter at lower end of pharynx |
| Palatopharyngeus (pharyngeal plexus) | Palatine aponeurosis | Thyroid cartilage | Elevates pharyngeal wall and pulls palatopharyngeal folds medially |
| Salpingopharyngeus (pharyngeal plexus) | Auditory tube | Merges with palatopharyngeus | Elevates pharynx and larynx |
| Stylopharyngeus (IX) | Styloid process of temporal bone | Thyroid cartilage | Elevates larynx during swallowing |

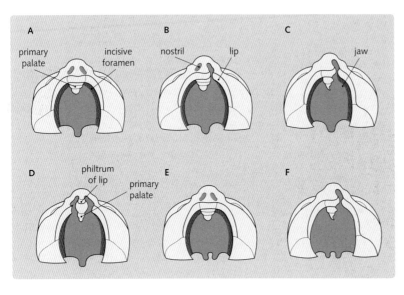

Fig. 2.16 Congenital abnormalities of the mouth and oropharynx. These result in variations of cleft palates and cleft lips. (A) Normal. (B) Unilateral cleft lip extending into the nose. (C) Unilateral cleft lip involving the lip and jaw and extending to the incisive foramen. (D) Bilateral cleft lip involving the lip and jaw. (E) Isolated cleft palate. (F) Cleft palate combined with unilateral anterior cleft. (Reproduced with permission from Sadler TW. Langman's Medical Embryology, 8th edn. Philadelphia, PA Lippincott, 2000.)

cleft lip, three a cleft palate and four have both. About 20% of babies with cleft lip or palate also have other malformations.

Unlike babies with a cleft lip, those with a cleft palate cannot be breastfed, but they may be given expressed breast milk or formula milk by a bottle with a special teat.

Median cleft lip is much rarer and is caused by incomplete fusion of the two medial nasal prominences in the midline. Infants with midline clefts often have brain abnormalities, including loss of midline structures. These defects occur early in neurilation (days 19–21). The infants are usually mentally retarded.

Failure of the maxillary prominence to merge with the lateral nasal swelling causes an oblique facial cleft, exposing the nasolacrimal duct.

Repair is surgical and is normally carried out after 3 months in the case of cleft lip and about 1 year in cleft palate. Genetic and environmental factors have been identified. Trisomy 13 (Patau's syndrome) and a number of teratogens (most notably anticonvulsants such as phenytoin and phenobarbital and also folic acid antagonists) are associated with both cleft lip and cleft palate.

# Infectious and inflammatory disease

The oral cavity and its mucosa are the target of many insults: infections, chemicals and physical agents. The oral mucosa is, therefore, affected by a number of inflammatory disorders, either restricted to the mouth, or as part of a systemic disease.

## Herpes simplex virus

Herpes simplex virus 1 (HSV-1) infection usually affects the body above the waist and herpes simplex virus 2 (HSV-2) below it. Changes in sexual practices, however, have led to an increase in HSV-1 infections below the waist and HSV-2 infections above it.

The primary infection may be asymptomatic or produce a severe inflammatory reaction. Presentation is usually with fever and painful ulcers in the mouth, which may be widespread and confluent.

The virus can remain latent in the trigeminal ganglia, but it may be reactivated by stress, trauma, fever and UV radiation. This recurrent form of the disease presents as cold sores.

About 70% of the population are infected with HSV-1 and recurrent infections are found in one third of those affected. Complications of HSV-1 include spread to the eye and acute encephalitis.

HSV infection in the immunocompromised, such as those undergoing cytotoxic chemotherapy for cancer, or those with human immunodeficiency virus (HIV) infection, is very dangerous. The infection can spread easily, leading to death in severe cases. Treat-ment for HSV involves topical or systemic administration of aciclovir, an antiviral drug.

## Oral candidiasis (thrush)

Candidiasis is caused by the yeast *Candida albicans*; it looks similar to leucoplakia (see later), but unlike leucoplakia it can be scraped off with a spatula. Although it is the most common fungal infection in humans, all the species that are pathogenic to humans are normal oropharyngeal and gastrointestinal commensals. Usually candidiasis is found in neonates, secondary to immunosuppression or a disturbance in the natural flora (e.g. after broad-spectrum antibiotic therapy). Therefore, these commensals can act as opportunists.

Candidiasis is common in acquired immune deficiency syndrome (AIDS) patients, in whom it may also cause lesions in the oesophagus.

Oral infections respond well to nystatin, oral amphotericin or miconazole. Systemic infections require parenteral therapy with amphotericin or ketoconazole for up to 3 weeks.

## Aphthous ulcers

Aphthous ulcers have a grey/white centre with a haemorrhagic rim, and usually heal spontaneously within a few days. Ulcers can occur for a number of reasons. The most common are minor aphthous ulcers, which recur, but have an unknown aetiology.

Sometimes nutritional deficiencies are found, such as iron, folic acid or vitamin $B_{12}$ (with or without gastrointestinal disorders). Trauma to the oral mucosa, infections and some drugs, e.g. antimalarials and methyldopa can also cause ulcers. Ulceration is also associated with inflammatory bowel diseases (Crohn's and ulcerative colitis; see Chapter 7) and coeliac disease.

## Glossitis

Glossitis is inflammation of the tongue. It may occur in anaemia and certain other deficiency states, most notably vitamin $B_{12}$ deficiency. It also occurs after trauma to the mouth from badly fitting dentures, jagged teeth, burns or the ingestion of corrosive substances.

The combination of glossitis, iron deficiency anaemia and an oesophageal web causing dysphagia occurs in Plummer–Vinson syndrome (Paterson–Brown–Kelly syndrome), most commonly seen in women with iron deficiency.

## Sialadenitis

Sialadenitis is inflammation of the salivary glands. This uncommon condition may be caused by infection or obstruction of salivary ducts. Mumps (infectious parotitis) can also be the cause.

Saliva has antibacterial properties but individuals with reduced amounts of saliva, e.g. in Sjögren's syndrome are at increased risk of sialadenitis.

## Oral manifestations of systemic disease

Many infections, dermatological conditions, haematological diseases and other disorders can present with oral manifestations.

As previously mentioned, ulcers can be indicative of inflammatory bowel disease. Other systemic diseases presenting this way include systemic lupus erythematosus, Behçet's disease, cyclic neutropenia and immunodeficiency disorders.

# Neoplastic disease

## Premalignant and benign neoplasms of the mouth

These include:

- Leucoplakia (hyperkeratosis and hyperplasia of squamous epithelium) – a premalignant condition that takes its name from the Greek for 'white patches' and is associated with excess alcohol, poor dental hygiene and, in particular, smoking.
- Erythroplakia (dysplastic leucoplakia) – lesions which have a higher malignant potential than leucoplakia.
- Squamous papilloma (nipple-like growth) and condyloma acuminatum (raised wart-like growth) – these are both associated with human papilloma viruses 6 and 11 and they are largely benign.

Leucoplakia and erythroplakia are more common in men, particularly those aged between 40 and 70 years.

## Malignant tumours of the mouth

In the UK, malignant tumours of the mouth account for 1% of all malignant tumours. Squamous cell carcinoma is by far the most common malignant tumour (95%); however, adenocarcinoma, melanomas and other malignant tumours may occur.

Alcohol and smoking predispose to squamous cell carcinoma; chewing tobacco even more so. The risk of a drinker who smokes developing squamous cell carcinoma is about 15 times that of the rest of the population.

Squamous cell carcinoma may arise in areas of leucoplakia and also on the lip, where it is associated with exposure to sunlight.

Treatment is by radiotherapy and/or surgery.

## Neoplasms of the salivary glands

Neoplasms of the salivary gland account for 3% of all tumours, worldwide. The majority occur in the parotid gland and pleomorphic adenomas are the most common, accounting for 2/3 of all salivary tumours. An adenoma is a benign epithelial growth derived from glandular tissue. Only 15% of pleomorphic adenomas (mixed tumours) become malignant.

Warthin's tumour (an adenolymphoma) is a tumour of the parotid salivary gland. It contains both epithelial and lymphoid tissues, with cystic spaces. It accounts for 5–10% of all salivary gland neoplasms.

# THE OESOPHAGUS

The oesophagus is a fibromuscular tube, approximately 25 cm in length, extending from the pharynx to the stomach. Its primary function is to convey food and fluids from the pharynx to the stomach during swallowing. It has cervical, thoracic and abdominal parts.

## Anatomy

The oesophagus begins in the neck, at the inferior border of the cricoid cartilage, where it is continuous with the pharynx (Fig. 2.17). Initially it inclines to the left, but is moved medially by the aortic arch at the level of T4. Inferior to the arch, it inclines to the left and passes through the diaphragm just left of the median plane.

In the superior mediastinum, it lies anterior to the first four thoracic vertebrae and posterior to the trachea, left main bronchus and the left recurrent laryngeal nerve. The azygos vein lies on the right of the oesophagus; the aortic arch and thoracic duct lie on the left.

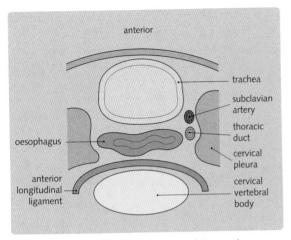

Fig. 2.17 Cross-section of the cervical region of the oesophagus, showing related structures at that level.

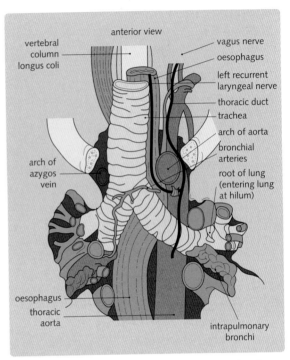

Fig. 2.18 Anterior view of the oesophagus, in relation to the other thoracic viscera.

Impressions or constrictions in the thoracic part of the oesophagus are made by the arch of the aorta, the point where the left main bronchus crosses the diaphragm as it passes through the oesophageal hiatus. This is a popular exam question!

At the level of T5, the oesophagus moves forward and to the left, accompanied by the right and left vagi to descend behind the fibrous pericardium and in front of the descending aorta. The oesophagus enters the abdomen through the oesophageal hiatus in the muscular part of the diaphragm, at the level of T10.

The abdominal part of the oesophagus is only about 2 cm long. It joins the stomach at the cardiac orifice, at the level of T11 (Fig. 2.18) and just posterior to the 7th costal cartilage. This part is also covered by peritoneum and encircled by the oesophageal plexus of nerves.

The oesophagus has two sphincters:

- The upper oesophageal sphincter, which is a striated muscular (anatomical) sphincter and part of the cricopharyngeus muscle. It is normally constricted to prevent air entering the oesophagus.
- The lower oesophageal sphincter, which is a physiological sphincter and made up of the lower 2–3 cm of oesophageal smooth muscle.

This is the intra-abdominal segment of oesophagus. It acts as a flap valve and with the muscosal rosette formed by folds of gastric mucosa, helps to occlude the lumen of the gastro-oesophageal junction. Normally there is tonic contraction of the circular muscles and the basal tone is regulated by vagal nerves.

Apart from the physiological lower oesophageal sphincter, the other factors which help prevent reflux of gastric contents are the abdominal pressure acting on the intra-abdominal part of the oesophagus, the valve-like effect of the oblique angle between the oesophagus and the stomach, the pinch-cock effect of the diaphragm on the lower oesophagus and the plug-like action of the mucosal folds.

## Blood supply

Blood supply is from the inferior thyroid artery, branches of the thoracic aorta and branches of the left gastric artery and left inferior phrenic artery (both ascend from the abdominal cavity).

## Venous drainage

Venous drainage is to both the systemic circulation (by the inferior thyroid and azygos veins) and the hepatic portal system (by the left gastric vein). It is a site of portosystemic anastomosis (see later).

## Innervation

The oesophagus is supplied by the vagus nerve and the splanchnic nerves (thoracic sympathetic trunks).

Striated muscle in the upper part is supplied by somatic motor neurons of the vagus nerve from the nucleus ambiguus, without synaptic interruption.

The smooth muscle of the lower part is innervated by visceral motor neurons of the vagus nerve that synapse with postganglionic neurons, whose cell bodies lie in the wall of the oesophagus and the splanchnic plexus. The oesophagus is also encircled by nerves of the oesophageal plexus.

## Embryology and development

At about 4 weeks of gestation, the respiratory diverticulum (lung bud) begins to form at the ventral wall of the foregut. The diverticulum becomes separated from the dorsal part of the foregut by the oesophagotracheal septum (Fig. 2.19).

The dorsal portion of the foregut becomes the oesophagus, which, although short initially, lengthens with the descent of the heart and lungs.

The ventral portion becomes the respiratory primordium and the surrounding mesenchyme forms the oesophageal muscle layers.

## Histology

The layers of the oesophagus are essentially the same as in other parts of the gastrointestinal tract (Fig. 2.20).

The serosa covers the oesophagus inside the abdominal cavity. In the neck and thorax it is referred to as the adventitia, and blends with the surrounding connective tissue.

The muscularis externa consists of an outer longitudinal and an inner circular layer, like the rest of the gastrointestinal tract.

The upper third of the oesophagus is striated muscle (a continuation of the muscular layer of the pharynx—the lowest part of cricopharyngeus forms the upper oesophageal sphincter). Striated muscle predominates here as the buccal phase of swallowing is voluntary, unlike the subsequent phases.

The middle third is made up of both striated and smooth muscle, while the lower third is entirely smooth muscle.

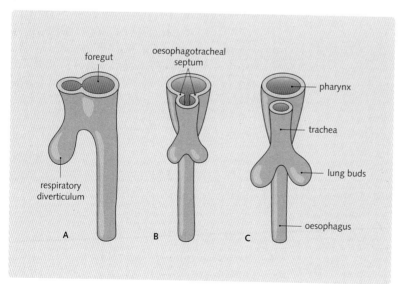

**Fig. 2.19** The development of the pharynx and oesophagus. (A) Development by end of week 3 of gestation. (B and C) Development in the course of week 4. Abnormalities at this stage of development can lead to atresia and fistulae, which can result in death for the infant.

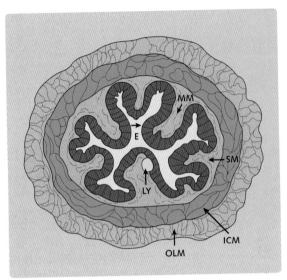

**Fig. 2.20** Cross-sectional view of oesophageal tissue. (LY = lymphoid nodule; E = epithelium; MM = muscularis mucosae; SM = submucosa; ICM = inner circular muscle layer; OLM = outer longitudinal muscle layer.)

The muscular layers of the upper 1/3 of the oesophagus are made up of striated muscle. The middle 1/3 has both striated (inner circular) and smooth (outer longitudinal) muscle and the lower 1/3 has only smooth muscle.

The submucosa contains numerous branched tubular glands, more abundant in the upper region, which produce mucus to lubricate the oesophagus. These are seromucous glands which are similar to the salivary glands. The submucosa also contains blood vessels, lymphatics and nerves in abundance.

The mucosa is lined by thick, non-keratinized stratified squamous epithelium and has a lamina propria similar to that in other parts of the body, but the muscularis mucosa is thicker than in the rest of the digestive tract. When relaxed, the mucosa is heavily folded. This allows for a great degree of distension when food is swallowed.

In the abdominal part, the mucosa is lined by columnar epithelium similar to that of the gastric cardiac region. This is the squamo-columnar junction. In reflux disease (see later), where the squamous epithelium of the lower oesophagus is exposed to gastric acid, the squamo-columnar junction moves higher up the oesophagus.

Numerous mucous glands are usually present in the uppermost part and mucus-producing 'cardiac glands' (resembling the glands in the cardiac region of the stomach) are found in the lowermost part.

The lumen appears branched in cross-section, because the oesophagus is usually collapsed antero-posteriorly.

# DISORDERS OF THE OESOPHAGUS

## Congenital abnormalities

### Atresia and tracheo-oesophageal fistulae

Atresia is the congenital absence or narrowing of a body opening. A fistula is an abnormal connection between two epithelial-lined surfaces (Fig. 2.21).

Atresia is a common condition, affecting 1/200 births and is caused by a failure of the oesophageal endoderm to grow quickly enough when the embryo elongates in week 5.

In 90% of cases, oesophageal atresia and tracheo-oesophageal fistula occur together, but either may occur without the other.

In the most common form of atresia, the upper part of the oesophagus has a blind ending but the lower end forms a fistulous opening into the trachea. This means that the infant cannot swallow milk or saliva and the diagnosis becomes apparent shortly after birth. The infant is at risk of aspiration pneumonia and of fluid and electrolyte imbalances.

Atresia should be suspected in a fetus where there is polyhydramnios (abnormally large amounts of amniotic fluid, i.e. over 2 L). Normally a fetus swallows amniotic fluid and some fluid is reabsorbed into the fetal circulation. Where there is atresia, the fetus cannot swallow, amniotic fluid is not reabsorbed and excess fluid thus accumulates, causing a distended uterus.

Treatment of atresia and fistulae is by surgery, with survival rates of more than 85%.

### Agenesis

This is the complete absence of an oesophagus and it is much rarer than atresia or fistula. Treatment is surgical.

### Stenosis

Stenosis is the abnormal narrowing of a passage or opening.

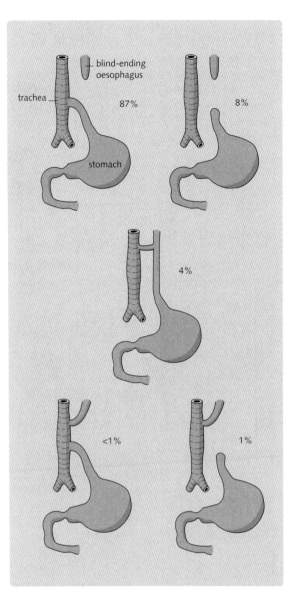

**Fig. 2.21** Different forms of oesophageal atresia and fistulae and their frequencies.

Congenital stenosis may occur, but acquired stenosis is more common (see later). Congenital stenosis is caused by incomplete recanalization during week 8, or from failure of development of blood vessels to the affected area. Usually the distal third is affected.

## Inflammatory disease

Oesophagitis (inflammation of the oesophagus) may be acute or chronic. Chronic oesophagitis is usually due to gastro-oesophageal reflux disease (GORD), which is common.

## Acute oesophagitis

Acute oesophagitis is more common in immunocompromised individuals, for example in HIV infection.

Oral and oesophageal candidiasis are common in AIDS patients, and may cause dysphagia or retrosternal discomfort. They give rise to white plaques with haemorrhagic margins.

Other causes are HSV and cytomegalovirus (CMV), which may also cause focal or diffuse ulceration of the gut. HSV ulceration is more common at the upper and lower ends of the gastrointestinal tract while CMV lesions are more common in the bowel, but either may affect any part of the tract from the mouth to the anus.

Acute oesophagitis may also be caused by the deliberate or accidental swallowing of corrosive substances.

## Gastro-oesophageal reflux disease (GORD)

Gastro-oesophageal reflux disease (GORD) is the reflux of acidic gastric content through the lower oesophageal sphincter. As mentioned earlier, it is the commonest cause of chronic oesophagitis and is highly prevalent, occurring in 30% of the general population.

### Aetiology

Factors associated with GORD are:

- Pregnancy or obesity.
- Fat, chocolate, coffee or alcohol ingestion.
- Large meals.
- Cigarette smoking.
- Anti-cholinergic drugs, calcium channel antagonists and nitrate drugs.
- Hiatus hernia (see later).
- Treatment for achalasia.

### Pathophysiology and clinical features

In GORD, one or more of the following mechanisms implicate the pathogenesis:

- The resting LOS tone is low or absent.
- The LOS tone fails to increase when lying flat, or when the intra-abdominal pressure has increased, e.g. during pregnancy or while wearing tight clothing.
- Poor oesophageal peristalsis leads to reduced clearance of acid in the oesophagus.
- A hiatus hernia can impair the function of the LOS and the diaphragm closure mechanism, as

the pressure gradient between the abdominal and thoracic cavities is diminished.

- Delayed gastric emptying increases the chance of reflux.

Most patients will complain of heartburn and 'acid regurgitation'. Some patients may be woken up at night if refluxed fluid irritates the larynx. Dysphagia and chest pain may be other presenting symptoms.

### Complications

The squamous mucosa of the lower oesophagus is not designed to cope with acid. Therefore, reflux causes injury to, and desquamation of, oesophageal cells. Normally the cells shed from the surface of the epithelium are replaced by basal cells, which mature and move up through the layers of squamous epithelium. Increased loss due to reflux is compensated

for by a proliferation of basal cells (basal cell hyperplasia) (Fig. 2.22).

Basal cell hyperplasia in reflux oesophagitis causes an elongation of the connective tissue papillae.

A number of inflammatory cells are usually present, which are a normal response to cell injury.

Ulcers form if basal cell formation cannot keep pace with cell loss. These may haemorrhage, perforate, or heal by fibrosis (sometimes forming a stricture) and epithelial regeneration. The premalignant disorder, Barrett's oesophagus (a columnar-cell-lined oesophagus) may also result.

### Treatment

Treatment for GORD includes losing weight, raising the head of the bed at night so that the patient does not lie flat and taking antacids. A reduction in the

**Fig. 2.22** Cell desquamation and proliferation in the normal oesophagus and in gastro-oesophageal reflux (GORD). Oesophagitis can be graded from I to IV; I being mild and IV being serious with danger of perforation. Often ulceration is seen with oesophagitis, and the premalignant disorder called Barrett's oesophagus may result.

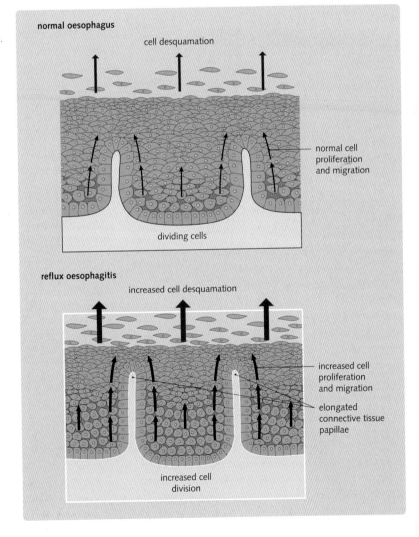

consumption of alcohol or other foods which precipitate an attack, as well as cessation of smoking is usually advised too.

The reduction of acid production can be achieved by using $H_2$-receptor antagonists and proton pump inhibitors (see Chapter 3). The former does not cure the oesophagitis associated with the disease, unlike the latter.

Metoclopromide, a motility stimulant (see Chapter 7), may enhance peristalsis and help acid clearance in the oesophagus.

Anti-reflux surgery (fundoplication) may be carried out in patients who fail to respond to medical treatment.

## Diseases associated with motor dysfunction

Motor dysfunction may be caused by:

- A failure of innervation.
- A defect in the muscle wall of the oesophagus.
- A combination of the two above.

### Achalasia

Achalasia is an uncommon condition (prevalence 1/100 000 in Western populations) which can present at any age, but it is rare in childhood. It involves the loss of coordinated peristalsis of the lower oesophagus and spasm of the lower oesophageal sphincter, thereby preventing the passage of food and liquids into the stomach. The aetiology is unknown.

It may be caused by damage to the innervation of the oesophagus, for example in Chagas' disease, where trypanosomes invade the wall of the oesophagus, damaging the intrinsic plexuses.

Degenerative lesions are found in the vagus nerve with a loss of ganglionic cells of the myenteric nerve plexus in the oesophageal wall. Two thirds of patients with achalasia have autoantibodies to a dopamine-carrying protein on the surface of the cells in the myenteric plexus.

Diagnosis is by radiography. A barium swallow shows dilatation of the oesophagus, with a beak deformity at the lower end, caused by a failure of relaxation of the lower oesophageal sphincter. Manometry shows an absence of peristalsis and a high resting lower oesophageal sphincter pressure.

The patient usually has a long history of sporadic dysphagia for both solids and liquids. Regurgitation of food is common, especially at night. Retrosternal chest pain is felt, due to the vigorous non-peristaltic contractions of the oesophagus.

Achalasia is a risk factor for squamous carcinoma of the oesophagus.

Treatment consists of endoscopic balloon dilatation of the lower oesophageal sphincter or surgery (Heller's cardiomyotomy/operation) to weaken the sphincter. Reflux is common after surgery unless a fundoplication is also performed.

### Hiatus hernia

Hiatus hernia describes the herniation of part of the stomach through the diaphragm. It is a common condition, occurring in 30% of those over the age of 50.

Hernias can be sliding, where the gastro-oesophageal junction slides through the hiatus and lies above the diaphragm, or rolling (para-oesophageal), where a part of the fundus of the stomach rolls up through the hernia next to the oesophagus (Fig. 2.23).

Sliding hernias are more common. Symptoms are usually associated with reflux, but many are asymptomatic.

Rolling hernias usually require surgical correction to prevent strangulation.

### Diverticula

Diverticula (out-pouchings) may form in the proximal or distal oesophagus, particularly where there is a disorder of motor function in the oesophagus. They may be due to pulsion, where pressure is raised due to muscle spasm, or to traction, where the diverticula result from 'pulling' due to fixation to other structures.

An example of a pulsion diverticulum is a pharyngeal pouch (Zenker's diverticulum). This may form in Killian's dehiscence, which is the area of weakness between the thyropharyngeus and cricopharyngeus, i.e. the two parts of the inferior pharyngeal constrictor (Fig. 2.14). Pharyngeal pouches are more common in elderly men. Food may collect in the pouch and later be regurgitated. Dysphagia (see Chapter 8) is common. A swelling may be felt in the neck.

Pharyngeal pouches are the only common diverticula of the oesophagus. Diagnosis is by barium swallow and treatment is surgical.

A traction diverticulum, which is very rare, may form in the lower oesophagus, particularly where fibrosis of the lower oesophagus has occurred.

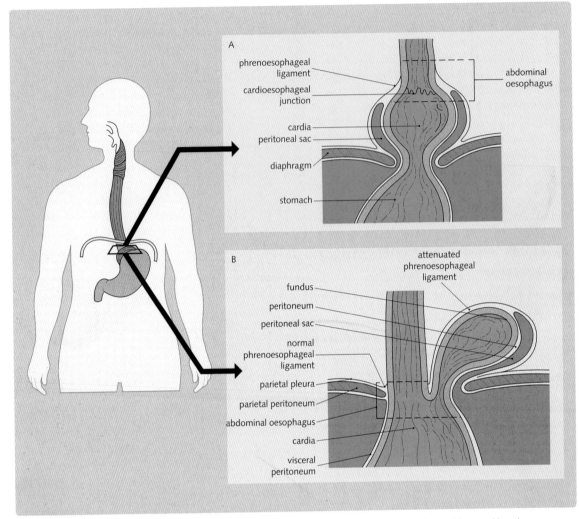

**Fig. 2.23** Sliding (A) and rolling (B) hiatus hernias. The sliding hernia is more common, especially in people over 50 years old, and can exacerbate reflux.

# Vascular disorders

## Oesophageal varices

Oesophageal varices are dilated veins at the junction of the oesophagus and the stomach. This is a site of a connection between the systemic and portal venous systems (porto-systemic anastomosis; see Chapter 4).

Normally, the connections are closed, but in patients with cirrhosis of the liver and portal hypertension the raised pressure in the portal system causes them to open up and enlarge.

The enlarged veins protrude into the lumen of the lower oesophagus (visible on endoscopy). They may burst, resulting in haematemesis, which may rapidly be fatal. Oesophageal varices are a common cause of upper gastrointestinal bleeding.

Prognosis following bleeding varices is poor, particularly when jaundice, ascites, encephalopathy or hypoalbuminaemia may be present. Overall, mortality from a first bleed from oesophageal varices is 40%.

Cirrhosis carries a particularly bad prognosis as clotting factors made in the liver are reduced as a result of cirrhotic damage.

Cirrhosis is the cause of 90% of varices in the UK, but schistosomiasis (bilharzia) is the major worldwide cause.

The management of acute variceal bleeding requires resuscitation involving restoring blood volume and taking measures to stop the bleeding. Urgent endoscopy is required and vasoconstrictor drugs (e.g. vasopressin and octreotide, a somatostatin analogue) can be given.

Sclerotherapy and banding are widely used techniques to stem the loss of blood. Both are performed by endoscopy and can help prevent rebleeding. Sclerotherapy involves injecting the varices with a sclerosing agent to produce vessel thrombosis and arrest bleeding.

Banding involves placing a tight-fitting band around the varix to stop it bleeding.

## Mallory–Weiss syndrome

Mallory–Weiss syndrome is haematemesis from a tear at the gastro-oesophageal junction (a Mallory–Weiss tear). It is caused by prolonged retching or coughing and a sudden increase in intra-abdominal pressure. It is most common in alcoholics.

# Neoplastic disease

## Barrett's oesophagus

Barrett's oesophagus is a premalignant condition resulting from prolonged reflux of the acid contents of the stomach into the oesophagus through an incompetent lower oesophageal sphincter. It occurs in approximately 20% of symptomatic cases of reflux and is most commonly seen in middle-aged men.

Diagnosis requires biopsies to be taken during endoscopy for analysis of any histological changes.

Normally the epithelium of the lower oesophagus is squamous but in cases of prolonged injury the normal epithelium may be replaced by columnar epithelium (a metaplastic change). This is believed to occur when prolonged injury to the lower oesophagus causes ulceration.

Pluripotent stem cells form a replacement epithelium. However, because acid contents are refluxing into the oesophagus, the pH in the area is lower than normal. This causes the stem cells to differentiate into the sort of epithelium seen in areas of low pH, such as gastric epithelium (found in the cardiac or fundic regions of the stomach) or intestinal epithelium. Macroscopically, this is seen as an abnormally high squamo-columnar junction, or Z-line.

Gastric and intestinal epithelium are more resistant to injury from the refluxing acid.

Adenocarcinoma is 30–40 times more likely to occur in a Barrett's oesophagus than in the normal oesophagus.

## Benign tumours

These are much less common than malignant tumours and account for only about 5% of all neoplasms of the oesophagus.

Leiomyomas are the most common of benign tumours but fibromas, lipomas, haemangiomas, neurofibromas and lymphangiomas may also arise.

## Malignant tumours

Cancer of the oesophagus is the eighth most common cancer in the world. It is found mainly in people 60–70 years of age.

Cancers in the upper third of the oesophagus are very rare. Tumours of the middle third are mainly squamous cell carcinomas and these account for 40% of oesophageal malignancy (Fig. 2.24).

Tumours in the lower third are adenocarcinomas, which comprise 45% of malignancies. These have usually developed from Barrett's oesophagus.

Clinical manifestations of oesophageal malignancies begin with persistent dysphagia and weight loss. Anorexia and lymphadenopathy are also common. Unfortunately, by the time symptoms are present, the carcinoma has usually spread and the 5-year survival is only about 5%.

**Fig. 2.24** Causes of squamous carcinoma of the oesophagus.

**Oesophageal disorders**
Chronic oesophagitis
Achalasia
Plummer–Vinson syndrome

**Predisposing factors**
Coeliac disease
Ectodermal dysplasia, epidermolysis bullosa
Tylosis
Genetic predisposition

**Dietary**
Vitamin deficiency (A, C, riboflavin, thiamine, pyridoxine)
Mineral deficiency (zinc, molybdenum)
Fungal contamination of foodstuffs
Nitrites/nitrosamines in foodstuffs

**Lifestyle**
Alcohol
Smoking

# Disorders of food intake

In Fröhlich's syndrome, a hypothalamic tumour causes obesity through excessive intake.

Anorexia nervosa is a potentially fatal psychiatric disorder, primarily of adolescent girls, in which patients persistently perceive themselves as overweight and, although obsessed with food, voluntarily starve.

Bulimia nervosa is another psychiatric eating disorder. It is characterized by binge eating and compensatory vomiting, purging or both.

## OVERVIEW

The stomach is a mobile, muscular organ that mixes food with digestive juices to form chyme. It receives food and fluid from the oesophagus, and releases its contents into the duodenum. Gastric contents are broken down both by the churning action of the stomach and by being squirted through the narrow pylorus.

The stomach acts as a reservoir for food as it is very distensible, with a capacity of up to 2–3 L. The wall of the stomach is impermeable to most substances, but alcohol, water, salts and some drugs may be absorbed through it. Most other substances are absorbed from more distal parts of the gastrointestinal tract.

## ANATOMY

The stomach lies between the oesophagus proximally and the duodenum distally. It varies widely in size and shape depending on body habitus, the food content and the posture of the body, hence its surface anatomy is variable. It is J-shaped normally and the pyloric part lies horizontally or ascends to meet the proximal part of the duodenum.

Anatomically, the stomach is divided into four parts (Fig. 3.1):

- Cardia – the region around the oesophagus. The cardiac orifice normally lies posterior to the 7th left costal cartilage at the level of T10 or T11 vertebra.
- Fundus – the superior part of the stomach, it lies above the imaginary horizontal plane passing through the cardiac orifice. Usually it is found posterior to the left 5th rib in the mid-clavicular line.
- Body – this lies between the fundus and the antrum, and is the largest part of the stomach.
- Pyloric part – this comprises the pyloric antrum and the narrower pyloric canal. It lies in the imaginary transpyloric plane at the level of L1 vertebra to the right of the angular notch (incisura angularis), which is the junction between the body and the pyloric part.

There are two sphincters at each of the gastric orifices. The physiological lower oesophageal sphincter (LOS) protects the oesophagus from reflux of the acidic gastric contents. The anatomical pyloric sphincter controls the flow of gastric contents into the duodenum.

The cardiac (gastro-oesophageal) orifice of the stomach lies behind the 7th left costal cartilage about

**Fig. 3.1** Structure of the stomach.

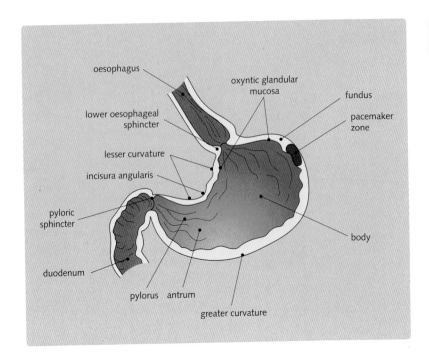

2–4 cm to the left of the median plane. The pylorus, which is the distal sphincteric region, has a variable location from L2–L4 vertebrae, but usually lies 1 cm to the right of the midline, in or below the transpyloric planes. It is joined to the cardiac orifice by the lesser curvature. The position of the greater curvature varies greatly. Fig. 3.2 shows the surface markings of the stomach.

## The omenta

The anterior and posterior surfaces of the stomach meet at the greater and lesser curvatures. The surfaces are covered by peritoneum except where blood vessels run on the curvatures and in a small area posterior to the cardiac orifice. The peritoneum is reflected at the greater curvature as the greater omentum. This is a fat-laden, apron-like double layer of peritoneum hanging off the stomach and the inferior border of the first part of the duodenum. It has a remarkable ability to stick to damaged or perforated parts of the gastrointestinal tract, sealing off leaks and giving some protection against peritonitis.

Excess fat may be stored in the greater omentum, especially in men, who have different distributions of fat from women. This is how the infamous beer belly came to be!

The lesser omentum is made up of peritoneum reflected at the lesser curvature to extend to the liver. The mucosa of the stomach is folded into large longitudinal rugae (wrinkles), which can be seen on radiographs after a barium meal. These permit the stomach to distend.

## Relations

The anterior surface is in contact with:

- The diaphragm (in the fundal region).
- The anterior abdominal wall.
- The left lobe of the liver.

The spleen lies posterolateral to the fundus.

The diaphragm, left adrenal gland, upper part of the left kidney, splenic artery, pancreas, transverse mesocolon and, in some people, the transverse colon lie posteriorly forming the stomach bed. They are separated from the stomach by the omental bursa (lesser sac of the peritoneum).

## Blood supply

There is a rich blood supply to the stomach (Fig. 3.3), derived from three branches of the coeliac trunk:

- The left gastric artery.
- The splenic artery.
- The common hepatic artery.

Fig. 3.2 Surface markings of the stomach.

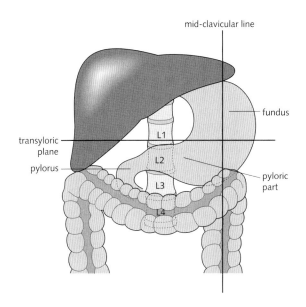

Fig. 3.3 The blood supply and lymphatic drainage of the stomach. The lymphatics follow the arteries. The lymphatics following the right gastric artery drain to the pyloric, hepatic and left gastric nodes. Those following the right gastroepiploic artery drain to the right gastroepiploic and pyloric nodes. Those following the left gastroepiploic and splenic arteries drain to the pancreaticosplenic nodes, and those following the left gastric artery drain to the left gastric nodes.

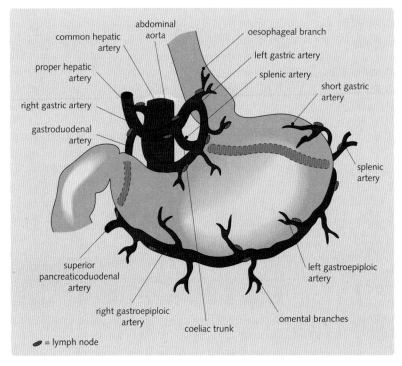

The left gastric artery supplies both anterior and posterior surfaces of the stomach, running along the lesser curvature. It anastomoses with the right gastric artery and also supplies the lower oesophagus.

The splenic artery follows a tortuous route across the posterior abdominal wall. It gives rise to the left gastroepiploic (gastro-omental) artery, which runs along the greater curvature and anastomoses with

43

the right gastroepiploic artery. Additionally, short gastric arteries to the fundus arise from the distal end of the splenic artery.

The common hepatic artery gives rise to the right gastric artery and the gastroduodenal artery. The gastroduodenal artery passes behind the first part of the duodenum and gives rise to the right gastroepiploic and the superior pancreaticoduodenal arteries. The latter, as its name suggests, supplies the pancreas and the duodenum and is not part of the arterial supply to the stomach.

Remember, there is a gastroduodenal artery that gives rise to the right gastroepiploic and superior pancreaticoduodenal arteries, but there is no gastroduodenal vein!

## Venous drainage

The stomach drains, like most of the alimentary system, to the hepatic portal system. The gastric veins accompany the arteries.

Drainage of specific veins is as follows:

- The right and left gastric veins drain into the portal vein itself.
- The short gastric and left gastroepiploic veins drain into the splenic vein and its tributaries.
- The right gastroepiploic vein usually drains into the superior mesenteric vein.
- Oesophageal tributaries of the left gastric vein form an important porto-caval anastomosis with tributaries of the azygos vein in the thorax.

## Lymphatic drainage

The lymphatics also follow the distribution of the arteries. There are four major groups of lymph nodes:

- The left gastric nodes.
- The pancreaticosplenic nodes.
- The right gastroepiploic nodes.
- The pyloric nodes.

Lymph drains from the anterior and posterior surfaces of the stomach towards its curvatures where many of the gastroepiploic nodes are situated.

These nodes all drain to the coeliac nodes and then to the cisterna chyli. From the cisterna chyli, lymph drains to the thoracic duct, which is the largest lymphatic vessel in the body and, unlike most of the lymphatic system, is visible to the naked eye. Knowledge of the lymphatic drainage is essential as in gastric carcinoma, the lymphatic drainage can spread metastases to the liver, pelvis and the rest of the body via the thoracic duct.

## Nerve supply

The stomach is supplied by both sympathetic and parasympathetic systems.

### Sympathetic supply

The sympathetic supply is from the autonomic coeliac plexus through the periarterial plexus, which runs along the arteries of the stomach. Presynaptic sympathetic fibres come from the splanchnic nerves (from T6 to T9 of the spinal cord).

It causes vasoconstriction of the gastric blood vessels, relaxation of the gastric muscles and decreased activity of gastric glands. These also carry pain fibres from the stomach.

### Parasympathetic supply

The parasympathetic supply is from the vagus nerve (Xth cranial nerve). Anterior and posterior vagal trunks from the oesophageal plexus pass through the diaphragm with the oesophagus and divide into anterior and posterior gastric branches on the anterior and posterior surfaces of the stomach. Posterior branches contribute to the coeliac plexus.

Gastric branches form Auerbach's and Meissner's intrinsic plexuses, described in the section on gastric histology. Upregulation of parasympathetic innervation causes an increase in gastric motility and secretion.

## EMBRYOLOGY AND DEVELOPMENT

The stomach develops from a fusiform dilatation of the foregut, which appears around the middle of week 4 of gestation (Fig. 3.4). Its appearance and position change greatly during development as it rotates around both a longitudinal and an anteroposterior axis.

The posterior wall grows faster than the anterior wall over the following two weeks and forms the greater and lesser curvatures.

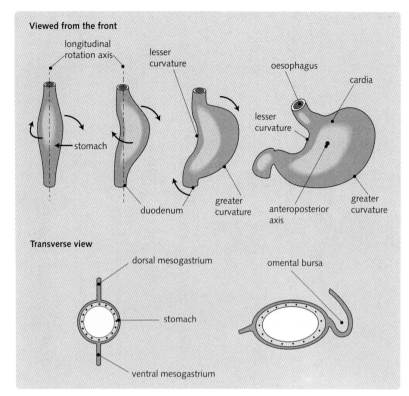

**Viewed from the front**

longitudinal rotation axis

lesser curvature

oesophagus

cardia

lesser curvature

stomach

greater curvature

duodenum

greater curvature

anteroposterior axis

**Transverse view**

dorsal mesogastrium

omental bursa

stomach

ventral mesogastrium

**Fig. 3.4** Development of the stomach. The stomach rotates 90° around its longitudinal axis, causing the left vagus to innervate the left, now anterior, surface and the right vagus to innervate the right, now posterior, surface. The longitudinal rotation also causes the formation of the space behind and to the left of the stomach, called the omental bursa (lesser sac), which is continuous with the coelomic cavity behind the stomach. (Redrawn with permission from Sadler TW. Langman's Medical Embryology, 6th edn. London: Williams & Wilkins, 1990.)

The stomach rotates 90° clockwise as it enlarges. There are three major consequences of this rotation:

- The greater curvature shifts to the left and the lesser curvature shifts to the right. The left side therefore forms the anterior surface and the right side the posterior surface. This explains why the left vagus nerve innervates the anterior surface while the right vagus nerve supplies the posterior surface.
- The cranial region becomes situated at the left and slightly inferiorly, while the converse is true for the caudal region. Before rotation, both the cranial and caudal ends are in the median plane.
- The long axis of the stomach becomes almost parallel with the long axis of the body.

## HISTOLOGY

All parts of the stomach have the same basic structural layers (Fig. 3.5):

- Mucosa.
- Submucosa.
- Muscularis externa.
- Serosa.

## Mucosa

The mucosa and submucosa are folded into longitudinal rugae when the stomach is empty. The mucosal surface is lined with simple columnar epithelium (which has a lifespan of about 1 week) and forms numerous gastric pits which are openings for the gastric glands. The mucous cells lining the gastric lumen secrete mucus as well as bicarbonate ions ($HCO_3^-$).

The depth of the gastric mucosa is divided into three histological zones (Fig. 3.6):

- A superficial zone (including the isthmus of the gland).
- A neck zone.
- A deep zone.

The upper superficial zone is composed of surface mucous cells with openings to the gastric pits, while the gland isthmus comprises mainly parietal cells.

The neck zone, between the superficial and deep zones, is composed of mostly immature stem cells, but has some neck mucous cells and parietal cells.

**Fig. 3.5** Cross-section of the stomach wall.

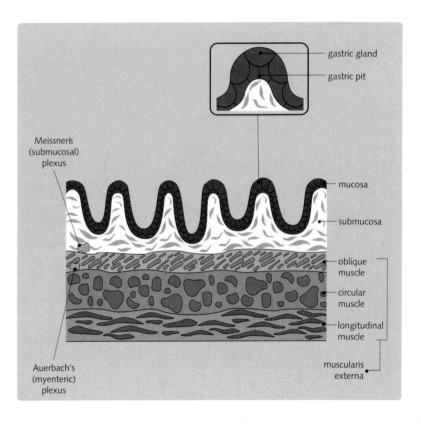

The immature stem cells eventually proliferate and move upwards to replace mucous cells in the superficial zone.

Stem cells are very important in the cell regeneration and healing of a gastric ulcer.

In the deep zone, glands are found. While the basic structure of any gastric gland is broadly similar, they also vary in structure according to where they are situated. Each of the three main areas of the stomach—the cardiac, fundus and body and the pyloric regions—have their own arrangement of gland (Fig. 3.6). The predominant cell types also vary according to region:

- Cardiac glands are predominantly composed of mucus-secreting cells.
- Glands in the fundus and body consist mostly of acid-secreting parietal cells and pepsin-secreting chief cells, along with some mucus-secreting cells.
- Pyloric glands are mostly composed of mucus-secreting cells and neuroendocrine cells which secrete the hormone gastrin.

The lamina propria contains numerous cells of the immune system, migrant cells from the blood and resident connective tissue cells. The muscularis mucosae consist of two thin layers of muscle.

## Submucosa

This is made up of collagen, fibroblasts and acellular matrix with blood vessels, nerves and lymphatics. It also contains autonomic ganglion cells and lymphoid aggregates, which make up the gut-associated lymphoid tissue (GALT). This structure is consistent throughout the digestive tract.

## Muscularis externa

Unlike the rest of the GI tract where the muscularis externa consists of two muscular coats, the gastric

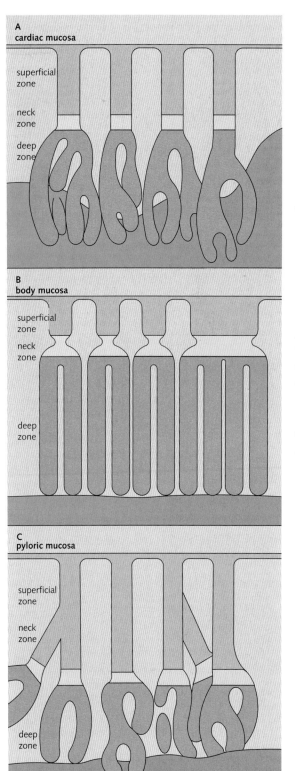

**Fig. 3.6** The different types of gland found in the stomach.
(A) Cardiac mucosa. (B) Body mucosa. (C) Pyloric mucosa.
(Redrawn with permission from Stevens A, Lowe J. Human Histology, 2nd edn. Edinburgh: Mosby, 1997.)

muscularis externa is comprised of three layers of smooth muscle:

- An outer longitudinal muscle layer (absent from much of the anterior and posterior surfaces of the stomach).
- A middle circular muscle layer (poorly developed in the paraoesophageal region).
- An inner oblique muscle layer.

## Serosa

This consists of an inner layer of connective tissue and an outer layer of simple squamous epithelium. It is also known as the visceral peritoneum and allows for frictionless movement of organs within their cavities.

## Gastric glands

As mentioned above, gastric glands vary according to their location, there being three main types which correspond roughly to the anatomical regions of the stomach.

### Gastric (body or fundic) glands

These are the most numerous and contain several types of cell:

- *Mucous neck cells* – These are found just below the gastric pits and contain numerous mucigen granules, a well-developed Golgi apparatus and rough endoplasmic reticula (RER). They are tall and columnar in shape, and stain poorly with haematoxylin and eosin (H&E) due to their mucin-containing vacuoles. They secrete $HCO_3^-$ ions into the mucous lining of the stomach wall.
- *Parietal (oxyntic) cells* – These are found deeper than mucous neck cells and are most plentiful in the gland isthmus. They are pyramidal cells which look triangular or rounded in section, with the apex pointing towards the gland lumen, and have a central spherical nucleus, which gives them a 'fried-egg' appearance. Parietal cells have eosinophilic cytoplasm and stain bright red with H&E, hence their alternative name, the oxyntic cell. They contain numerous mitochondria to provide energy for HCl production. They secrete HCl and intrinsic factor, which is needed for vitamin $B_{12}$ absorption. Parietal cells are absent in achlorhydria ('absence of acid'); thus, no intrinsic factor is

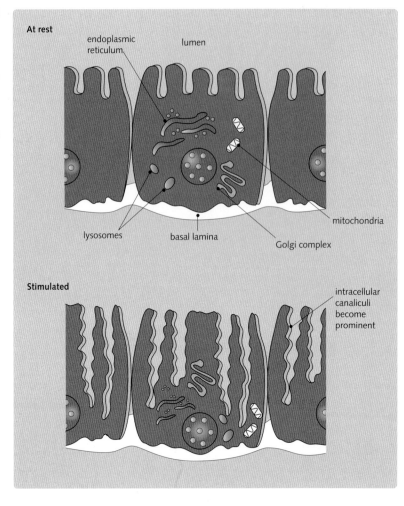

**Fig. 3.7** Morphological changes in parietal cells. At rest, the parietal cells have numerous tubulovesicles derived from smooth endoplasmic reticulum (SER). These contain H+ pumps and do not connect with the apical surface membrane. After stimulation of acid secretion, the tubulovesicles merge and become deep trough-like invaginations of the apical surface, called secretory canaliculi. These communicate with the lumen of the gland. The surface area is also increased by numerous microvilli.

produced in this condition, which if prolonged will cause vitamin B$_{12}$ deficiency and a macrocytic anaemia. Their internal appearance changes when food has been eaten (Fig. 3.7).

- *Chief (zymogen) cells* – These are found in the deepest part of gastric glands and are typical protein-secreting cells. They secrete pepsinogen, the inactive precursor of pepsin (a proteolytic enzyme), which is converted to pepsin by acid. They are rich in mitochondria, Golgi bodies and RER, which are required for the production of pepsinogen. The enzyme precursor is delivered to the lumen by exocytosis. Histologically, they have condensed nuclei which are basally located, and highly basophilic cytoplasm due to their numerous ribosomes.
- *Neuroendocrine (enteroendocrine) cells* – These are also called APUD cells (amine precursor uptake and decarboxylation cells) and are part of the diffuse neuroendocrine system. They are found on the epithelial basement membrane and secrete peptide hormonal substances, such as vasoactive intestinal polypeptide (VIP) and somatostatin. In the gastric region, the most common type of endocrine cell is the enterochromaffin-like (ECL) cell. These are 20 times smaller than parietal cells and secrete histamine into the lamina propria of the mucosa.
- *Undifferentiated stem cells* – Stem cells are precursors of all the mucosal epithelial cells. When undifferentiated, they show no cytoplasmic specialization and are capable of becoming any of the cell types present in the gastric mucosal glands. They are usually located in the neck zone. Histologically, they are most easily identified in mucosal sections by their mitotic figures after mucosal damage, as this is when they divide most actively.

## Cardiac glands

Cardiac glands are mostly mucus-secreting, coiled tubular glands, but they may be branched. The superficial and deep zones are about equal in thickness. Some undifferentiated stem cells are present in the neck region. Neuroendocrine (APUD) cells and parietal cells are scattered throughout, increasing in number nearer the junction with the body. The muscularis mucosae below the cardiac glands is thick and often interdigitates with the glands.

## Pyloric glands

The pyloric glands are coiled (but less so than cardiac ones) and often branched, with the superficial zone being slightly thicker than the deep zone. They contain mainly mucous cells, but they have parietal, enteroendocrine and stem cells scattered throughout.

In particular, the enteroendocrine cells secrete gastrin in this area. These cells are called G cells, because they secrete gastrin. D cells, another type of enteroendocrine cell, secrete somatostatin in paracrine fashion. Nearer the pyloric sphincter, parietal cells become more numerous. The cell types found in each region of the stomach are summarized in Fig. 3.8.

## Nerve fibres

There are two major networks of intrinsic nerve fibres:

- Auerbach's (myenteric) plexus, between the inner oblique and the middle circular muscle layer.
- Meissner's (submucous) plexus, between the inner oblique muscle layer and the mucosa.

Both plexuses are interconnected and contain nerve cells with processes that originate in the wall of the gut or mucosa.

The mucosa has mechanoreceptors and chemoreceptors, which are sensitive to stretch of the gut wall and composition of the stomach contents, respectively.

Nerve cells innervate hormone-secreting cells (see next section) and all the muscle layers in the mucosa.

The plexuses are sometimes described as a third division of the autonomic system—the enteric nervous system.

**Fig. 3.8** Types of gastric cell. (APUD cells = amine precursor uptake and decarboxylation cells; VIP = vasoactive intestinal polypeptide).

| Cell type | Area of stomach | | Function |
|---|---|---|---|
| Mucous cells | Cardiac | Many | Secrete mucus to protect the epithelium from acid secretions |
| | Gastric | Fewer | |
| | Pyloric | Many | |
| Parietal cells (oxyntic cells) | Cardiac | Few | Secretion of HCl and intrinsic factor (for vitamin $B_{12}$ absorption) |
| | Gastric | Many | |
| | Pyloric | More near the pyloric sphincter | |
| Chief cells (zymogen cells) | Cardiac | Many | Secretion of pepsinogen, the precursor of pepsin, a proteolytic enzyme |
| | Gastric | Few | |
| | Pyloric | | |
| Enteroendocrine (APUD cells) | Cardiac | Few | Secretion of protein hormones such as VIP and somatostatin (gastrin is secreted in the pyloric region) |
| | Gastric | Many | |
| | Pyloric | Few | |
| Stem cells | Cardiac | Present | These give rise to new cells to replace the old mucosal and glandular epithelial cells |
| | Gastric | Present | |
| | Pyloric | Present | |

# FUNCTIONS AND PHYSIOLOGY

## Storage of food

The stomach acts as a reservoir for food, releasing the gastric contents into the duodenum at a steady rate. Relaxation of the LOS and arrival of food in the stomach is followed by a receptive relaxation of the fundus and body of the stomach.

This is mediated by a vagal reflex, which inhibits the smooth muscle tone in this area (via the vagal inhibitory fibres with release of VIP and nitric oxide). The vagal inhibitory fibres cause relaxation by inducing hyperpolarization.

The muscle wall is thinner in the fundus and body, resulting in generally weaker muscle contractions than in the antral area. These factors allow the fundus and body of the stomach to store food and accommodate up to 1.5 L without a marked increase in intragastric pressure.

The muscles in the antral region contract vigorously, mixing the food with gastric secretions to continue digestion. Salivary digestion is still occurring, particularly at the centre of the mass. The smooth muscle in the antral area has a higher resistance to stretch than that of the fundus and body.

Food may remain in the stomach, unmixed, for up to 1 hour. Fats form an oily layer on top of other gastric contents. A fatty meal delays gastric emptying but liquids generally empty more quickly.

> Rennin is an enzyme produced in neonatal stomachs, which converts caseinogen (milk protein) to insoluble casein. This ensures the milk stays in the stomach for as long as possible, to be digested by other enzymes.

## Gastric secretions

The average adult produces 2–3 L of gastric juice every 24 hours. Gastric juice contains mucus, digestive enzymes (pepsinogen and lipase), HCl and intrinsic factor.

## Resting juice

Resting juice is an isotonic juice secreted by the *surface cells*. It is similar to plasma, but it has an alkaline pH of 7.7 and a higher concentration of $HCO_3^-$.

## Mucus

Mucus is secreted by *goblet cells* of the surface epithelium and *mucus neck cells*, especially in the pyloric antrum.

The alkaline mucus of the stomach is a thick, sticky mucopolysaccharide. It is secreted with $HCO_3^-$ ions, which are exchanged for $Cl^-$ ions by the epithelial cells. It plays an important role in the protection of the stomach against its acid contents.

Mucus forms a water-insoluble gel that adheres to the surface of the stomach lumen. It reduces the flow of $H^+$ ions and acts as a barrier to pepsin. Although pepsin can degrade mucus, the $HCO_3^-$ secretions increase the pH and make the enzyme less active.

## Pepsin

Pepsin is secreted from the *chief cells* in the gastric pits in the form of its precursor, pepsinogen. HCl activates pepsinogen (42 kDa) by cleaving off nine amino acid residues to form pepsin (37.5 kDa).

Pepsin is a proteolytic enzyme that acts on proteins and polypeptides, by hydrolysing internal peptide bonds.

## Lipase

Gastric lipase is an enzyme that acts on triglycerides to produce fatty acids and glycerol. It is useful in facilitating subsequent hydrolysis by pancreatic lipases, but it is of little physiological importance except in pancreatic insufficiency.

## Intrinsic factor

Intrinsic factor (IF) is made in the *parietal* cells of the stomach; it is a glycoprotein vital for the absorption of vitamin $B_{12}$ via receptors for IF-$B_{12}$ in the terminal ileum. Without intrinsic factor, vitamin $B_{12}$ is digested in the intestine and not absorbed.

R-proteins in the saliva and stomach protect vitamin $B_{12}$ until it is absorbed. Upon absorption, it is bound to transcobalamin II, which serves to transport it in plasma.

Most diets contain excess vitamin $B_{12}$ and stores are built up in the liver. These stores last for 2–3 years; thus, it takes considerable time for a dietary deficiency to produce symptoms. However, once body stores have been used up, pernicious anaemia develops.

## Hydrochloric acid

HCl is produced by the parietal (oxyntic) cells. The concentration of HCl depends on:

- The rate of HCl secretion.
- The amount of buffering provided by the resting juice, ingested food and drink and the alkaline secretion of the pyloric glands, duodenum, pancreas and bile.
- Gastric motility.
- The rate of gastric emptying.
- The amount of diffusion back into the mucosa.

The pH of the contents of the stomach after feeding is normally about 2–3.

Gastric HCl is not essential for life, but it has a number of important functions. It provides a defence mechanism that is non-specific in killing ingested microorganisms. It also aids protein digestion (by enabling the activation of pepsin from pepsinogen) and stimulates the flow of bile and pancreatic juice.

The secretion of HCl by parietal cells is stimulated by histamine, acetylcholine and gastrin (Fig. 3.9). It is also stimulated by caffeine, through the activation of cyclic AMP. Both $H^+$ and $Cl^-$ are actively transported by different ion pumps in the parietal cell membrane.

> Because alcohol and caffeine are substances which promote the secretion of HCl, patients with peptic ulcers or underlying gastric hypersecretion should avoid beverages which contain these two chemicals.

Secretion is inhibited by vagotomy (which removes acetylcholine stimulation) and pharmacologically, the latter of which is covered in the next section.

## Pharmacology of gastric acid secretion

The key points to note are:

- The three main factors which stimulate acid production are gastrin, histamine and acetylcholine.

Fig. 3.9 Stimulation of secretion of HCl by parietal cells. (ACh = acetylcholine; AC = adenylate cyclase; ECL = enterochromaffin-like; $IP_3$ = inositol triphosphate; PLC = phospholipase C; cAMP = cyclic AMP; ATP = adenosine triphosphate; GR = gastrin receptor; MR = muscarinic receptor; $H_2R$ = histamine-2 receptor.)

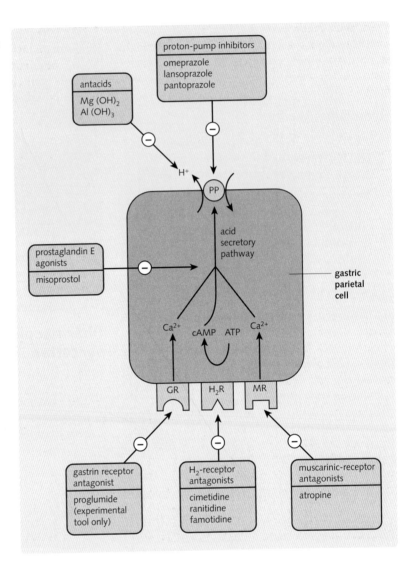

**Fig. 3.10** Sites and mechanisms of action of drugs which inhibit gastric acid secretion and drugs which protect the gastric mucosa. (GR = gastrin receptor; H$_2$R = histamine-2 receptor; MR = muscarinic receptor; PP = proton pump; cAMP = cyclic AMP; ATP = adenosine triphosphate.)

- Acid secretion can be modified by extrinsic neural factors (vagus nerve) and intrinsic neural reflexes.
- The terminal step in the pathway is H$^+$/K$^+$-ATPase.

As such, these factors, or their receptors, are possible sites of action for drugs which inhibit gastric acid secretion. There are also drugs which act to neutralize secreted acid.

However, no drugs which act on muscarinic or gastrin receptors are currently licensed for clinical use to inhibit gastric acid secretion, although a muscarinic blocker such as atropine will have this effect. Proglumide is a gastrin receptor blocker, but it is an experimental tool only.

Fig. 3.10 summarizes the gastric pharmacology relevant to the scope of this book.

## H$_2$-receptor antagonists

These block H$_2$-receptors on the gastric parietal cell, preventing intracellular cAMP synthesis and thus reducing acid secretion. Additionally, they also inhibit gastrin-stimulated acid secretion and decrease acetylcholine-stimulated secretion, as a result of which pepsin secretion also decreases due to the reduction in volume.

As such, they promote healing of duodenal ulcers, but relapses are likely when treatment is stopped. Common examples of $H_2$-receptor antagonists are cimetidine, ranitidine, nizatidine and famotidine.

## Proton-pump inhibitors (PPIs)

PPIs are irreversible inhibitors of $H^+/K^+$-ATPase, also known as the proton pump. As stated above, the proton pump is the final step in the acid secretory pathway. PPIs are so far the most effective and powerful drugs in reducing gastric acid secretion. Examples of PPIs are omeprazole, lansoprazole, pantoprazole and rabeprazole.

PPIs are weak bases inactive at neutral pH, and they therefore accumulate and are activated in the acidic environment of the parietal cell canaliculi. This preferential accumulation causes PPIs to have a specific effect on the parietal cells. They are the drug of choice in drug-resistant peptic ulceration and in hypersecretion caused by the Zollinger–Ellison syndrome.

PPIs are the most effective class of drug at reducing gastric acid secretion as they are irreversible inhibitors of $H^+/K^+$-ATPase, thus acid production can continue only when new enzymes have been synthesized.

## Antacids

Antacids neutralize gastric acid and therefore cause a rise in gastric pH. They thus cause inhibition of peptic activity, as secretion ceases at pH 5. Common antacids are salts of aluminium and magnesium, for example aluminium hydroxide and magnesium hydroxide. It is important to note that magnesium salts cause diarrhoea while aluminium salts cause constipation, therefore mixtures of the two types of salts are used to ensure normal bowel function.

Alginates may be combined with antacids, an example of which is Gaviscon. These are used in oesophageal reflux. The alginic acid, when combined with saliva, forms a raft which floats on the gastric contents, thus protecting the oesophageal mucosa during reflux.

# Control of gastric secretion

The control of gastric secretion is brought about by a combination of nervous, hormonal and paracrine messages. There are three phases of stimulation (Fig. 3.11):

- The cephalic phase.
- The gastric phase.
- The intestinal phase.

## The cephalic phase

The cephalic phase is the shortest phase and is initiated by the sight, smell and taste of food. It usually begins before the meal and lasts up to 30 minutes into the meal. This allows the stomach to prepare itself for the imminent arrival of food.

It is mediated entirely by the vagus nerve, hence vagotomy of the stomach leads to cessation of the cephalic phase and was performed in the past to reduce acid secretion before pharmacological means were available.

Acid secretion is upregulated by acetylcholine (ACh) released from neurons of the intramural plexus acting:

- Directly, by stimulation of the parietal cells.
- Indirectly, by causing release of gastrin from antral G cells, which stimulates the parietal cells too. The mediator at the G cell is gastrin-releasing peptide (GRP).
- Indirectly, by causing the release of histamine from ECL cells, which also upregulates acid production.

## The gastric phase

This is the longest phase, lasting for up to $2\frac{1}{2}$ hours after the start of the meal. It is triggered by the presence of food causing distension of the stomach, and the presence of amino acids and peptides (products of pepsin degradation). Alcohol and caffeine are also pro-secretory factors. Most acid secretion in response to a meal takes place during the gastric phase.

Distension of the body or antrum of the stomach stimulates mechanoreceptors that cause local (enteric) and central vago-vagal cholinergic reflexes.

Amino acids and peptides activate vagal chemoreceptors and also antral G cells, which are sensitive to peptides. These secrete gastrin in response.

Gastrin and acetylcholine then activate ECL cells to produce histamine, which further increases acid secretion from the parietal cells.

A

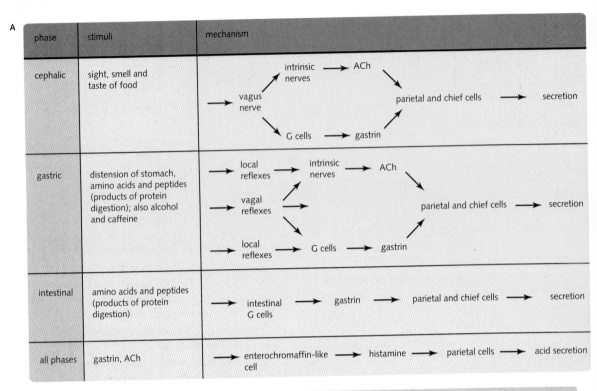

| phase | stimuli | mechanism |
|---|---|---|

**Fig. 3.11** The three phases of gastric secretion. (A) Control mechanisms for each phase of gastric secretion. (ACh = acetylcholine.) (B) Graphical representation of the three stages.

B

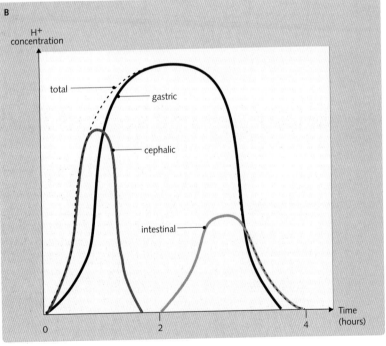

Vago-vagal reflexes, as found in the gastric phase of the control of gastric secretions, are so named because both afferent and efferent impulses are carried by neurons in the vagus nerve.

## The intestinal phase

The intestinal phase is brought about by the presence of chyme in the duodenum. It has both excitatory and inhibitory components. In the excitatory component, amino acids and peptides in chyme stimulate intestinal gastrin release. This is carried via the blood to the stomach and thus contributes to serum gastrin levels during a meal.

The inhibitory phase, however, predominates, as the same factors, i.e. acid (with a pH less than 2), fat, hypertonicity and distension have the following effects in the duodenum:

- Somatostatin is released from D cells. This acts directly on the parietal cells to inhibit acid secretion.

- Acid mediates the release of secretin into the bloodstream. This inhibits the release of gastrin by G cells and reduces the response of parietal cells to gastrin.
- Fatty acids (from triglyceride digestion) in the duodenum and proximal jejunum cause the release of gastric inhibitory polypeptide (GIP) and cholecystokinin (CCK), which both act to inhibit secretion of acid by parietal cells. GIP also suppresses gastrin release.

Secretin, GIP and CCK are collectively called enterogastrones, because they have an inhibitory effect on gastric secretion. Hypertonic solutions in the duodenum also suppress gastric secretion. This is mediated by an unidentified enterogastrone. The inhibition of gastric secretions is also controlled by an enteric reflex, which is integrated with higher controls from the medulla oblongata.

The loss of volume in the stomach and the distension of the duodenum (as chyme passes from one to the other), both activate the local enteric reflex, via mechanoreceptors. Chemoreceptors in the duodenum can also activate the reflex ion response to irritants, reduced pH and hypertonic solutions. The mechanisms for inhibiting acid secretion are summarized in Fig. 3.12.

**Fig. 3.12** Mechanisms inhibiting gastric acid secretion.

| Stimulus | Mediator | Action |
|---|---|---|
| Acid (pH <2) | Somatostatin | Directly inhibits parietal cells |
| | Secretin | Inhibits gastrin release Decreases response of parietal cells to gastrin |
| | Enteric reflex | Directly inhibits parietal cells |
| Fatty acids | Gastric inhibitory peptide (GIP) | Directly inhibits parietal cells Inhibits gastrin secretion from G cells |
| | Cholecystokinin (CCK) | Adds to the inhibition of parietal cells |
| Hypertonic solutions | Unidentified enterogesterone | Inhibits acid secretion |
| | Enteric reflex | Inhibits acid secretion |
| Distension of duodenum | Mechanoreceptor initiated enteric reflex | Decreases acid secretion |
| Emptying of stomach | Enteric reflex | Decreases acid secretion |

# Gastric motility and emptying

Gastric motility and emptying are carefully regulated to ensure that chyme is delivered to the duodenum at a rate at which it can be absorbed.

## Gastric motility

Motility in the stomach is initially brought about by reflex receptive relaxation, which allows food to enter from the oesophagus. This process is mediated by vagal inhibitory fibres.

Mixing of the food with gastric secretions follows and takes place in the distal body and antrum of the stomach (the caudal region). The muscularis externa is thicker in this area of the stomach. The contractions involved in mixing and emptying the stomach contents are brought about by the three smooth muscle layers, which are coordinated by intrinsic and extrinsic nerves.

The most prominent plexus is Auerbach's plexus, situated in a three-dimensional matrix between the layers of smooth muscle in the stomach wall. It receives innervation from both sympathetic and parasympathetic systems. Axons from the plexus innervate both muscle fibres and glandular cells.

Interneurons connect intrinsic afferent sensory fibres with efferent neurons of smooth muscle and secretory cells, to ensure that gastric activity is fully coordinated, even in the absence of external innervation. Cholinergic (parasympathetic) stimulation from the vagus increases gastric motility and secretion, but adrenergic (sympathetic) stimulation in the coeliac plexus has the opposite effect.

### The mechanics of gastric motility

When the stomach is full of food, it undergoes a 'lag' phase. During this time, the stomach is not contracting, but intense secretions are digesting the food down to basic components to form chyme. Once the lag phase is over, there is a reversal of vagal discharge. There is an upregulation in vagal excitatory fibre activation and a decrease in vagal inhibitory fibre activation.

The contractions break off small boluses of food, carrying them towards the pylorus. Large pieces of food are refluxed back towards the gastric body for further degradation. This process is termed retropulsion and allows for the thorough mixing and mechanical breakdown of solid food material (Fig. 3.13).

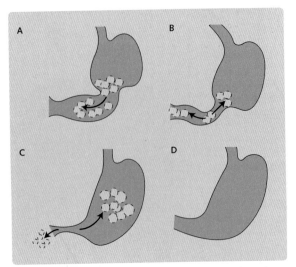

Fig. 3.13 Effects of gastric peristaltic contractions on intraluminal contents. (Redrawn with permission from Johnson LR. Physiology of the Gastrointestinal Tract, 4th edn. New York: Raven Press, 2000.)

The force and frequency of contractions depends on:

- The neural activity of intrinsic and extrinsic nerves.
- The myogenic properties of smooth muscle.
- The properties of paracrine and endocrine agents (gastrin and motilin upregulate the force of gastric contraction, but secretin inhibits it).

The cephalad region of the stomach (fundus and corpus) is the area for storage and the caudad region (distal corpus and antrum) is the area for mixing food.

### The basic electrical rhythm of the stomach

The pacemaker zone of the stomach is located in the fundus on the greater curvature. The cells in the pacemaker zone spontaneously depolarize, setting the basic electrical rhythm (BER) of the stomach. This depolarization occurs continuously. Depending on the excitability of the gastric smooth muscle at the time, the BER may trigger large peristaltic contractions. These sweep down towards the antrum where the amplitude of contraction is greatest, due to its thicker muscle layers (the smooth muscle of the fundus and body is much thinner). The contractions occur at a rate of 3 per minute, and last between 2 and 20 seconds (Fig. 3.14).

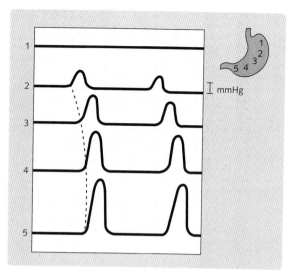

**Fig. 3.14** Intraluminal pressures recorded from five areas in the stomach. (Redrawn with permission from Johnson LR. Physiology of the Gastrointestinal Tract, 4th edn. New York: Raven Press, 2000.)

Between contractions, the pressure in the caudal region of the stomach nearly equals intra-abdominal pressure.

## Gastric emptying

Emptying of gastric contents into the duodenum is part of the continuum of gastric motility. As retropulsion occurs, the pyloric sphincter opens by a coordination of antral and duodenal contractions. Small digested particles are squirted through the sphincter into the duodenum. The rate at which the stomach empties depends on:

- *The type of food eaten.* Carbohydrates are emptied most quickly, proteins more slowly and fatty foods even more so to ensure that food is released into the duodenum at a rate at which it can be absorbed. Fatty acids or monoglycerides in the duodenum decrease the rate of gastric emptying by increasing the contractility of the pyloric sphincter. The presence of acidic contents with a pH of less than about 3.5 in the duodenum also slows gastric emptying, as may amino acids and peptides.
- *The osmotic pressure of the contents of the duodenum.* Duodenal osmoreceptors initiate a decrease in gastric emptying in response to hyperosmolar chyme.

- *Vagal innervation.* Antral and duodenal overdistension activates mechanoreceptors that stimulate a vago-vagal reflex. This acts to inhibit gastric contractile activity by vagal inhibitory fibres. Vagotomy results in a marked decrease in the rate of gastric emptying.
- *The release of somatostatin, secretin, CCK and GIP by the duodenum,* in response to the presence of chyme. These all inhibit gastric emptying.

## Protection of the gastric mucosa

The gastric mucosa is frequently subjected to the corrosive secretions of HCl and pepsin. Several mechanisms exist to prevent tissue damage by the gastric juices:

> When the stomach is empty, it is small and relaxed. Peristaltic contractions are weak, but as hunger sets in, the muscle contractions increase in size and frequency. The tetanic contractions last for 2–3 min. Hunger pangs usually begin 12 hours after the previous meal. Low blood sugar increases the contractions.

> Liquids empty from the stomach at a faster rate than solids, unless they have a high lipid content. Solids and semi-solids undergo a lag phase of intense secretion before the stomach begins to empty.

- *Mucus,* secreted by neck and surface mucous cells in the body and fundus and similar cells elsewhere in the stomach, forms a water-insoluble gel that coats the mucosa (Fig. 3.15). Prostaglandins stimulate mucus production.
- *The surface cells secrete $HCO_3^-$ which, together with the mucus, forms an adherent layer.* This raises the pH around the mucus layer, thus making pepsin less active and preventing the enzymes degrading the mucus.
- *The surface membranes of the mucosal cells, the tight junctions between them and the ability to form a fibrin coat* protect the cells.

Fig. 3.15 Protection of gastric mucosa from low pH by mucus layer. (Redrawn with permission from Underwood JCE. General and Systematic Pathology, 4th edn. Edinburgh: Churchill Livingstone, 2004.)

- *Prostaglandins*, especially those of the E and I series, inhibit acid secretion by enhancing blood flow to the mucosa which in turn encourages mucus production.

Several factors cause a breakdown of the mucosal protection or an increase in acid production and predispose to gastric irritation and peptic ulceration:

- Acid secretion (from the parietal cells) is stimulated by histamine, acetylcholine and gastrin (Fig. 3.9).
- *Non-steroidal anti-inflammatory drugs (NSAIDs) and aspirin* reduce mucus secretion and decrease bicarbonate secretion by inhibiting prostaglandin production.
- In the Zollinger–Ellison syndrome, gastrin-secreting adenomas result in marked hyperacidity. The adenomas are usually found in the pancreas and present as gastric or duodenal ulcers. The syndrome is rare.
- *Helicobacter pylori* (see later).
- *Hyperparathyroidism* predisposes to ulcer formation because increased levels of calcium stimulate acid production.
- Chronic exposure to nicotine from smoking causes an increase in acid secretion.
- Stress may also result in ulcer formation (this is rare).

# Pharmacology of gastric mucosal protection

As mentioned above, prostaglandins are protective against gastric mucosal ulceration. Prostaglandin analogues have the same effect. Misoprostol, which is a stable analogue of $PGE_1$ protects the mucosa by inhibiting gastric acid secretion, enhancing or maintaining the blood flow to the mucosa and increasing the secretion of bicarbonate and mucus. It is used to prevent gastric ulceration due to long-term use of non-steroidal anti-inflammatory drugs (NSAIDs), which also act through the arachidonic acid/prostaglandin pathway.

Sucralfate is a complex of sulphated sucrose and aluminium hydroxide. In acidic conditions under pH 4, it forms a polymerized gel with mucus. The gel is believed to decrease mucus degradation as well as limit hydrogen ion diffusion. In addition, it stimulates mucus and bicarbonate production as well as prostaglandin secretion.

Bismuth chelate protects the mucosa by coating the bases of peptic ulcers, adsorbing pepsin and increasing bicarbonate and prostaglandin secretion. More importantly, it has toxic effects on *H. pylori* and may be used as part of triple therapy to eradicate the bacterium. Bismuth may cause blackening of the faeces and tongue.

# Gastric defences against infection

The stomach has a number of defence strategies. Gastric acid and pepsin secretions act to kill aerobic micro-organisms (they require oxygen) and other ingested bacteria, preventing infection of the gastric mucosa.

The intestines are colonized with millions of commensal anaerobic microorganisms. These prevent other organisms colonizing and causing damage or inflammation. However, because of the presence of these commensals, rupture of the stomach or intestines may lead to peritonitis.

Other factors preventing infection include:

- Mucus production.
- Peristalsis and fluid movement.
- Seamless epithelium with tight junctions.
- A fast cell turnover.
- IgA secretions at mucosal surfaces.

# DISORDERS OF THE STOMACH

## Congenital abnormalities

### Diaphragmatic hernia

The diaphragm develops from:

- The septum transversum.
- The pleuroperitoneal membranes.
- The dorsal mesentery of the oesophagus.
- Muscular components of the body wall.

The pleuroperitoneal folds appear at the beginning of week 5. They fuse with the septum transversum and the oesophageal mesentery in week 7, separating the abdominal and thoracic cavities. This primitive diaphragm then fuses with a ring of muscle that develops from the body wall.

If there is incomplete fusion, the contents of the abdomen may push up into the pleural cavity, forming a diaphragmatic hernia (usually on the left side), pushing the heart forwards and compressing the lungs. The incidence is about 1 in 2000 births and treatment is surgical.

### Hypertrophic pyloric stenosis

Pyloric stenosis (narrowing) occurs in about 1 in 150 male infants and 1 in 750 female infants. A genetic factor is involved.

Stenosis is caused by hypertrophy of the circular muscles of the pylorus, obstructing the pyloric canal and the flow of contents from the stomach into the duodenum. Typically, it presents 4–6 weeks after birth with projectile vomiting within half an hour of a feed. Note that there is no bile in the vomit because the obstruction is proximal to the ampulla of Vater.

Peristaltic waves are visible in the child, a sausage-shaped mass (the enlarged pylorus) can be felt in the right upper quadrant and the hypertrophied pyloric muscle can be observed using ultrasonography. Treatment is surgical.

Stenosis may also be acquired in adult life, usually caused by scarring from peptic ulceration or because of malignancy obstructing the outflow. It is diagnosed by barium meal and gastroscopy.

> When treating a patient who is vomiting, always test the vomit for the presence of bile. Bile joins the intestinal contents at the ampulla of Vater. Vomit will only contain bile if the lesion is below the ampulla.

# Gastritis (inflammation of the stomach)

Inflammation of the stomach (gastritis) may be acute or chronic.

## Acute gastritis

This involves an acute inflammatory reaction at the superficial mucosa, with the infiltration of neutrophils. Acute gastritis is almost always caused by drugs (especially NSAIDs such as aspirin) or by alcohol (the most common cause) causing chemical exfoliation of the surface epithelial cells and decreasing the secretion of protective mucus.

The causative drugs or chemicals often inhibit prostaglandins, which protect the gastric mucosa by stimulating mucus and $HCO_3^-$ production and inhibiting acid secretion (despite their role in inflammation). The degree of damage depends on the amount of toxic substance and the time it has been there. It also varies from erosions (acute erosive gastritis, see below) to ulcers (involving the full thickness of the mucosa). *H. pylori* has been implicated in both acute and chronic gastritis.

Acute erosive gastritis is typified by a partial loss of gastric mucosa. It is caused by shock, severe burns and toxic substances and alcohol as mentioned above. Discomfort (dyspepsia) and vomiting are typical symptoms; if ulceration is severe there may be haematemesis.

Severe necrotizing ulcerative gastritis occurs when strong acids or alkalis are ingested.

NSAIDS, such as aspirin, inhibit the enzyme cyclooxygenase (COX), which is necessary for prostaglandin production. Concurrent therapy with a proton-pump inhibitor can prevent gastritis and ulcer formation.

## Chronic gastritis

Chronic inflammatory changes in the mucosa cause atrophy and epithelial metaplasia (which may develop into carcinoma). Chronic gastritis is classified as:

- Type A (autoimmune).
- Type B (bacterial infection).
- Type C (reflux).

An aid to remembering the different types of gastritis: A is for autoimmune, B for bacterial and C for chemical (reflux).

### Type A gastritis

Inflammation is caused by antibodies against gastric parietal cells (90%) and intrinsic factor (60%). Intrinsic factor is needed to absorb vitamin $B_{12}$. In its absence, macrocytic anaemia develops once liver stores of vitamin $B_{12}$ have been used up.

Pernicious anaemia occurs where autoimmune gastritis and macrocytic anaemia exist together. It is associated with other autoimmune diseases such as thyroid disease, vitiligo, Addison's disease and myxoedema. Pernicious anaemia is a risk factor for carcinoma of the stomach.

The body of the stomach is always affected and often this type of gastritis involves the entire stomach.

Vitamin $B_{12}$ is needed for the synthesis of DNA. Normally, the nucleus is extruded from red blood cells before they are released into the peripheral blood from the bone marrow. In vitamin $B_{12}$ deficiency, however, maturation of the nucleus is delayed relative to the cytoplasm and macrocytic blood cells are seen in the peripheral blood.

### Type B gastritis

*Helicobacter pylori* infection is present in about 90% of cases of active chronic type B gastritis. It provokes an acute inflammatory response and the release of proteases, which destroy gastric glands, leading to atrophy. There is a mixed acute and chronic inflammatory reaction in the epithelium and lamina propria.

Type B gastritis usually begins in the antrum, but it may cause atrophy, fibrosis and intestinal metaplasia of the entire stomach, where the normal gastric mucosa is replaced with epithelium similar to that found in the small intestine.

### Type C gastritis

Also known as reflux or reactive gastritis, this is caused by regurgitation of duodenal contents into the stomach through the pylorus and is more common where pyloric or duodenal motility has been compromised, for example after surgery to the pyloric part. This type of gastritis is caused by irritants such as NSAIDs, alcohol and biliary reflux, and may present with dyspepsia and bilious vomiting.

### Helicobacter pylori

*Helicobacter pylori* is a Gram-negative spiral-shaped bacillus with the ability to penetrate the gastric mucus lining. It is a common pathogen, with more than half of adults over the age of 50 in the UK being infected, but the incidence in younger groups is falling. In developing countries the infection rate is far higher, with rates of up to 90% in some countries, and patients usually acquire the infection during childhood. However, most infected patients are asymptomatic.

The bacterium is highly pathogenic and has many virulence factors which allow it to survive in the hostile environment of the stomach:

- Its *motility* allows it to penetrate close to the epithelium, where the pH is near-neutral.
- It produces the enzyme *urease*, which converts urea to ammonia, which buffers the gastric acid with the concurrent production of carbon dioxide. This is a highly effective virulence factor, as urea channels in the inner cell membrane of the bacterium open at pH levels less than 6.5, delivering urea to the bacterial urease. The activity of *H. pylori* urease is the basis for the urea breath test to detect the bacterium (see Chapter 10).

- The *vacuolating toxin* (VacA) alters intracellular vesicular trafficking in gastric cells, leading to the formation of large vacuoles.
- The *cytotoxin-associated antigen* (CagA) is an immunodominant antigen which elicits a strong serological response. It has been shown to be involved in pathogenesis via the insertion of pathogenicity islands.
- Other virulence factors include *adhesin, phospholipases and porins.*

Fortunately, *H. pylori* can be eradicated pharmacologically with a combination of a PPI plus two antibiotics (triple therapy). Current examples are:

- Omeprazole, amoxycillin and metronidazole.
- Lanzoprazole, clarithromycin and tinidazole.

Adherence to treatment, resistance to metronidazole and side-effects are the main determinants of success with triple therapy. Quadruple therapy, with the addition of bismuth chelate (see above) should be offered to patients in whom triple therapy is unsuccessful. Note that metronidazole should not be given during the first trimester of pregnancy and interacts adversely with alcohol.

When prescribing metronidazole, advise patients to avoid alcohol. Metronidazole has a disulfiram-like effect and patients will feel severely ill if they drink alcohol at the same time. Disulfiram inhibits acetaldehyde dehydrogenase, an enzyme in the pathway for alcohol metabolism. In this situation acetaldehyde builds up which can cause unpleasant flushing and nausea. Unless they are warned, they will understandably think the symptoms are caused by the drug and stop taking it.

## Peptic ulcer disease

Ulcers arise when damaging factors, particularly gastric secretions, overwhelm the natural protection of the mucosal lining of the gastrointestinal tract. They can result from a decrease in protective factors, an increase in damaging factors, or both.

Peptic ulcers can be divided into acute and chronic forms. The former are usually caused by the same factors as acute erosive gastritis, and in the same locations. Severe stress and trauma, such as after burns (Curling's ulcer), head trauma (Cushing's ulcer) and ischaemia of the gastric mucosa are other causes.

Chronic peptic ulcers occur in the upper gastrointestinal tract where gastric acid and pepsin are present. They are caused by hyperacidity, *H. pylori* infection (the commonest cause), reflux of duodenal contents, NSAIDs and smoking. Genetic factors play a role, as peptic ulceration is more common in patients with blood group O and first-degree relatives of people with duodenal ulcers are three times more likely to develop them themselves. Males are three times more likely to develop chronic ulcers than females. They are an example of a chronic inflammatory process (Fig. 3.16).

Peptic ulcers are most common in:

- The duodenal cap.
- The stomach (especially at the junction of the antrum and body).
- The distal oesophagus, particularly in a Barrett's oesophagus.
- A Meckel's diverticulum (particularly where ectopic gastric mucosa is present).
- Where a gastroenterostomy has been performed.

Duodenal ulcers (DU) are two to three times more common than gastric ulcers (GU), occurring in about 15% of the population. There is an increase in incidence of peptic ulcer above the age of 45 years. Both duodenal and gastric ulcers are common in the elderly.

About 90% of DU and 70% of GU are associated with *H. pylori*. NSAID treatment is associated with the rest.

Gastric ulcers may also occur in response to acute gastritis or extreme hyperacidity, as in Zollinger–Ellison syndrome. Excess gastrin secretion in this syndrome may also cause hypertrophy of the rugae, which may be mistaken for a tumour on a radiograph.

Zollinger–Ellison syndrome is a rare condition due to gastrin-secreting pancreatic adenomas causing excess acid production. It can lead to acute ulcers in the antrum, duodenum and, in severe cases, the jejunum.

Complications of chronic peptic ulcer include:

- Haemorrhage.
- Perforation, leading to peritonitis.
- Penetration, where the ulcer penetrates through the stomach or duodenal wall into underlying tissue. Usually it is the pancreas or liver which is affected.

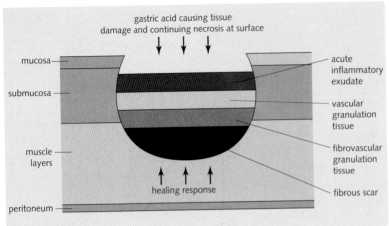

**Fig. 3.16** Structure of a peptic ulcer. The interplay between the opposing forces of continuing tissue damage and healing with scar formation is the cause of chronic inflammation. (Redrawn with permission from Stevens A, Lowe J. Human Histology, 2nd edn. Edinburgh: Mosby, 1997.)

- Stricture, causing acquired pyloric stenosis in the stomach, or oesophageal stricture which is more common.
- Malignant change, which is rare.

Endoscopy and tests for the presence of *H. pylori* are the usual investigations performed when peptic ulcer disease is suspected.

## Vascular disorders

### Angiodysplasia

Angiodysplasia is a rare cause of upper gastro-intestinal bleeding, which may range in severity from occult to massive. It is a condition where there is one or more malformed blood vessels (typically veins) in the mucosa or submucosa. These can be found anywhere in the gastro-intestinal tract. The vessels are dilated, thin-walled and look like 'cherry spots'. They are normally asymptomatic.

A Dieulafoy lesion is an example of angiodys-plasia. It is a large ulcerated submucosal vessel. Because of the ulceration, it may bleed heavily. It is associated with chronic gastritis.

### Gastric varices

Gastric varices are uncommon, but they may occur in submucosal veins below the gastro-oesophageal junction as a result of portal hypertension.

Like oesophageal varices, they should never be biopsied or they will haemorrhage with potentially fatal consequences.

Treatment includes injecting with a sclerosing agent to arrest bleeding by thrombosis or banding

to cut off the blood flow to the damaged vessel. Bleeding ulcers can be injected with adrenaline (epinephrine) or a sclerosing agent.

## Delayed gastric emptying

Gastric emptying can be delayed by mechanical or non-mechanical obstructions.

Mechanical obstructions include tumours, duodenal, gastric or pyloric stenosis, and bezoars (a mass of swallowed foreign material, which has collected and is obstructing emptying).

Non-mechanical delayed gastric emptying is known as gastroparesis. This is an uncommon complication of diabetes, but it can also occur due to gastric arrhythmias, myotonic dystrophy, collagen-vascular diseases, neuropathies and after vagotomy.

Mechanical delayed gastric emptying must be excluded before non-mechanical aetiologies can be explored. Quite often, the cause is unknown and the problem is called idiopathic gastroparesis, but is probably due to gastric arrhythmias. Diabetic gastroparesis is associated with peripheral neuropathy.

Patients can be asymptomatic, or they may have a combination of symptoms, including bloating, abdominal pain, persistent belching, nausea (with or without vomiting), anorexia, early satiety and weight loss.

Treatment includes:

- Nutritional supplementation.
- Prokinetic drugs, e.g. metoclopramide – see Chapter 7.
- Surgery.

# Neoplastic disease

## Benign neoplasms

These include:

- Leiomyomas, arising from smooth muscle, which may bleed from ulceration. These are the most common benign gastric tumours.
- Adenomas (benign tumours of glandular origin) make up 5–10% of polypoid lesions in the stomach and may contain proliferative dysplastic epithelium with the potential for malignant transformation. They are much more common in the colon but, if present in the stomach, are usually in the antrum. They may be pedunculated (with a stalk) or sessile (without a stalk) and are more common in males. The incidence of adenomas increases with age.
- Hyperplastic polyps (regenerative polyps) are elongated gastric pits separated by fibrous tissue, usually found in association with *H. pylori* infection in the antrum.
- Simple fundic polyps (glandular cystic dilatation in the body of the stomach).
- Hamartomas (overgrowth of mature tissue, displaying disordered arrangement and proportion) are most commonly seen in Peutz–Jeghers syndrome, a hereditary disorder.
- Ectopic (heterotopic) pancreatic tissue.
- Fibromas and neurofibromas, which are connective tissue tumours.
- Haemangiomas, which are highly vascular in nature.

## Malignant neoplasms

### Aetiology

Adenocarcinoma is the most common gastric neoplasm and accounts for 90% of all malignant neoplasms in the stomach. Malignant lymphomas account for 5% of gastric malignant neoplasms, and other malignancies such as carcinoid and malignant spindle cell tumours occur rarely.

In the UK, 15 in 100 000 men are affected each year with gastric carcinoma and the incidence increases with age, affecting men more than women. It is the fifth biggest cause of death due to malignancy, surpassed only by lung, colorectal, breast and prostate carcinoma. Nevertheless, the incidence is falling in both Europe and the USA, although it remains high in the Far East, for example in Japan.

A number of conditions are premalignant, such as atrophic gastritis, some chronic gastric ulcers, pernicious anaemia, and post-gastrectomy (carcinomas often develop 15–20 years after surgery).

Genetic factors may be involved, as the incidence is slightly higher in blood group A as well as in patients with hereditary non-polyposis colorectal cancer, but a decrease in gastric acid secretion and corresponding increase in bacteria (which are normally killed by gastric acid), particularly *H. pylori*, are common predisposing factors.

*Helicobacter pylori* infections cause chronic gastritis, which occasionally becomes atrophic gastritis, leading to metaplasia, dysplasia and ultimately carcinoma.

Dietary factors may act to initiate or promote carcinogenesis. A diet high in salt increases the risk. Also, dietary nitrates are converted to carcinogenic nitrosamines by bacteria. Therefore, diets high in nitrates predispose to carcinoma. The incidence is high in Japan but much lower amongst Japanese living in the USA. Diets high in fruit and vegetables can help protect against cancer because of the antioxidants they contain.

### Pathology

Four different macroscopic appearances may be recognized:

- *Malignant ulcers* with raised, everted edges.
- *Polypoid tumours*—these tend to present early with discomfort, as they protrude into the lumen and so are subject to trauma. It has the best prognosis of all the pathological types as it is most suitable for surgical excision.
- *Colloid tumours*—these are large tumours which appear gelatinous.
- *Diffuse infiltrative tumours* (linitis plastica, or 'leather bottle' stomach, so named because the stomach becomes small, thick and contracted)—these present very late and so have a poor prognosis, metastatic spread usually having occurred at the time of diagnosis. Unfortunately, they comprise a third of all gastric carcinomas. Symptoms are usually non-specific, including loss of appetite and food intolerance as the capacity of the stomach is reduced. Histology shows sheets of anaplastic cells, many with a single vacuole displacing the nucleus to one side, giving them the name 'signet-ring cells'.

Carcinomas may spread through:

- The lymphatic system.
- The bloodstream.
- Direct spread locally.
- Transfusion through a body cavity (transcoelomically).

Metastases can occur in the liver, bone, brain and lung. Through peritoneal seeding, metastases can also be found in the ovary (Krukenberg tumour).

### Clinical features

Presentation is often late, with a correspondingly poor prognosis.

Signs and symptoms include:

- Epigastric pain.
- Nausea and vomiting (especially if the tumour is at the pylorus, causing obstruction).
- Anorexia.
- Anaemia from occult bleeding.
- Haematemesis.
- Weight loss.
- Palpable epigastric mass (in 50% of patients).
- Abdominal tenderness.

Generally, the 5-year survival rate is less than 10%, but it is much better for diagnosis of early carcinoma, i.e. neoplasms confined to the mucosa and submucosa. Treatment includes radiotherapy and surgery to excise the tumour and any affected lymph nodes.

Partial or total gastrectomy may be necessary in some cases. Screening is important for patients who have had a previous gastrectomy for peptic ulceration.

Never ignore it if one of the supraclavicular lymph nodes on the left side of the body is enlarged. Lymph from the cardiac region of the stomach drains to these nodes and they may become enlarged due to metastatic spread from gastric carcinoma (Virchow's node, also called Troisier's sign).

After reading this chapter, you should be able to:

- Describe the anatomy of the liver, with regard to its macroscopic structure, relations, arterial supply, venous and lymphatic drainage, and nerve supply.
- Outline the embryological development of the liver.
- Describe the histological structure of the liver, and understand the function of its different cell types.
- Outline and reproduce the structure of a classic liver lobule, a portal lobule and an acinus, and understand the basis of this classification.
- Outline the functions of the liver.
- Outline the functions of bile, and understand the factors controlling its production.
- Explain the term 'enterohepatic recycling'.
- Describe the limited responses of the liver to injury.
- Define the term 'cirrhosis'.
- Outline the clinical features of liver failure.
- Define 'jaundice', and explain the pathophysiological mechanisms which cause it.
- Describe the complications of portal hypertension.
- Describe the effects of alcohol on the liver.
- Describe the different types of hepatitis viruses.
- Outline the following types of hepatic disorders: congenital abnormalities, infections and inflammatory disease, vascular disease and neoplastic disease.

## OVERVIEW

The liver is the largest abdominal organ and also the largest gland in the body. It is vital for life, and it has many metabolic, endocrine and detoxifying functions.

The biliary system removes waste products from the liver and carries bile salts to the intestine where they aid digestion.

## ANATOMY

The liver is a soft reddish-brown organ, weighing about 1.5 kg and situated under the diaphragm. It is surrounded by a capsule of strong connective tissue (Glisson's capsule).

It lies in the right upper quadrant and occupies most of the right hypochondriac region, extending into the left hypochondriac and epigastric regions (see Fig. 1.1).

The liver is protected by the rib cage and moves during respiration, owing to its attachment to the diaphragm by the falciform, coronary and triangular ligaments (Fig. 4.1).

**Fig. 4.1** Summary table of ligaments attaching the liver to the diaphragm.

| Ligament | Attachments |
|---|---|
| Falciform ligament (remnant of the ventral mesentery of the abdominal foregut) | Attaches the anterior and superior surfaces of the liver to the anterior abdominal wall and the diaphragm |
| Coronary ligament | Attaches the posterior surface of the right lobe to the diaphragm |
| Right triangular ligament | An extension of the coronary ligament |
| Left triangular ligament | Attaches the posterior surface of the left lobe to the diaphragm |

The lesser omentum connects the stomach to the liver, and it is continuous with the left triangular ligament.

The liver has diaphragmatic and visceral (posteroinferior) surfaces. The sharp inferior border separates the two surfaces.

The visceral surface is related to:

- The abdominal oesophagus.
- The fundus and body of the stomach (the gastric area).
- The lesser omentum.
- The gallbladder.
- The superior part of the duodenum (the duodenal area).
- The transverse colon, including the hepatic flexure (the colic area).
- The right kidney and associated adrenal gland (the renal area).

In life, the liver is soft and jelly-like.
In death, the capsule of connective tissue (Glisson's capsule) gives it a definite shape, as seen in the cadaver.

Peritoneum covers the visceral surface (except the gall bladder and porta hepatis) and the superior part of the liver, except the posterior part known as the bare area. This area is in direct contact with the diaphragm and is situated between the reflections of the coronary ligament. The inferior vena cava and the right adrenal gland also lie next to the bare area (Fig. 4.2).

Macroscopically and functionally, the liver is comprised of two 'true' lobes, the left and the right, by the plane joining the tip of the gall bladder and the groove of the inferior vena cava. This division is made on the basis of the blood supply (Fig. 4.3) and bile drainage. There are also two minor lobes (used for descriptive purposes) called the caudate and quadrate lobes. The left lobe includes the caudate lobe and most of the quadrate lobe.

In terms of blood supply that can be surgically isolated, the liver has eight segments (of Couinaud) which may be an important consideration when resection for primary or metastatic cancer is being contemplated. The segments can be mapped onto the lobes (Fig. 4.4).

The space between the visceral surface of the right lobe and the right kidney is the hepatorenal recess; the diaphragmatic recess separates the diaphragmatic surface from the diaphragm.

## Blood supply

The liver has a very rich blood supply from two main sources:

- *The hepatic artery* (a branch of the coeliac trunk), which divides into left and right branches to supply the left and right lobes. This supplies about 30% of the blood to the liver.
- *The portal vein*, which carries venous blood rich in products of digestion from the gastrointestinal (GI) tract. It supplies 70% of the blood to the liver, and divides into left and right branches to supply the two functional lobes. An accessory left hepatic artery, often arising from the left gastric artery, may be found. Variations in the hepatic arterial supply are common. The arterial blood connects to the central vein of each liver lobule.

The main branches of the hepatic artery and portal vein divide each lobe into the vascular segments mentioned earlier. There are eight segments in the whole of the liver.

The hepatic veins drain from the central veins of each lobule into the inferior vena cava.

## Lymphatic drainage

The lymphatics of the liver drain to deep and superficial vessels.

The deep vessels come together at the porta hepatis and end in the hepatic lymph nodes scattered along the hepatic vessels, e.g. the cystic lymph node near the neck of the gall bladder. These then drain to the coeliac lymph nodes to enter the thoracic duct.

Some deep lymph vessels follow the hepatic veins through the diaphragm to end in the phrenic lymph nodes.

The superficial lymph vessels follow the same drainage as the deep vessels, but they can also drain to the mediastinal lymph nodes.

## Nerve supply

The liver receives both sympathetic and parasympathetic innervation. The nerve fibres reach the liver

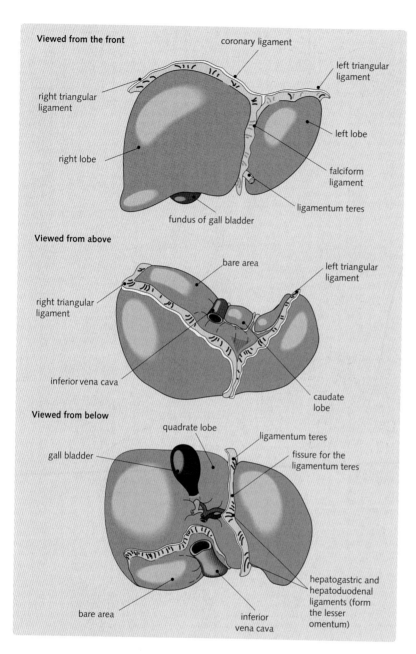

**Fig. 4.2** Three different views of the liver, showing the anterior, superior, and inferior sides. The bare area on the posterior part of the liver is not covered with peritoneum.

**Viewed from the front**

coronary ligament

left triangular ligament

right triangular ligament

left lobe

right lobe

falciform ligament

ligamentum teres

fundus of gall bladder

**Viewed from above**

bare area

left triangular ligament

right triangular ligament

inferior vena cava

caudate lobe

**Viewed from below**

quadrate lobe

ligamentum teres

gall bladder

fissure for the ligamentum teres

bare area

inferior vena cava

hepatogastric and hepatoduodenal ligaments (form the lesser omentum)

via the hepatic plexus, which is derived from the coeliac plexus. It also receives parasympathetic innervation from the right phrenic nerve and left and right vagi (Xth cranial nerves).

The hepatic nerves follow the blood supply of the liver and enter at the porta hepatis.

The porta hepatis is a deep fissure on the visceral surface of the liver, and it contains the hepatic artery, portal vein, hepatic nerve plexus, hepatic ducts and lymphatic vessels.

**Fig. 4.3** The hepatic portal venous system. (Redrawn with permission from Hall-Craggs ECB. Anatomy as a Basis for Clinical Medicine. London: Waverly Europe, 1994.)

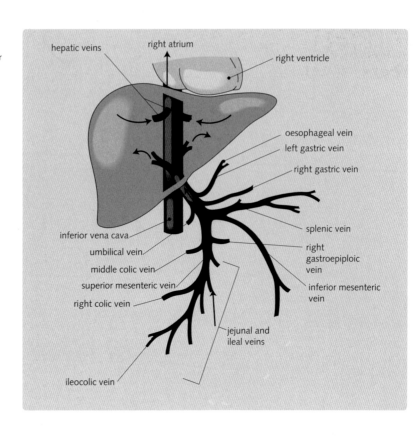

**Fig. 4.4** Anterosuperior view of the liver showing the correlation between lobes and vascular segments. Segment I corresponds to the caudate lobe, segments II, III and IV to the left lobe and segments V, VI, VII and VIII to the right lobe. The segments are organized according to the divisions of the hepatic artery and portal vein. (Reproduced with permission from O'Grady J, Lake J, Howdle P. Comprehensive Clinical Hepatology. London: Mosby, 2000.)

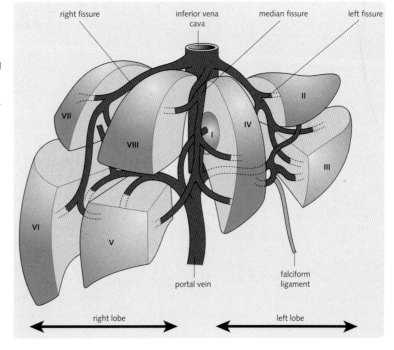

# EMBRYOLOGY AND DEVELOPMENT

The liver develops from the liver bud (hepatic diverticulum) that appears as an outgrowth of the endodermal epithelium at the distal end of the primitive foregut in the middle of the 3rd week (Fig. 4.5).

The liver bud is composed of rapidly proliferating cells, which penetrate the mesodermal septum transversum. The connection between the liver bud and the foregut (duodenum) narrows and forms the bile duct.

A small ventral outgrowth from the bile duct gives rise to the gallbladder and cystic duct. The structure of the liver is formed by epithelial liver cords that mix with the vitelline and umbilical veins to give rise to hepatic sinusoids.

The liver cords differentiate into the hepatocytes (parenchyma), the bile canaliculi, and the hepatic ducts. The mesoderm of the septum transversum gives rise to:

- Haematopoietic cells.
- Kupffer cells.
- Connective tissue cells.

The liver is the major haematopoietic organ in the embryo, and by the 4th week, haematopoiesis has already begun.

The lesser omentum and the falciform ligament are both also derived from the mesoderm of the septum transversum, located between the foregut and liver, and the ventral abdominal wall and the liver, respectively.

The rotation of the stomach, liver and spleen occurs between the 6th week and 11th week of embryonic development (Fig. 4.6).

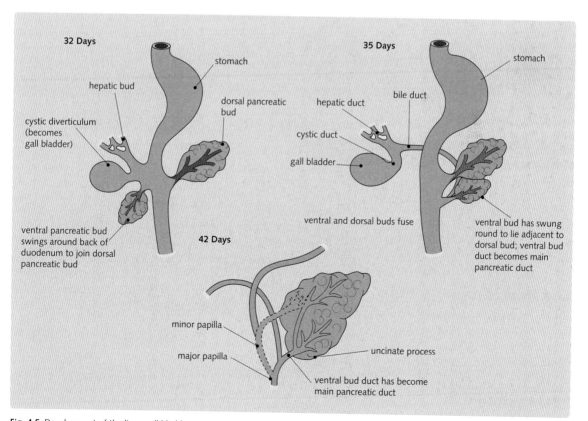

**Fig. 4.5** Development of the liver, gall bladder and pancreas. (Redrawn with permission from Hall-Craggs ECB. Anatomy as a Basis for Clinical Medicine. London: Waverly Europe, 1994.)

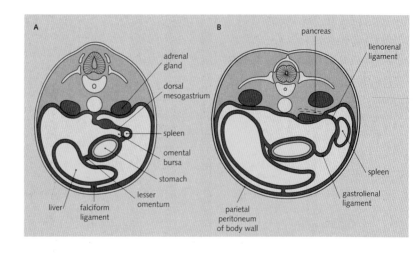

**Fig. 4.6** Rotation of the stomach and liver during the 6th week of embryonic development, shown in transverse section. (Reproduced with permission from Sadler TW. Langman's Medical Embryology, 8th edn. Philadelphia: Lippincott, 2000.)

At about the 12th week, the hepatocytes begin to form bile. This is able to enter the duodenum, as the biliary tract and gallbladder are both fully formed.

Hepatocytes are highly metabolically active and rich in cytoplasmic organelles, especially mitochondria.

## HISTOLOGY

Traditionally, there are three ways of describing the structural units of the liver (Fig. 4.7):

- Classical lobule.
- Portal lobule.
- Acinus.

## Classical (simple) lobule

Each lobule may be thought of as a hexagon with a central vein at its centre and a portal triad at its outer corners. A portal triad consists of a branch of the hepatic artery, a branch of the portal vein and a bile duct.

## Portal lobule

This views the liver as being made up of a series of triangles with a central vein at each corner and a portal triad at the centre, and it emphasizes exocrine function.

## Acinus

This is a more accurate description of the functional unit within the structure of the liver parenchyma. An acinus is an elliptical unit with a portal triad at the centre and a central vein at each pole, and it emphasizes endocrine function.

It reflects the gradient of metabolic activity found in the liver, and is divided into three zones for descriptive purposes:

- The periportal zone (zone 1).
- The midzone (zone 2).
- The centrilobular zone (zone 3).

Most oxygenated blood is found in the centre of the acinus around the portal triad (zone 1); this zone is adjacent to the portal canal and receives the most blood from the hepatic artery and portal vein. Therefore, it is most susceptible to damage from toxins carried to the liver in the hepatic portal vein and toxins absorbed from the alimentary tract, e.g. in paracetamol poisoning. Most of the metabolic activity of the liver takes place here. This zone makes up the limiting plate.

Conversely, zone 3, being furthest from the portal triad and closest to the central vein, is most susceptible to ischaemic damage, e.g. in heart failure.

**Fig. 4.7** Structural units of the liver.

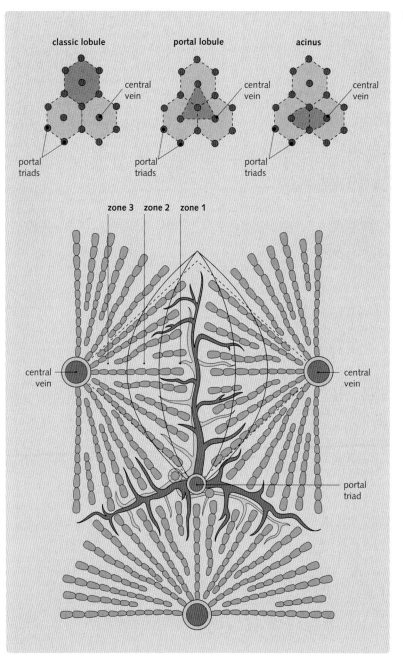

## Types of cell

Different types of cell make up the architecture of the liver: hepatocytes, Kupffer cells, haematopoietic cells and perisinusoidal cells.

The functions of these cells are summarized in Fig. 4.8.

## Sinusoids, perisinusoidal spaces and bile canaliculi

The hepatocytes are arranged in 'cords', which radiate out in a spoke-like fashion from the central vein (Fig. 4.9). They are large, eosinophilic cells with round nuclei. An interesting feature is that more than half

**Fig. 4.8** Cell types of the liver.

| Cell type | Function |
|---|---|
| Kupffer cells | Phagocytosis, found in sinusoids |
| Hepatocytes | Perform most of the functions of the liver (Fig. 4.11) |
| Ito cells (perisinusoidal cells) | Replace damaged hepatocytes and secrete collagen |
| Endothelial cells | Scavenger cells for denatured collagen, harmful enzymes, and pathogens they line the sinusoids |
| Haematopoietic cells | Haematopoiesis in the fetus, and in adults with chronic anaemia |

In between the hepatocytes and the sinusoidal endothelial cells is the perisinusoidal space (of Disse). This contains perisinusoidal cells (stellate, or Ito, cells) which secrete collagen, providing a supportive mesh. It is these cells which contribute to fibrosis in liver damage (see later).

At their sinusoidal surface, the hepatocytes have numerous short microvilli, which extend into the perisinusoidal space. Between the bases of the microvilli lie coated pits that are used for endocytosis.

The microvilli increase the surface area for the transfer of digestive products, nutrients, oxygen, and other substances between the blood in the sinusoids and the hepatocytes.

Two surfaces of each hepatocyte communicate with a space of Disse and two surfaces communicate with a bile canaliculus (Fig. 4.10).

Bile canaliculi are formed by a groove between surfaces of adjacent hepatocytes. The canaliculi are about 0.5–2.5 mm in diameter and they are sealed by zonulae occludentes, which prevent leakage of bile into the intercellular spaces.

The canaliculi form rings around the hepatocytes and approach the bile ductules in the portal tracts by opening into canals (of Hering).

of the cells are tetraploid, i.e. they have four times the number of normal chromosomes. They have a network of capillaries, or sinusoids, between them, which are lined with discontinuous fenestrated endothelium, stellate cells and phagocytic Kupffer cells. Kupffer cells are part of the monocyte–macrophage system and phagocytose old erythrocytes and other cellular debris from the circulation.

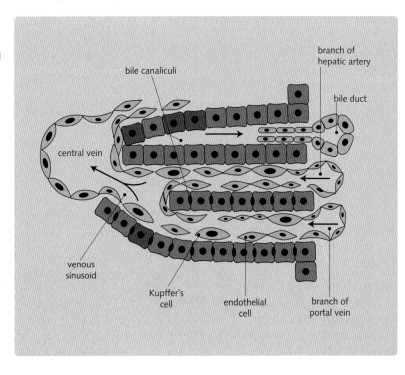

**Fig. 4.9** Cords of hepatocytes radiating out from the central vein. The space of Disse (the perisinusoidal space) is located between the hepatocytes and the fenestrated endothelial cells, interspersed with Kupffer cells, that line the sinusoids. Perisinusoidal cells (Ito cells) reside here and secrete collagen. (Redrawn with permission from Marshall W. Clinical Chemistry, 3rd edn. London: Mosby.)

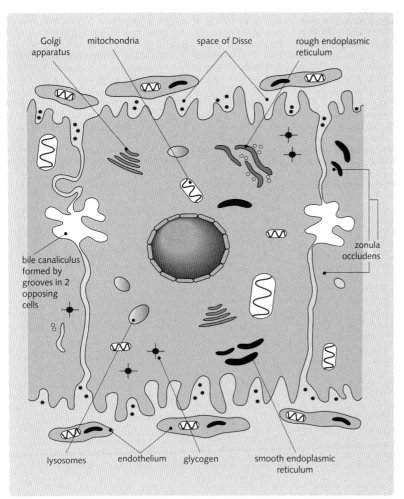

**Fig. 4.10** Two sides of each hepatocyte communicate with a sinusoid (via the space of Disse), and bile canaliculi are formed by a groove between adjacent hepatocytes.

Labels in figure:
- Golgi apparatus
- mitochondria
- space of Disse
- rough endoplasmic reticulum
- zonula occludens
- bile canaliculus formed by grooves in 2 opposing cells
- lysosomes
- endothelium
- glycogen
- smooth endoplasmic reticulum

These are short corridors lined with cuboidal cells that drain bile into the ductules of the portal tracts.

In the fetal liver, islands of haematopoietic cells are found within the spaces of Disse for the production of blood cells.

## Portal canal and limiting plate

The portal canal consists of the portal triad (hepatic portal vein, hepatic artery and bile duct) surrounded by connective tissue.

A small space (the space of Mall) exists between the connective tissue covering and the surrounding hepatocytes. Lymph is thought to originate in the space of Mall.

The limiting plate (the hepatocytes of the peri-portal zone), which surrounds the portal tract, makes up a protective layer of cells, which are first to be exposed to toxins in the systemic or portal blood. Breaching the plate can lead to liver damage, in particular cirrhosis.

The gallbladder epithelial cells are highly specialized for absorption. They have a brush border of microvilli, are rich in mitochondria, and have numerous $Na^+/K^+$ ATPase transporters at their lateral surfaces.

## FUNCTIONS AND PHYSIOLOGY

The liver performs many functions vital for life, and it has a substantial capacity to regenerate after injury. The main functions of the liver are metabolism of protein, fat and carbohydrate; bile production; storage of vitamins, minerals, and glycogen; biotransformation; and detoxification and protection (by filtration of portal blood). These are summarized in Fig. 4.11.

**Fig. 4.11** The main functions of the liver and hepatocytes.

| Function | Processes involved |
|---|---|
| Protein metabolism | Synthesis and secretion of albumin<br>Synthesis of plasma proteins<br>Formation of urea from ammonia<br>Deamination of amino acids<br>Synthesis of coagulation factors, e.g. factors V, VII, IX, X and prothrombin<br>Metabolism of polypeptide hormone |
| Fat metabolism | Formation of lipoproteins and fatty acids<br>Synthesis of cholesterol<br>Conversion of cholesterol to bile salts<br>Conversion of carbohydrates and protein to fat<br>Ketogenesis<br>Metabolism and excretion of steroid hormones |
| Carbohydrate metabolism | Gluconeogenesis<br>Synthesis and breakdown of glycogen |
| Bile secretion | Production of bile salts<br>Elimination of bilirubin |
| Storage | Glycogen<br>Vitamins (A and $B_{12}$) |
| Biotransformation and detoxification | Drugs and exogenous substances<br>Gonadal hormones<br>Aldosterone<br>Glucocorticoids<br>Nitrogenous gut toxins |
| Protection | Filtration of portal blood<br>Removal of bacteria/antigens by Kupffer cells (phagocyctosis) |
| Haematopoiesis | The fetal liver is the major source of blood cell production |

To maintain these functions, the liver must receive 25% of the cardiac output through the portal vein and hepatic artery. Nutrients and other substances are absorbed from the sinusoids into the hepatocytes.

The varied nature of hepatic function requires that the hepatocytes differ functionally from each other. The functional differences correspond to the zones of the liver acinus (see earlier). The cells in each zone differ in ultrastructure, function, and distance from the blood supply, with zone 1 being nearest to the arterial supply and zone 3 the furthest.

Functional differences include:

- The periportal hepatocytes take up bile under normal circumstances, but during bile overload, this function is also adopted by the centrilobular (perivenous) hepatocytes.
- The centrilobular hepatocytes contain enzymes required in esterification, but the periportal hepatocytes are rich in oxidative enzymes.

## Carbohydrate metabolism

In the normal individual, blood glucose levels are carefully regulated. The liver plays an important role in glucose homeostasis.

Blood glucose levels rise transiently after a meal but the liver takes up the glucose and converts it to glycogen.

In the fasting state, glycogen is converted to glucose (glycogenolysis) and released into the bloodstream to keep levels within the range 3.5–5.5 mmol/L.

The liver contains approximately 80 g of glycogen. This is enough to keep blood glucose levels within the normal range for approximately 24 hours at rest, but for less time during heavy exercise.

The peptide hormones insulin and glucagon, both produced by the pancreas, control the levels of plasma glucose. Insulin promotes synthesis of glycogen, protein and fat, while inhibiting gluconeogenesis and lipolysis.

Glucagon acts on the liver primarily and has no effect on muscle. It upregulates gluconeogenesis and ketogenesis.

In diabetes, the utilization of carbohydrates is impaired and ketone bodies are formed in the liver from $\beta$-oxidation of fatty acids.

Ketones are released from hepatocytes and carried to other tissues where they are metabolized.

In prolonged starvation, ketone bodies and fatty acids are used as alternative sources of fuel, and body tissues (except the brain) adapt to a lower glucose requirement.

> The liver also contains the hydrolytic enzyme glucose-6-phosphatase, which allows for release of glucose from cells. This enzyme is absent in the brain and muscle so that, in effect, the liver is the only organ which can release glucose into the bloodstream to maintain blood sugar levels.

## Lipid metabolism

Most of the fat (lipids) in the diet is in the form of triglycerides (esters of fatty acid and glycerol). The digestion and absorption of dietary lipids is described in Chapter 7.

Lipids are insoluble in water, and they are assembled into lipoproteins (complexes of lipid and protein) in the liver, for transport in the blood (Fig. 4.12). Depending on their composition, lipoproteins are classified into chylomicrons (the lowest density), very-low-density, intermediate-density, low-density, and high-density lipoproteins (Fig. 4.13).

Low-density lipoproteins (LDLs) have been implicated in atheroma and their level in the plasma should be kept low. Conversely, high-density lipoproteins (HDLs) have a protective function and their levels should be higher.

The apoprotein element of the polar coat is made in the liver and intestine, and defects in its synthesis have important effects on lipid metabolism.

apolipoprotein    triglyceride
free cholesterol    cholesteryl ester
phospholipid

**Fig. 4.12** Structure of a lipoprotein particle. Lipoproteins are complexes of lipids and proteins. They have a triglyceride and cholesterol ester middle and a polar coat, made up of phospholipids, apoproteins and unesterified cholesterol. (Reproduced with permission from Gaw A et al. Clinical Biochemistry: An Illustrated Colour Text, 2nd edn. Edinburgh: Churchill Livingstone, 1999.)

**Fig. 4.13** The density classes of plasma lipoproteins.

| Class | Abbreviation | Sources | Mean diameter (nm) |
|---|---|---|---|
| Chylomicrons | CHYLO | Intestine | 500 |
| Very-low-density lipoproteins | VLDL | Liver | 43 |
| Intermediate-density lipoproteins | IDL | Catabolism of very-low-density lipoproteins lipoproteins and chlomicrons | 27 |
| Low-density lipoproteins | LDL | Catabolism of very-low-density lipoproteins | 22 |
| High-density lipoproteins | HDL | Catabolism of chylomicrons and very-low-density lipoproteins; liver and intestine | 8 |

Cholesterol is needed for the manufacture of steroid hormones and bile acids, and can be synthesized in the liver. It is also a component of most diets, and it is found in all animal products, especially eggs.

It is easy to remember the ideal levels of circulating lipoproteins. Low-density ones should be LOW and high-density ones should be HIGH.

## Protein metabolism

The liver synthesizes all the plasma proteins except γ-globulins. Amino acids from the intestines and muscles enter the liver and by controlling their metabolism (especially via transamination and gluconeogenesis) the plasma protein concentrations can be regulated.

The protein concentration of plasma is 60–80 g/L and is made up of mainly albumin, globulin and fibrinogen. The plasma proteins synthesized by the liver are summarized in Fig. 4.14.

## Urea metabolism

Amino acids are transaminated and deaminated via oxidative pathways in the liver to form ammonia, which is converted to urea via the urea (ornithine) cycle. This occurs mainly in the periportal cells (hepatocytes adjacent to the portal canals).

The cycle occurs partly in the mitochondria and partly in the cytoplasm, so the enzymes are situated in one or the other, according to their function in the cycle.

In liver failure, there is decreased synthesis of urea and increased levels of ammonia—a toxic product. Ammonia can depress cerebral blood flow and cerebral oxygen consumption. Ammonia toxicity is usually due to cirrhosis, but it is also seen in inherited deficiencies of urea cycle enzymes.

Transamination of amino acids is the interconversion of amine ($-NH_2$) groups from amino acids to $\alpha$-ketoacids, to produce different amino acids. This is catalysed by transaminase in the liver.

**Fig. 4.14** Plasma proteins synthesized by the liver.

| Protein | Function |
|---|---|
| Albumin | Maintain colloid osmotic pressure Transport of hydrophobic substances, e.g. bilirubin, hormones, fatty acids, drugs |
| Lipoprotein | Transport of lipids in the blood |
| Transferrin | Carrier molecule for iron |
| Caeruloplasmin | Carrier molecule for copper |
| Globulins (not γ-globulins) | Antibody functions Transport of lipids, Fe or Cu in the blood |
| $\alpha_1$-antitrypsin | Protein inhibitor of the enzyme trypsin |
| $\alpha_1$-fetoprotein | Secreted by yolk sac and embryonic liver epithelial cells In adults is produced by proliferating liver cells and can be used as an indicator of liver cancer |
| Fibrinogen | |
| Prothrombin | Blood clotting factors |
| Factors V, VII, IX, X, XII (not VIII) | |
| Complement cascade proteins | Immune function upregulators and coordinators Inflammatory functions |

## Vitamin metabolism

The liver is the main store of the fat-soluble vitamins (A, D, E and K). Vitamin deficiency may occur when there is malabsorption of fat, due to a variety of hepatic and extrahepatic causes.

Vitamin $B_{12}$ is absorbed from the diet in the terminal ileum, provided intrinsic factor is made by the parietal cells of the stomach, and enough is stored in the liver to last 2 or 3 years. Deficiency eventually leads to megaloblastic anaemia (pernicious anaemia).

The liver stores folate and converts it to its active form, tetrahydrofolate. Folate is needed as a coenzyme for the transfer of 1-carbon groups and its deficiency also leads to megaloblastic anaemia, but more quickly than vitamin $B_{12}$ deficiency because body stores of folate are only sufficient for a few months. Folate deficiency in early pregnancy may also lead to neural-tube defects in the fetus.

Dietary deficiency of folate is much more common than vitamin $B_{12}$ deficiency, and it is seen in alcoholics and others on a poor diet or suffering from a severe illness where folate utilization is increased, e.g. in cancer.

In general, a deficiency of any substance may result from:

- Increased utilization.
- Increased excretion.
- Decreased manufacture.
- Decreased absorption.

## Storage

The liver acts as a store for, among others, glycogen, fat and fat-soluble vitamins, folate, iron and copper. This storage function is important as it enables the body to withstand periods of insufficient intake of the stored nutrients.

Some stores are large enough to sustain the body's needs for a few years, e.g. stores of vitamin $B_{12}$ are sufficient for about 3 years; folate stores can last a few months.

## Drug and hormone metabolism

The liver metabolizes drugs and hormones via biotransformation in three stages:

- Phase I (oxidation).
- Phase II (conjugation).
- Phase III (elimination).

These processes are useful, in conjunction with the filtering action of the portal blood supply (see later) in allowing the body to detoxify or degrade toxins or waste products.

Phase I reactions often produce more active metabolites, e.g. they can change prodrugs into the active drugs. Phase II reactions make the substrate more water soluble to facilitate phase III. Phase III occurs via ATPase pumps.

### Phase I reactions

The mixed function oxygenase system of the hepatocyte smooth endoplasmic reticulum catalyses oxidation reactions. Several enzymes are involved, most notably those of the cytochrome $P_{450}$ family.

Oxidation may also be carried out by other enzymes such as xanthine oxidase and monoamine oxidase, present in other tissues as well as the liver.

A number of drugs induce microsomal enzymes, affecting the metabolism of other drugs taken at the same time, and this should be borne in mind when deciding what dose to prescribe.

Notable examples of enzyme-inducing drugs include phenobarbital, ethanol and phenylbutazone.

### Phase II reactions

A number of groups are conjugated with drugs or their metabolites in the liver, including glucuronyl, acetyl, methyl, glycyl, sulphate and glutamyl groups, of which glucuronyl is the most common.

Conjugation is important in the metabolism of paracetamol. It is inactivated by conjugation to form a glucuronide or sulphate, but the liver has a limited capacity.

If the normal conjugation pathway is saturated, mixed-function oxidases form a toxic metabolite instead. The toxic metabolite is itself inactivated by conjugation with glutathione, but stores of glutathione are limited.

In paracetamol overdose, the saturation of liver enzymes and depletion of glutathione lead to liver necrosis and damage to kidney tubules by toxic metabolites. Treatment is with N-acetylcysteine, which increases the formation of glutathione, or with methionine.

Paracetamol has a narrow therapeutic index, i.e. the difference between a beneficial and a toxic dose is small, hence paracetamol overdose is common. Symptoms of liver damage may not be apparent immediately, but when they do occur it is often too late, with fatal consequences.

### Phase III reactions

The elimination of conjugated substances is via the blood, which then results in excretion through the kidneys, or via bile through the intestines.

ATPase pumps are required to actively transport the substance out of the hepatocyte. Some pumps are specific for the conjugating molecule, e.g. glutathione.

Some drugs are rapidly inactivated by the liver, e.g. propranolol. The amount of active drug reaching the circulation is reduced and the drug is said to undergo significant first-pass metabolism. Drug metabolism in the liver is summarized in Fig. 4.15.

## Defence

The portal blood supply to the liver allows for toxins and microorganisms to be filtered out before the blood returns to the systemic circulation. This protects the rest of the body from any harmful substances that may have breached the gut defence mechanisms. Kupffer cells in the sinusoids facilitate this, via phagocytosis.

## Haematopoiesis

In embryonic life, the liver is the main site of haematopoiesis. This occurs from the 2nd to 7th months, but ceases before birth.

By 5 months of gestation, the bone marrow is supplementing the liver in this function.

Between conception and the 2nd month, haematopoiesis takes place in the yolk sac. The liver and spleen can resume their haematopoietic role (extramedullary haematopoiesis) if necessary.

## Bile production and function

Bile is an aqueous, alkaline, greenish-yellow liquid produced by the liver to:

- Eliminate endogenous and exogenous substances from the liver.
- Emulsify fats in the small intestine and facilitate their digestion and absorption.

Bile consists of bile acids, cholesterol, phospholipids, bile pigments (bilirubin and biliverdin), electrolytes ($Na^+$, $K^+$, $Ca^{2+}$, $Cl^-$, $HCO_3^-$) and water.

Waste products found in bile include cholesterol and the bile pigments, bilirubin and biliverdin, which give bile its colour.

Bile passes out of the liver through the bile ducts, and it is concentrated and stored in the gall bladder. During and after a meal, it is excreted from the gall bladder by contraction and passes into the duodenum through the common bile duct.

Most of the bile acids are reabsorbed from the terminal ileum and recycled by the liver (see later). Bile pigments are normally excreted in the faeces, which they colour dark brown.

### Bile acids

Bile acids (also called bile salts) are detergents which emulsify lipids. They have a hydrophobic and a hydrophilic end, and they form micelles in aqueous solutions.

Bile acids are synthesized in hepatocytes from cholesterol and excreted into bile. They account for approximately 50% of the dry weight of bile.

The principal primary bile acids are cholic acid and chenodeoxycholic acid. They are made more soluble by conjugation with taurine or glycine.

Of the bile acids excreted into the intestine, 95% are reabsorbed (mostly in the terminal ileum) and recycled by the liver. This is termed enterohepatic recycling (Fig. 4.16). The total pool of bile acids is recirculated six to eight times a day. Reabsorption through enterohepatic recirculation means we only need a small pool of bile acids. Normally about

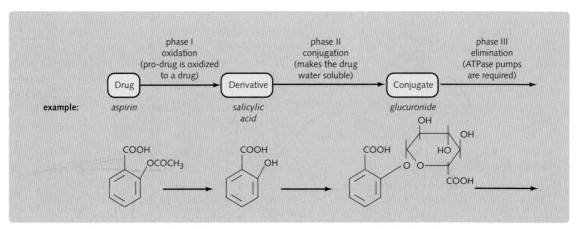

Fig. 4.15 Drug metabolism in the liver. (Adapted from Rang et al. Pharmacology, 5th edn. Edinburgh: Churchill Livingstone, 2003.)

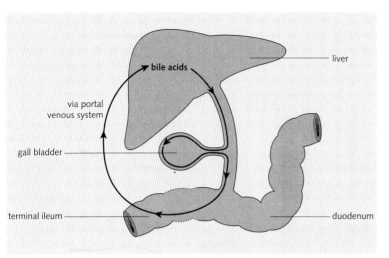

Fig. 4.16 Enterohepatic recycling of bile acids.

liver

bile acids

via portal venous system

gall bladder

terminal ileum

duodenum

250–500 mg of bile acids are produced a day, which replaces the amount excreted in the faeces.

The main functions of bile acids are:

- *Triglyceride assimilation*—bile acids emulsify lipids with the aid of lecithin (found in high concentrations in bile) and break them down to 1 mm diameter droplets. This provides a large surface area for digestive enzymes to act on.
- *Lipid transport*—bile acids form mixed micelles with the products of lipid digestion and facilitate transport to the brush border, where they are absorbed.
- *Bile flow induction*—bile acids stimulate the flow of bile by osmotically attracting water and electrolytes as they are secreted. It is also thought that some bile acids are secreted in an unconjugated form. They are absorbed without water and electrolytes from the bile ducts to be quickly carried back to the liver for resecretion.
- *Regulation of bile acid synthesis*—normal reabsorption of bile acids from the intestines inhibits hepatic synthesis of bile acids. Not all bile acids are equally effective: chenodeoxycholic acid and lithocholic acid significantly reduce cholic acid formation. It is thought that the feedback mechanism acts on the rate-limiting step of bile acid synthesis.
- *Water and electrolyte secretion*—if bile acids are present in the colon, they stimulate water and electrolyte secretion. This can result in diarrhoea. A deficiency of bile acids results in malabsorption of fat.

## Bilirubin

This yellow pigment, which gives bile its colour, is the principal constituent in bile. Knowledge of bilirubin metabolism is essential to understanding the pathophysiology behind jaundice (see later).

Most bilirubin is formed by the breakdown of haemoglobin from worn-out red cells (Fig. 4.17), but about 15% results from the breakdown of other haem-containing proteins such as myoglobin, cytochromes and catalases.

Bilirubin is insoluble and is transported to the liver in the plasma, bound to albumin. There, most of it dissociates from albumin, and is extracted from the blood in the sinusoids by the hepatocytes. It binds to cytoplasmic proteins in the hepatocytes, and is conjugated with glucuronic acid to form bilirubin diglucuronide (a reaction catalysed by glucuronyl transferase, found mainly in smooth endoplasmic reticulum).

Bilirubin diglucuronide is water soluble, unlike bilirubin, and is actively transported against its concentration gradient into the bile canaliculi. A small amount escapes into the blood, where it is transported bound to albumin, and then excreted in the urine.

The intestinal mucosa is permeable to unconjugated bilirubin and to urobilinogen (a colourless derivative of bilirubin produced by intestinal flora); some of the bile pigments and urobilinogens are reabsorbed from the gut into the portal circulation. The intestinal mucosa is relatively impermeable to conjugated bilirubin.

Some of the reabsorbed substances are excreted again by the liver, but small amounts of urobilinogens enter the general circulation and are excreted in the urine.

Figs 4.17 and 4.18 summarize the production and excretion of bilirubin.

## Control of bile production

There are two different mechanisms of control of bile production (Fig. 4.19):

- Bile acid-dependent.
- Intrahepatic bile-duct-dependent.

The bile acid-dependent mechanism describes how water and electrolytes passively follow the movement of bile acids, which have been actively transported into the bile canaliculi and ducts. Movement of water and electrolytes is achieved by tight junctions between hepatocytes.

The tight junctions can become more permeable in response to bile acids, vasopressin, epinephrine

**Fig. 4.17** Production and fate of bilirubin.

**Fig. 4.18** The fate of bilirubin after processing in the hepatocyte. (From Sanford PA. Digestive System Physiology, 2nd edn. London: Edward Arnold, 1992. Reproduced by permission of Hodder/Arnold Publishers.)

and angiotensin II. It is thought that bile acids are secreted across the canalicular membrane into bile by protein-mediated facilitated transport, driven partly by the electrochemical difference across the membrane.

The intrahepatic bile duct mechanism describes the aqueous secretion that makes up 50% of the total volume of bile.

The solution is secreted by epithelial cells lining the bile ducts, and is isotonic, with sodium and potassium concentrations similar to those of plasma. It has a higher concentration of bicarbonate and a lower concentration of chloride.

## Control of bile acid synthesis and secretion

Cholecystokinin increases the rate of bile acid secretion during the intestinal phase of digestion.

High concentrations of bile acids in the portal blood stimulate bile acid secretion and inhibit its synthesis during the intestinal phase.

Conversely, low levels of bile acids in the portal blood during the interdigestive phase stimulate the synthesis and inhibit the secretion of bile acids.

Secretin stimulates secretion by the bile duct epithelium and this effect is strongly potentiated by cholecystokinin. Secretin alone has no effect on the concentration of bile acids in bile.

# PATHOLOGICAL MANIFESTATIONS OF LIVER DAMAGE

The liver is essential to life and has a remarkable capacity to regenerate. Damage from whatever cause (apart from trauma) results in similar pathology but

**Fig. 4.19** The control of bile acid synthesis and secretion. This involves bile acid-dependent, bile acid-independent and intrahepatic bile duct-dependent control. (From Sanford PA. Digestive System Physiology, 2nd edn. London: Edward Arnold, 1992. Reproduced by permission of Hodder/Arnold Publishers.)

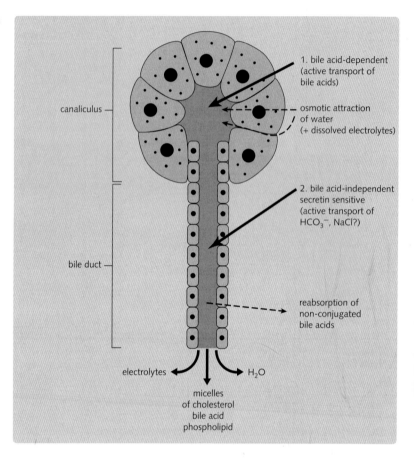

following certain patterns which are dependent on the aetiology. Nevertheless, there is usually an inflammatory reaction, some attempt at regeneration, and, if unsuccessful, cell death. The patterns of injury are elaborated upon in the next section.

The causes of liver injury can be classified into five main groups: infection, drugs and toxins, tumours, metabolic diseases and vascular disorders. Damage may be acute or chronic, and the same agents may result in either.

Because the processes underlying liver injury are similar, the resultant clinical picture will be one of the following types, which represent stages in the progression of liver damage:

- Acute hepatitis.
- Chronic hepatitis.
- Liver fibrosis.
- Cirrhosis, which is the end-point of chronic liver damage.
- Complications of the necro-inflammatory or cirrhotic process.

# Histopathological patterns of liver injury

These are the different ways in which injury to the liver manifests itself at the tissue level, and should not be confused with the clinical pictures mentioned above.

## Necrosis

Hepatic necrosis can be described in a number of ways (Fig. 4.20):

- *Apoptotic necrosis* describes necrosis of individual hepatocytes. It is caused by several diseases, including acute viral hepatitis. Complete recovery with no long-term sequelae is the norm. The dead hepatocytes form eosinophilic Councilman bodies.
- *Focal or spotty necrosis* describes small groups of necrotic hepatocytes. Macrophages and lymphocytes tend to accumulate around them in an effort to localize damage or infection.

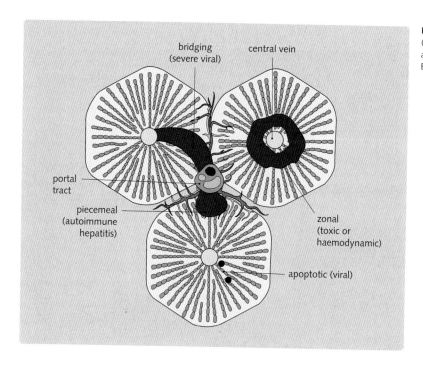

**Fig. 4.20** Patterns of hepatic necrosis. (Redrawn from Underwood JCE. General and Systematic Pathology, 2nd edn. Edinburgh: Churchill Livingstone, 1996.)

This type of necrosis is seen in acute viral or drug-induced hepatitis.

- *Zonal necrosis* describes destruction of hepatocytes within a particular zone of the liver acinus. Haemodynamic necrosis is a type of zonal necrosis because concentric bands of necrotic hepatocytes are seen around the central vein. This occurs in cardiac failure, stasis of hepatic venous blood and poisoning. Zone 3 (the centrilobular zone) is most affected by necrosis, e.g. due to paracetamol overdose, and necrosis of zone 2 is rare, but seen in yellow fever.
- *Confluent bridging necrosis* involves a large number of hepatocytes in a 'band' of necrosis stretching between hepatic venules (central to central) or between hepatic venules and portal tracts (central to portal). This pattern of necrosis is caused by severe drug- or viral-induced hepatitis.
- *Piecemeal necrosis* occurs in chronic liver disease. It describes the necrosis of hepatocytes at the interface between the parenchyma and fibrous tissue. Lymphocytes, particularly plasma cells, infiltrate the area.
- *Submassive or panacinar necrosis* affects the entire acinus. Massive necrosis affects the entire liver. Both are caused by viral- or drug-induced injury.

Massive necrosis can result in fulminant hepatic failure.

## Degeneration

Degeneration is less serious than necrosis and is characterized by swollen, oedematous hepatocytes (*ballooning degeneration*) with irregularly clumped cytoplasm and large clear spaces. Diffuse, foamy, swollen hepatocytes suggest cholestasis.

## Inflammation

In inflammation of the liver (hepatitis), an influx of acute or chronic inflammatory cells may occur secondary to hepatocellular necrosis.

## Regeneration

Regeneration is the norm following injury. Hyperplasia and hypertrophy are common after injury. Hepatocyte proliferation results in a thickening of the cords radiating out from the central vein. The architecture may be disturbed unless the connective tissue framework remains intact.

The normal liver can restore its original weight, even if up to two thirds of the liver is removed. This allows for recovery from numerous injuries and even extensive surgical removal of tumours.

## Fibrosis

Fibrosis from inflammation or a direct toxic insult may occur around the portal tracts, the central vein or within the spaces of Disse, disrupting the normal architecture and interfering with liver function. In severe cases, cirrhosis results.

## Cirrhosis

Cirrhosis is a diffuse and irreversible condition that results from necrosis of hepatocytes followed by the formation of regeneration nodules separated by fibrosis.

Cirrhosis has three key characteristics:

- *Chronic hepatocyte necrosis.*
- A *chronic inflammatory process* which encourages fibrosis.
- *Nodules* caused by *hepatocyte regeneration.*

The process causes architectural disturbances and interferes with normal liver blood flow and function.

Cirrhosis may be micronodular (nodules less than 3 mm in diameter), macronodular (diameters greater than 3 mm) or mixed (both forms coexisting). However, this classification has little clinical significance.

The causes of cirrhosis are summarized in Fig. 4.21, and the complications in Fig. 4.22. Many of the complications are similar to those of liver failure, as cirrhosis is a major cause of hepatic failure.

### Treatment of cirrhosis

After performing a number of investigations, including liver function tests, liver biopsy, ultrasound and computed tomography (CT) imaging, the severity and type of cirrhosis can be determined.

Treatment depends on the diagnosis and any complications that accompany the cirrhosis. Certain drugs are contraindicated in liver disease, and these should be avoided.

Broadly, treatment for cirrhosis may be divided into two categories:

- *Treatment of the underlying cause,* i.e. to stop the pathological process. Depending on the cause, this may include alcohol abstention, antiviral therapy, immunosuppression or withdrawal of drugs.
- *Management of complications,* for example ascitic taps and treatment of hepatic encepalopathy (see later).

**Fig. 4.21** Causes of cirrhosis.

Unknown (10% of cases)

Alcohol (50% of cases)

Hepatitis B (±D) and C

Iron overload (haemochromatosis)

Gallstones

Autoimmune liver disease

Wilson's disease (leading to deposition of copper in the liver)

$\alpha_1$-antitrypsin deficiency

Type IV glycogenosis

Galactosaemia

Tyrosinaemia

Biliary cholestasis

Budd–Chiari syndrome

Drugs, e.g. methotrexate

Biliary cirrhosis

Hepatic venous congestion

Cystic fibrosis

Glycogen storage disease

Patients require 6-monthly checks, involving ultrasound and serum $\alpha$-fetoprotein measurements. These will enable early detection of hepatocellular carcinoma development.

# Systemic and organic manifestations of liver damage

## Portal hypertension

The normal pressure in the hepatic portal vein is about 7 mmHg, but this increases two- to threefold in portal hypertension.

Liver disease is the most common cause, but it is not the only one as many diseases and disorders can result in this condition. Broadly, the causes of portal hypertension may be classified as:

- *Prehepatic* – a blockage of the portal vein before the liver.
- *Hepatic* – a disruption or change of the liver architecture.
- *Posthepatic* – a blockage in the venous system after the liver.

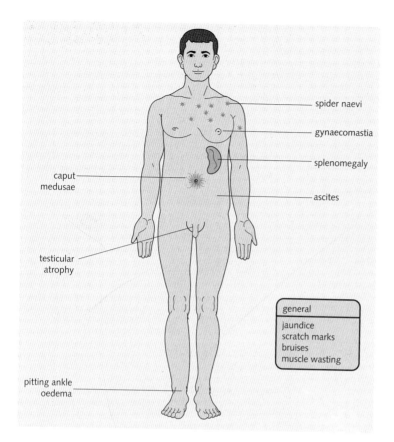

Fig. 4.22 Consequences of cirrhosis.

spider naevi

gynaecomastia

splenomegaly

ascites

caput medusae

testicular atrophy

pitting ankle oedema

general

jaundice
scratch marks
bruises
muscle wasting

Prehepatic causes include:

- Portal vein thrombosis.
- Arteriovenous fistula.
- Increased splenic bloodflow, secondary to splenomegaly or arteriovenous fistulae.

Hepatic causes include:

- Cirrhosis.
- Schistosomiasis.
- Sarcoidosis.
- Miliary tuberculosis (granulomata).
- Massive fatty change.
- Nodular regenerative hyperplasia.
- Alcoholic hepatitis.

Posthepatic causes include:

- Budd–Chiari syndrome (a rare condition caused by hepatic vein obstruction, sometimes associated with the oral contraceptive) (see later).

- Veno-occlusive disease (see later).
- Severe right-sided heart failure (very rare with modern cardiac treatment).
- Constrictive pericarditis (very rare with modern cardiac treatment).

Cirrhosis results in disruption of the normal liver architecture, which increases hepatic vascular resistance and causes intrahepatic arteriovenous shunting. It is the most common cause of portal hypertension in the UK. Worldwide, however, cirrhosis due to viral hepatitis is the main cause of portal hypertension.

Many patients with portal hypertension are asymptomatic, and they are picked up incidentally with low platelet or white cell count related to splenomegaly. Clinical features related to complications include haematemesis or melaena (from ruptured gastro-oesophageal varices), ascites and encephalopathy. The complications of portal hypertension are described below.

## Ascites

Ascites is the abnormal collection of fluid in the peritoneal cavity, and is a common complication of portal hypertension secondary to cirrhosis.

It may form as a result of:

- Na$^+$ and water retention, due to peripheral arterial vasodilatation particularly of the splanchnic circulation. This reduces effective blood volume and activates the renin–angiotensin system and sympathetic nervous system (both upregulate water and salt retention).
- A local hydrostatic pressure increase due to the portal hypertension, resulting in an increased production of lymph in the hepatic and splanchnic regions. Transudation of the fluid into the peritoneal cavity causes ascites.
- Low serum albumin levels (hypoalbuminaemia), due to decreased liver synthesis, causing a low plasma oncotic pressure.
- Secondary hyperaldosteronism with reduced catabolism of this salt-retaining hormone. The aldosterone antagonist spironolactone is thus often used to treat ascites.

These mechanisms can occur simultaneously.

Clinically, ascites may be detected by abdominal swelling, some abdominal pain, a shifting dullness, and a fluid thrill. Many patients also have peripheral oedema, due to hypoalbuminaemia.

It should be managed by reducing sodium intake and increasing renal sodium excretion with diuretics such as spironolactone and/or amiloride. Fluid may be removed by paracentesis (drainage via a needle through the abdominal wall). However, there is a risk that fluid will accumulate again in the peritoneal cavity at the expense of the systemic circulation. This leads to shock, so intravenous albumin should also be given.

A peritoneovenous shunt (a catheter from the peritoneal cavity into the internal jugular vein) may be used to return the fluid to the systemic circulation. This is used in rare cases when diuretic therapy fails.

If the portal pressure rises above 12 mmHg, then dilatation of the venous system causes collateral vessels to form. These are connections between the portal and systemic venous systems, and are found mainly at the gastro-oesophageal junction, rectum, diaphragm, left renal vein, the retroperitoneum and the umbilical region of the anterior abdominal wall and are described further in the next section.

Oesophageal varices can rupture, causing haematemesis and sometimes fatal consequences (oesophageal varices are described in Chapter 2). Enlargement of veins at other sites of portosystemic anastomoses may also occur, forming caput medusae around the umbilicus and rectal varices (see later).

### Dilatation of portosystemic anastomoses

These occur at four sites in the body (Fig. 4.23):

- The lower end of the oesophagus, between the left gastric vein (portal) and the azygos vein (systemic): when dilated, they are called *oesophageal varices*.
- The lower part of the rectum, between the superior (portal), middle and inferior (systemic) rectal veins: when dilated, they are called *rectal varices*.
- The umbilical region of the anterior abdominal wall, between the paraumbilical veins in the falciform ligament of the liver (portal) and the epigastric veins (systemic): when dilated, they are called *caput medusae*.
- *The bare areas of the gastrointestinal tract and its related organs*, e.g. veins between the bare area of the liver and the diaphragm.
- Additionally, some patients with liver disease who have had intestinal surgery – e.g. colectomy for ulcerative colitis associated with sclerosing cholangitis – can have varices form at the site of the surgical anastomosis or the stoma site and these can subsequently bleed.

These anastomoses may enlarge if the portal vein is obstructed by a thrombus or the venous flow through the liver is impeded by cirrhosis.

Oesophageal varices are clinically the most important cause of bleeding in portal hypertension and are diagnosed by endoscopy.

The locations of the porto-systemic anastomoses is a popular anatomy exam question – make sure you know them. Interestingly, caput medusae at the umbilicus is so-called because it looks like the serpents on the head of Medusa!

### Splenomegaly

Splenomegaly is the term used to describe an enlarged spleen. It can be massive (extending into the right iliac fossa), and has a large number of causes.

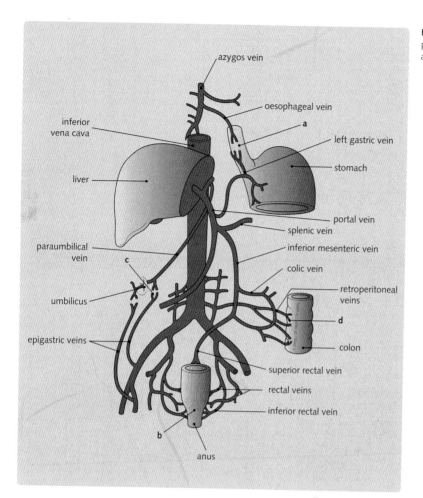

**Fig. 4.23** Diagram showing the sites of portosystemic anastomoses, indicated by a–d.

azygos vein

oesophageal vein

inferior vena cava

a

left gastric vein

stomach

liver

portal vein

splenic vein

paraumbilical vein

inferior mesenteric vein

c

colic vein

umbilicus

retroperitoneal veins

d

epigastric veins

colon

superior rectal vein

rectal veins

inferior rectal vein

b

anus

Normally the spleen weighs about 200 g; it is oval in shape and found between the 9th and 11th ribs. It plays an important role in immune defence and the removal of expired or abnormal blood cells.

Portal hypertension may cause moderate congestive splenomegaly, as may thrombosis of the extrahepatic portion of the portal vein or of the splenic vein.

A raised pressure in the inferior vena cava may be transmitted to the spleen through the portal vein, and is a cause of posthepatic splenomegaly; other causes include decompensated right-sided heart failure and pulmonary or tricuspid valve disease.

Splenomegaly may cause abdominal discomfort, and an enlarged spleen may occasionally rupture following minor trauma. Additionally, it can cause excess removal of blood cells leading to pancytopenia. This is called hypersplenism.

Splenomegaly is easily detected on examination of the abdomen, as it is dull to percussion.

Do not forget that other non-hepatic causes of splenomegaly include infections and inflammatory and haematological diseases, such as TB, infectious mononucleosis, septic shock, malaria, rheumatoid arthritis and haemolytic anaemia.

## Jaundice and cholestasis

Clinical jaundice (icterus) is caused by plasma levels of bilirubin exceeding 50 μmol/L, and it presents as a yellow pigmentation of skin, sclera and mucosa. The colour of the sclera is the best indicator, but it must be examined in good white light. Biochemical jaundice has a much lower threshold, and is simply a plasma bilirubin level above the normal range of 18–24 μmol/L.

Jaundice may be classified by its cause in relation to the hepatocyte as:

- Prehepatic.
- Hepatic.
- Posthepatic.

## Prehepatic jaundice

This describes conditions giving rise to jaundice where the mechanism occurs before the bilirubin gets to the hepatocyte, but its clinical usefulness is extended by considering it as all steps up to conjugation of bilirubin. Disorders of conjugation such as Gilbert's syndrome are thus included under this heading, although strictly speaking they are due to hepatic causes.

Bilirubin is formed from the breakdown of haemoglobin and, normally, is conjugated with glucuronic acid by hepatocytes when it reaches the liver. This makes it more soluble. Unconjugated bilirubin remains in the circulation only when the liver is unable to conjugate all the bilirubin that is delivered to it.

However, increased haemolysis, e.g. in haemolytic anaemias such as sickle-cell disease or haemolytic disease of the newborn, may cause an excess of bilirubin, and this can overcome the liver's capacity to conjugate it. Congenital hyperbilirubinaemias are another cause.

Therefore, haemolytic jaundice results in raised levels of unconjugated bilirubin. This is particularly dangerous in neonates, as the unconjugated bilirubin can cross the blood–brain barrier and cause brain damage (kernicterus).

Because unconjugated bilirubin is not soluble, it does not pass into the urine, so this type of jaundice is often called 'acholuric jaundice'. The urinary urobilinogen is elevated due to increased resorption from the gut, as the total bilirubin load is raised.

The congenital hyperbilirubinaemias are rare, and you do not need to know them in detail at this stage, with the possible exception of Gilbert's syndrome which is relatively more common.

### Gilbert's syndrome

This congenital disorder is caused by patients having a reduced amount of the enzyme UDP-glucuronyl transferase (UGT-1), which conjugates bilirubin with glucuronic acid. It is due to an abnormally long gene promoter sequence (TATA box) resulting in deficient trancription but the RNA sequence and enzymatic protein are normal.

This affects between 2% and 7% of the population, and is not a serious disease. The reticulocyte (immature red blood cell) count is normal, and there is only a slight increase in serum bilirubin (unconjugated), often after prolonged starvation or intercurrent illness.

The syndrome is asymptomatic, although some patients complain of fatigue. Treatment is not usually required but carbohydrate loading can help.

### Crigler–Najjar syndrome

This is an extremely rare disease due to more severe abnormalities in the translated gene sequence of UGT-1, resulting in total absence of enzyme (type I) or an abnormal but functional enzyme (type II); both types are autosomal recessive.

Type II patients have a decreased level of UDP-glucuronyl transferase and, therefore, they can survive into adulthood. This form is thought to be very similar to Gilbert's syndrome.

Type I patients lack the enzyme altogether, and they do not survive, unless they undergo liver transplantation. Both types of patient have high serum levels of unconjugated bilirubin.

## Hepatic jaundice

This type of jaundice describes mechanisms which occur within the hepatocyte, or more specifically, after the bilirubin conjugation stage. It therefore includes some rare congenital hyperbilirubinaemias and hepatocyte transport 'exporter protein' defects, as well as diseases resulting in hepatocellular damage and cholestasis (loss of bile flow).

### Dubin–Johnson syndrome

This is an autosomal recessive disorder in which the liver fails to excrete conjugated bilirubin (caused by a mutation in the canalicular multispecific organic anion transporter, CMOAT). It results in jaundice, and the liver appears black because of deposits of a melanin-like pigment.

### Rotor syndrome

This is very similar to Dubin–Johnson syndrome, with a defect in intracellular binding proteins for bilirubin. There is no pigment deposit.

### Hepatocellular jaundice

Damage to the hepatocytes and the intrahepatic biliary tree leads to an increase in both unconjugated and conjugated serum levels of bilirubin. There is an increase in clotting time, serum alanine amino-transferase and serum aspartate aminotransferase because of the hepatocellular damage.

Clinically, features of a conjugated hyperbilirubinaemia predominate, as excretion, not conjugation is the rate-limiting step in the metabolism of bilirubin, hence this hepatocellular jaundice can be categorized as a form of cholestatic jaundice.

Viruses such as the hepatitis A, B, C and E, and Epstein–Barr viruses, can lead to hepatocellular jaundice, as can leptospirosis (Weil's disease), a bacterial infection spread by infected rat urine.

Autoimmune or drug-induced damage, as well as cirrhosis and tumours, can cause hepatocellular jaundice.

Haemochromatosis, an autosomal recessive disorder of iron metabolism, can lead to cirrhosis, jaundice and liver failure if untreated.

Wilson's disease, an autosomal recessive disorder of copper metabolism, leads to cirrhosis and jaundice.

## POSTHEPATIC JAUNDICE

Normally, conjugated bilirubin passes from the liver to the gallbladder where it is stored and then released into the duodenum following a fatty meal.

In the terminal ileum, intestinal flora convert it first to urobilinogen (some of which is reabsorbed and excreted in the urine) and then to stercobilinogen, which is excreted in the faeces (giving them their brown colour).

In posthepatic jaundice, the passage of conjugated bilirubin through the biliary tree is blocked, and it leaks into the circulation instead. It is soluble and excreted in the urine, making it dark. However, the faeces are deprived of their stercobilinogen and are pale. These are key symptoms in the history.

There is no problem with the synthesis of any of the bile products in posthepatic obstructive jaundice, only its release into the duodenum. Obstruction also results in cholestasis. Therefore, bile salts, along with conjugated bilirubin, escape into the circulation, and this causes itching (pruritus), another important symptom.

Causes of posthepatic cholestatic jaundice include gallstones, biliary stricture, congenital biliary atresia (complete blockage from birth), carcinoma of the pancreas or bile ducts and pancreatitis.

The symptoms and causes of jaundice are summarized in Fig. 4.24.

One clinical question can be used to separate prehepatic jaundice from the other causes, i.e. whether the patient has pale stools and dark urine. This is a symptom of cholestatic rather than prehepatic jaundice – note that it does not imply obstruction, as obstruction is only one cause of cholestasis. One simple test can be used to identify posthepatic jaundice, i.e. an ultrasound scan.

The types of jaundice can be correlated as follows: prehepatic jaundice is where bilirubin is unconjugated, posthepatic jaundice is where bilirubin is conjugated and hepatic jaundice gives a mixed picture.

### Further investigations for jaundice

Investigations other than liver function tests, a full blood count, serum bilirubin levels, virology screening and urinanalysis that can be performed are:

- Ultrasound.
- Liver biopsy.
- Endoscopic ultrasound (EUS).
- Endoscopic retrograde cholangio-pancreatography (ERCP).
- Magnetic resonance cholangio-pancreatography (MRCP).

Lack of bile salts and, therefore, a lack of fat absorption, causes the slow clotting time associated with jaundice. Vitamin K (a clotting factor) is a fat-soluble vitamin which requires fat for absorption from the gut. In jaundice: decreased fat absorption = low vitamin K concentrations = slow clotting.

## Hepatic failure

Despite its large capacity to regenerate after injury, the liver can sometimes fail due to severe acute liver

**Fig. 4.24** The classification of the different types of jaundice, showing the causes and symptoms or clinical signs. (AST = serum aspartate aminotransferase; ALT = serum alanine aminotransferase; EBV = Epstein–Barr virus; γ-GT = γ-glutamyl transferase; AP = alkaline phosphatase.)

| Type of jaundice | Cause | Signs |
|---|---|---|
| Prehepatic | Haemolysis<br>Ineffective erythropoiesis | Increased concentrations of unconjugated bilirubin (no bilirubin in the urine because it is insoluble) |
| Hepatic (congenital and hepatocellular) | • Gilbert's syndrome<br>• Grigler–Najjar syndrome<br>• Rotor syndrome<br>• Dubin–Johnson syndrome<br>• Viral infection, (e.g. Hep. A, B, C, E, and EBV)<br>• Cirrhosis<br>• Drugs<br>• Autoimmune disease<br>• Weil's disease<br>• Wilson's disease | • Increased clotting time<br>• Increased ALT and AST<br>• Hepatocellular damage |
| Posthepatic (obstrutive or cholestatic) | • Pancreatitis<br>• Primary biliary cirhosis<br>• Gallstones<br>• Drugs<br>• Carcinoma (of head of pancreas or bile duct)<br>• Biliary stricture<br>• Congenital biliary atresia | • Dark urine (with bilirubin, no urobilinogen)<br>• γ-GT and AP increase due to damage to the biliry tree<br>• Pale stools<br>• Itching |

injury, e.g. in viral hepatitis or drug toxicity, or chronic liver disease, e.g. cirrhosis. Liver failure can therefore be acute or chronic.

The liver has a large number of vital functions, and its failure to perform these can lead to systemic consequences, from neurological problems to decreased coagulation or renal failure.

## Acute (fulminant) liver failure

Fulminant means developing suddenly (from the Latin for 'lightning') and fulminant liver failure is the development of hepatic encephalopathy within 2–3 weeks of the first symptoms of hepatic insufficiency. Viral infection is the most common cause.

Clinical features are subtle initially, and are those of hepatic encephalopathy (see below). There is usually jaundice, unless the cause is Reye's syndrome (see later), and the liver is enlarged only in the initial stages, being impalpable after that.

The prognosis depends on the health and age of the patient, as in many other diseases.

Hepatic encephalopathy that takes longer to develop (2–12 weeks) is called subfulminant hepatitis.

### Hepatic encephalopathy

This is a neurological disorder caused by metabolic failure of the hepatocytes and the shunting of blood around the liver (due to cirrhosis or after portocaval anastomosis).

It may occur in both chronic and acute liver failure, and results in the exposure of the brain to abnormal metabolites, causing oedema and astrocyte changes.

Normally the liver eliminates the toxic nitrogenous products of gut bacteria. In liver failure, their elimination is reduced and some of them act as false transmitters (mimicking the normal neurotransmitters of the central nervous system). This results in central nervous system disturbances.

Other factors may play a part in the pathology, including ammonia and electrolyte disturbances, hypotension, changes in vascular permeability and increased cerebral sensitivity due to the metabolic disturbances.

Symptoms include:

- Disturbances in consciousness (ranging from confusion to coma and death).
- Asterixis (a flapping tremor of outstretched hands).
- Fluctuating neurological signs (muscular rigidity and hyperreflexia).

There is no specific treatment, except to restrict protein intake (to reduce uraemia and endogenous protein breakdown), treat any infection, empty the bowels of nitrogen-containing material and correct the metabolic and coagulation disturbances. Flumazenil, a benzodiazepine receptor antagonist, can improve the encephalopathy in the short term.

## Chronic liver failure

This refers to the situation in which the functional capacity of the liver is unable to maintain normal physiological conditions. 'Decompensated liver disease' is a synonymous term.

Clinical features are similar to those of cirrhosis (Fig. 4.22). However, it must be noted that cirrhosis and chronic liver failure are not the same; cirrhosis may cause chronic liver failure but not vice-versa. Infection and hepatic vascular disease may precipitate chronic liver failure, with cirrhosis being a possible step in the pathogenesis.

Management involves treating the underlying cause, treating the symptoms and maintaining normal nutritional status. Liver transplantation (see later) may be an option.

The prognosis is poor, with a 25% 5-year survival rate.

> Cirrhosis and chronic liver failure are very closely related because any condition which may lead to death of hepatocytes and thus predispose to chronic liver failure may also cause cirrhosis. Examples include viral hepatitis, vascular diseases such as the Budd–Chiari syndrome and metabolic diseases affecting the liver. The association with cirrhosis is also why the liver becomes impalpable over the course of the disease, as progressive hepatocyte death and fibrosis cause the liver to shrink.

## Hepatorenal syndrome

This is the combination of renal failure in a previously normal kidney and severe liver disease. However, kidney function improves dramatically if the liver failure is reversed.

Renal failure is caused by a drop in renal blood flow and glomerular filtration rate, causing a fall in urine output and increased retention of sodium by the kidney. These mechanisms are brought about by upregulation of the renin–angiotensin–aldosterone system, norepinephrine and vasopressin. It may be fatal.

Treatment includes the use of dopamine to increase renal blood flow, and protein restriction.

## Liver transplantation

Liver transplantation is increasingly used in the treatment of:

- Acute and chronic liver disease.
- Alcoholic liver disease (provided the patient has given up drinking and is well motivated).
- Primary biliary cirrhosis, when serum bilirubin rises above 100 mmol/L.
- Chronic hepatitis B and C when complications ensue.
- Primary metabolic disease with end-stage liver disease, e.g. Wilson's disease and $\alpha_1$-antitrypsin deficiency.
- Other conditions, including sclerosing cholangitis or rarely hepatocellular carcinoma.

Absolute contraindications are active sepsis outside the hepatobiliary tree and metastatic malignancy. If the patient lacks psychological commitment, as might occur in alcoholic liver disease, then transplantation is not an option. Complications increase and recovery is impeded with advancing years over 70.

Most organs are taken from cadavers, but a relative may donate a single lobe to an infant.

The liver is less aggressively rejected than other organs but early (reversible), or late (irreversible) rejection may occur. Acute (cellular), or early rejection occurs within 5–10 days after the transplant. The patient develops pyrexia, general malaise, and abdominal tenderness due to hepatomegaly. This is caused by an inflammatory reaction.

Immunosuppressive therapy works very well in this situation.

Chronic (ductopenic) rejection occurs 6 weeks to 9 months after the transplant. This type of rejection cannot be reversed with immunosuppressive drugs and retransplantation is the only treatment. Graft-versus-host disease is very rare.

Ciclosporin has proved useful, but most patients require more than one immunosuppressant. However, 5 years after the transplant, 20–30% of patients no longer receive immunosuppressants.

# DISORDERS OF THE LIVER

As the liver, gallbladder and biliary tract are anatomically and functionally connected, diseases and disorders which affect one part of the hepatobiliary system may therefore have an impact on the other components. It is important to bear this in mind when thinking about the pathological processes that can occur in these organs.

## Congenital abnormalities

### Polycystic liver disease

In polycystic liver disease, the liver has numerous cysts, lined with flattened or cuboidal biliary epithelium and containing straw-coloured fluid. This is an autosomal dominant condition.

The cysts are not connected to the biliary tree, and they do not contain pigmented bile.

The number of cysts varies from just a few to several hundred, and the cysts themselves vary in diameter from 0.5 cm to 4.0 cm.

They may cause discomfort or pain if the patient stoops, and rupture of a cyst may cause acute pain. Asymptomatic cysts do not need treatment; painful ones may require aspiration.

Polycystic liver disease may be associated with polycystic kidney disease, which may lead to renal failure, in which case the prognosis is worse.

### Congenital hepatic fibrosis

Congenital hepatic fibrosis is inherited as an autosomal recessive disorder. It may present with complications of portal hypertension and, perhaps most importantly, with bleeding varices (a medical emergency).

The liver is divided into irregular islands by bands of collagenous tissue that enlarge the portal tracts and form septa.

Abnormally shaped bile ducts are scattered throughout the fibrous tissue and the septal margins contain bile duct remnants.

Associated conditions include polycystic kidneys and medullary sponge kidneys.

Diagnosis is by wedge biopsy. This allows differentiation between fibrosis and cirrhosis.

## Disorders of metabolism

Haemochromatosis and hyperlipidaemias are relatively the most common of these diseases; the others are rare.

### Haemochromatosis

Primary haemochromatosis is an autosomal recessive disorder characterized by the absorption of too much iron, which then accumulates (as haemosiderin) in the liver, pancreas, heart, pituitary and joints.

A gene defect near the HLA region on chromosome 6, called the HFE gene, results in a loss of regulation of iron absorption from the small intestine even when the iron-binding protein, transferrin, is fully saturated. Iron stores may be many times greater than normal levels, rising from about 1 g to as much as 20 g.

Heterozygotes have only modest increases in absorption but generally they have normal iron stores. It can take decades for sufficient iron to accumulate to cause organ damage so that most cases present after the age of 40. Symptoms are rare in women of child-bearing age as menstrual losses and pregnancy compensate for the excess iron absorption. The presenting complaint in men is often loss of libido and hypogonadism, secondary to dysfunction of the pituitary gland, but the commonest presentation now is an incidental finding of abnormal liver enzymes or raised ferritin level.

The clinical features include:

- Liver enlargement.
- Fibrosis and cirrhosis.
- Bronze discolouration of the skin.
- Diabetes mellitus in two-thirds of cases (hence the alternative name, bronze diabetes).
- Cardiac arrythmias, cardiomyopathy and heart failure.
- Arthritis in hands and knees.

Untreated, the condition may lead to liver failure and primary hepatocellular carcinoma. Early in the disease, iron is deposited in periportal hepatocytes (as haemosiderin) and then in Kupffer cells, bile duct epithelium and portal tract connective tissue. There is hepatocyte necrosis possibly due to free-radical generation, and cirrhosis occurs as the disease progresses.

Diagnosis is by blood tests (which characteristically show raised ferritin with transferrin saturation of 100%) and liver biopsy showing heavy deposits of iron (as haemosiderin) in hepatocytes.

Treatment is by phlebotomy (venesection) once or twice a week for a year or more until iron levels return to normal, and then three or four times a year.

Chelation therapy (a drug that complexes with a metal ion for its removal) can be used in patients who cannot have venesection due to cardiac disease or anaemia. Desferrioxamine can be given continuously subcutaneously, or as and when required.

Secondary haemochromatosis (haemosiderosis) may result from iron overload, e.g. in thalassaemia patients after repeated blood transfusions or from excess iron absorption, e.g. in congenital haemolytic anaemias.

## Wilson's disease

Wilson's disease (hepatolenticular degeneration) is a rare, autosomal recessive disorder in which copper accumulates in the liver and the basal ganglia of the brain. The cause is a mutation in a copper transport ATPase gene located on chromosome 13.

Normally copper is secreted into bile, but in Wilson's disease biliary copper excretion is low. In the liver, a chronic hepatitis results, which leads to cirrhosis. Signs and symptoms may appear in patients at any age from about 5 years to 50 years, and they include hepatic and neurological abnormalities. Faint, brown (Kayser–Fleischer) rings may appear in the eye at the junction of the cornea and sclera in Descemet's membrane. They are diagnostic but usually require slit-lamp examination. Psychiatric symptoms may be seen as a result of copper deposition in the brain.

Diagnosis is by measurement of the copper-binding protein caeruloplasmin in the blood. This is low in Wilson's disease because the non-functioning copper transport protein does not allow copper to stimulate its production. Special staining of liver biopsy tissue will show an excess of copper. Twenty-four hour urinary copper concentrations are normally raised in Wilson's disease.

Treatment is with penicillamine, a chelating agent that binds to copper and enables it to be excreted.

Prognosis depends on the stage at which treatment is begun. If started early, before significant amounts of copper have been deposited, prognosis is good. Neurological damage may be irreversible, and in hepatic failure or cirrhosis, the only treatment is transplantation. Thus although rare, a high index of suspicion is necessary for Wilson's disease due to the serious consequences.

## $\alpha_1$-antitrypsin deficiency

$\alpha_1$-antitrypsin is a serum protein that is produced in the liver and has anti-protease effects, e.g. on pulmonary neutrophil elastase, thus preventing emphysema. It is part of the serine protease inhibitors (SERPIN) superfamily of enzymes. One in ten northern Europeans carry a deficiency gene, which is autosomal recessive in inheritance.

The protease inhibitor (Pi) gene controlling its production is located on chromosome 14 and a number of variants exist. The normal variant is M allele, and the most important abnormal one is the Z allele.

Symptoms include emphysema in about 75% of homozygotes and liver cirrhosis in approximately 10%. Heterozygotes have an increased risk of developing emphysema if they smoke.

In the livers of homozygotes, $\alpha_1$-antitrypsin accumulates by polymerization in hepatocytes, shown by PAS (periodic acid–Schiff)-positive intracellular globules on liver biopsy. There is a chronic inflammatory picture leading to cirrhosis, but the exact mechanisms causing the cirrhosis are unknown.

Diagnosis is by measurement of serum $\alpha_1$-antitrypsin and by liver biopsy.

Treatment is symptomatic, and patients should be advised to stop smoking.

## Reye's syndrome

Reye's syndrome is a rare disorder affecting children up to 15 years of age. It is characterized by acute encephalopathy and infiltration of fatty microvesicles in the liver (steatosis), and typically occurs during recovery from upper respiratory tract infections, influenza or chickenpox.

The encephalopathy and hepatic microvesicular steatosis are caused by inhibition of β-oxidation and the uncoupling of oxidative phosphorylation in mitochondria. Aspirin has been implicated as a precipitating factor.

There is rapid progression to hepatic failure with neurological deterioration and eventual coma.

Histologically, the liver shows a foamy accumulation of triglycerides and alterations in the mitochondria; this is also seen in the brain.

Treatment is supportive, with corticosteroids and mannitol (to reduce brain swelling) and dialysis or transfusion to correct chemical imbalances resulting from liver damage.

Prognosis is poor, with an overall mortality of about 50%, mainly due to cerebral oedema.

## Hyperlipidaemias

Hyperlipidaemias are a group of metabolic disorders characterized by high levels of lipids (chiefly cholesterol, triglycerides and lipoproteins) in the blood. Several types of hyperlipidaemia have been described, depending on levels of which lipid are raised.

Disorders resulting in hyperlipidaemia can stem from:

- Abnormal expression of genes encoding apoproteins.
- Lipoprotein lipase deficiency.
- Low-density lipoprotein (LDL)-receptor defects.

Hyperlipidaemia is closely associated with atheroma and cardiovascular disease, particularly in the West, where diets contain too much fat.

Treatment includes the use of bile acid binding resins such as cholestyramine and colestipol. These prevent the reuptake of bile acids from the terminal ileum and result in a greater de novo synthesis by the liver, using up cholesterol and lowering its circulating levels.

HMG-CoA reductase inhibitors or 'statins', e.g. pravastatin and simvastatin, inhibit the rate-limiting step in cholesterol synthesis and can reduce LDL cholesterol by up to 40%.

Other treatments include fibrates, e.g. gemfibrozil and ciprofibrate, nicotinic acid and omega-3 marine triglycerides, which limit hepatic triglyceride synthesis, reduce free fatty acid concentrations, and reduce hepatic very low density lipoprotein (VLDL) secretion respectively.

## Neonatal hepatitis

Neonatal hepatitis is the end-result of a range of injurious processes including:

- Congenital infection with rubella.
- Cytomegalovirus and toxoplasmosis.
- $\alpha_1$-antitrypsin deficiency.
- Tyrosinaemia.
- Cystic fibrosis.
- Storage disorders.
- Galactosaemia.
- Hepatitis A and B viruses.

The histological picture may include multinucleate giant cells and cholestasis or hepatocellular necrosis, and inflammatory infiltrates in the portal tracts and lobules. Hyperbilirubinaemia is present.

The condition is often familial, inheritance being autosomal recessive. It is very difficult to find the precise aetiology behind neonatal hepatitis.

## Glycogen storage diseases

There are many different types of glycogen storage diseases, each caused by a different enzyme defect. All of these diseases are autosomal recessive, except type IX B, which is X-linked.

Hepatocytes are involved in types I, II, III, IV, VI and VIII, with a different site for glycogen storage in each. Most patients present in childhood with hepatomegaly.

Patients with type I may develop hepatocellular adenoma. Type IV predisposes to cirrhosis and usually results in death by the age of 5 years. The heart and skeletal muscle can be involved, resulting in myopathies and possible cardiac failure.

Treatment varies according to the type of glycogen storage disease. Extreme exercise must be avoided, and oral glucose and fructose maintain blood glucose concentrations. Liver transplantation is a very successful treatment for glycogen storage diseases.

## Lysosomal storage diseases

There are a number of lysosomal storage diseases, all of which have a specific enzyme defect. This results in the abnormal accumulation of the enzyme substrate in lysosomes.

Gaucher's disease (a deficiency of glucocerebrosidase) is the most common type of lysosomal storage disease. This leads to the abnormal storage of glucocerebroside (glycosylceramide) in reticuloendothelial cells (macrophages and monocytes) found in the liver, spleen and bone marrow.

Its incidence is high in Ashkenazi Jews (1 in 2000) and it usually presents in childhood with splenomegaly, hepatomegaly, anaemia and elevated levels of serum aminotransferases.

Liver failure is rare and treatment includes splenectomy, bone marrow transplantation and replacement enzyme therapy (with alglucerase). If there is neurological involvement, then the outlook is poor.

# Infectious and inflammatory disease

## Viral hepatitis

Viral hepatitis is a common cause of liver injury. The most common causes by far are the hepatitis viruses (A, B, C and E ). Rarer causes are cytomegalovirus (CMV), Epstein–Barr virus (EBV, hepatitis D and G and arboviruses, e.g. in yellow fever.

Acute viral hepatitis may be asymptomatic or symptomatic, with or without jaundice and itching. Asymptomatic infection is common particularly in hepatitis A acquired by children and more than 50% of those suffering from hepatitis B and C.

Symptoms are similar, regardless of the infecting virus and present as a non-specific influenza-like illness, or with symptoms of gastroenteritis. Hepatitis B infection may lead to arthritis or arthralgia with a rash (caused by immune complexes). Liver function tests are abnormal, with raised serum transaminases indicative of hepatocyte damage. Occasionally, fulminant hepatic failure may occur.

Infection with hepatitis A and E does not result in chronic infection. Hepatitis A, C, D and E are all RNA viruses; hepatitis B is a DNA virus (Fig. 4.25).

### Hepatitis A

This disease is caused by an RNA picornavirus which is found worldwide, especially where there is poor sanitation and hygiene, and it is spread by the faecal–oral route through contaminated food and water, e.g. eating contaminated shellfish or swimming in sewage-polluted water. It may cause outbreaks, and is very resistant to heat and disinfectants.

The incubation period is 2–4 weeks, and infection may be asymptomatic (as in most childhood infections) or cause fever, malaise or a gastro-enteritis-like illness followed by jaundice for 1–3 weeks. Diagnosis is by virus-specific IgM. Neither

carrier states nor chronic infections occur (Fig. 4.26), but virus is present in the stools of patients about 2 weeks before and up to about a week after jaundice is apparent.

### Hepatitis B

Infection with hepatitis B virus (HBV) may lead to a chronic carrier state, liver cancer or cirrhosis. HBV is a DNA virus belonging to the hepadna group.

Transmission is through contaminated blood or blood products, body fluids, sexual contact and vertical transmission from mother to baby during parturition. It is also secreted in breast milk.

HBV is found worldwide, and is especially endemic in Southeast Asia, China and tropical Africa. Eastern Europe, Central and South America, and the Mediterranean are areas of intermediate endemicity.

Areas of low endemicity include Northern Europe, North America and Australia. Infection in these areas is associated with high-risk activities such as intravenous drug use, unprotected male homosexual contact, tattoo and acupuncture practices and the use of blood products by haemophiliacs.

Incubation is 2–6 months and over 50% of cases are asymptomatic.

Of infected adults, 90–95% recover completely and become immune, the remaining 5–10% become carriers (either asymptomatic carriers, or suffering from chronic hepatitis which may lead to cirrhosis). About 1% develop fulminant acute hepatitis (a cause of acute liver failure – see above), which has a very high mortality rate. Infants infected perinatally have a worse prognosis: 70–90% become carriers. This may be due to their relatively underdeveloped immune systems.

Complications of chronic carriage include chronic active hepatitis, cirrhosis and hepatocellular carcinoma.

The intact HBV, also called the Dane particle, has a number of antigens. The viral coat contains surface antigen (HBsAg), while the core contains the core antigen (HBcAg) and the e antigen (HBeAg) as well as the viral DNA.

All carriers have HBsAg and anti-HBc. A carrier state is defined as one in which HBsAg persists for 6 months or longer (Fig. 4.27). Immune people (those who have recovered from the infection and those vaccinated against it) have anti-HBs and anti-HBc antibodies.

Previously, the e antigen (HBe) used to be a good determinant of infectivity: it is present in highly

**Fig. 4.25** Viral hepatitis. (HAV IgM = hepatitis A virus immunoglobulin M; HBsAg = hepatitis B virus surface antigen; HBeAg = hepatitis B virus e antigen; HBc IgM = hepatitis B virus core immunoglobulin M; anti-HCV = anti-hepatitis C virus; PCR = polymerase chain reaction; HDD Ag = hepatitis D virus antigen; HDV IgM = hepatitis virus immunoglobulin; HEV IgG = hepatitis E virus immunoglobulin G; HBIG = hepatitis B immunoglobulin; HNIG = human normal immunoglobulin.) (Data courtesy of Dr Tilzey, St Thomas's Hospital, London.)

| Type | Virus | Spread | Incubation period | Carrier state/ chronic infection | Diagnosis of acute infection | Specific Prevention | Treatment |
|---|---|---|---|---|---|---|---|
| A | Picornavirus | Faecal–oral | 2–3 weeks | No | HAV IgM | Vaccine HNIG | N/A |
| B | Hepadnavirus | Contaminated blood and body fluids:<br>• percutaneous<br>• sexual<br>• mother to baby | 2–6 months | Yes<br>Adults 5–10%<br>Neonates 70–90% | HBsAg<br>HBeAg<br>HBc IgM | Vaccine, HBIG | α-interferon |
| C | Flavivirus | Contaminated blood and body fluids:<br>• percutaneous<br>• sexual<br>• mother to baby | 6–8 weeks | Yes<br>Adults 60–90% | Anti-HCV<br>PCR | N/A | α-interferon |
| D | Defective RNA virus coated with HBsAg | Contaminated blood and body fluids:<br>• percutaneous<br>• sexual<br>Note: requires HBsAg for propagation and hepatotropism | N/A | Yes | HDV AG<br>HDV IgM<br>(up to 6 wks)<br>HDV IgG<br>(after 6 wks) | Prevent HBV | N/A |
| E | Calicivirus | Faecal–oral | 2–9 weeks | No | HEV IgG | N/A | N/A |

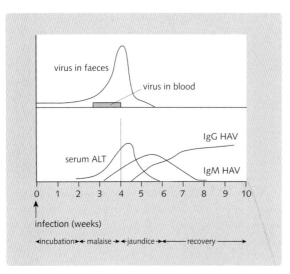

**Fig. 4.26** The sequence of events in hepatitis A infection. (ALT = serum alanine aminotransferase; IgG HAV, IgM HAV = antibodies to hepatitis A virus – immunoglobulins G and M.)

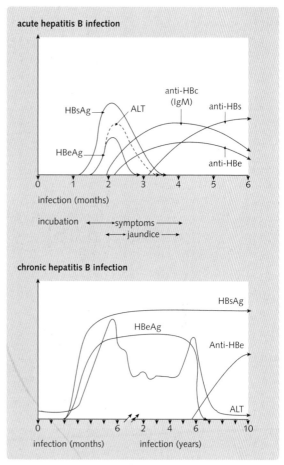

**Fig. 4.27** Time-course of infective markers in acute and chronic hepatitis B infection. (ALT = serum alanine aminotransferase; HBc = hepatitis B core; HBs = hepatitis B surface.) (Redrawn with permission from Kumar P, Clarke M. Clinical Medicine, 3rd edn. London: Saunders, 1994.)

infectious carriers, carriers without e antigen are intermediately infective, and anti-e antibody means a person has low infectivity. However, HBe-negative but replication-competent mutants have been detected. This means that a patient infected with the mutant virus will, under the old standards, be classified as having low infectivity and a low risk of developing chronic liver disease when this is not the case. Infection with HBe-negative mutants should be suspected if HBV DNA is present in the blood but HBe antigen is negative.

Other important mutants include 'escape variants' such as those with a mutation in the gene for HBs which enables them to 'escape' neutralization by antibodies.

It is no longer true that hepatitis B patients without the e antigen (HBeAg) do not have high infectivity. This is because HBeAg-negative mutants which are able to replicate have been detected. If in doubt, request a viral DNA assay.

Carriers are defined as people in whom hepatitis B surface antigen has been detected for more than 6 months.

The risk of contracting hepatitis B from a needle contaminated with e antigen positive, i.e. highly infectious, blood following a needlestick injury is 30%.

Those who should receive hepatitis B vaccination are:

- All healthcare workers.
- Members of emergency and rescue teams.
- Haemophiliacs.
- Homosexual and bisexual men and prostitutes.
- Long-term travellers.
- Children in high-risk areas.
- Morticians/embalmers.

## Hepatitis C

Hepatitis C virus (HCV) is the major cause of post-transfusional hepatitis. It is an RNA flavirus.

HCV may be transmitted parenterally, from mother to baby or through sexual contact, but because blood viral titres are much lower, these routes of transmission are uncommon (unlike hepatitis B). It has a low incidence rate at sexually transmitted disease (STD) clinics, suggesting that transmission via sexual contact is uncommon.

HCV shows much genetic diversity, with six genotypes and more than 100 subtypes. However, all are equally pathogenic. It is found worldwide, particularly in Japan, parts of South America, the Mediterranean, Africa and the Middle East.

The UK, Northern Europe and North America are areas of low seroprevalence, and most infection is associated with high-risk activity (intravenous drug abuse or multiple blood transfusions).

The incubation period is 6–8 weeks and infection is asymptomatic in about 90% of cases. However, unlike hepatitis B, only 15% of patients recover fully, with 60–90% of people becoming chronic carriers with a risk of developing chronic active hepatitis, cirrhosis or hepatocellular carcinoma. Less than 1% will develop fulminant acute hepatitis.

## Hepatitis D

Hepatitis D virus (HDV) is a defective RNA virus that can cause infection and replicate only in conjunction with hepatitis B.

It has a worldwide distribution, and is particularly prevalent in the Middle East, parts of Africa and South America.

Infection in Northern Europe is mainly confined to high-risk behaviour (intravenous drug abuse and multiple blood transfusions). Transmission is mainly parenteral. Hepatitis D may infect at the same time as hepatitis B or infect someone already chronically infected with hepatitis B (superinfection).

Infection with HDV rarely resolves and most patients will develop cirrhosis, some within the span of a few years.

## Hepatitis E

This is especially common in Asia, Africa and the Middle East.

It is spread by the faecal–oral route. The incubation period is 2–9 weeks (usually 6 weeks). Clinically, the infection is mild but jaundice is apparent.

High-risk age groups include those aged 15–40 years, and it has a 15–20% mortality rate in pregnant women as it may cause fulminant acute hepatitis in this group. It does not lead to chronic infection.

## Treatment of viral hepatitis

The treatment for viral hepatitis depends on the specific infecting virus. Prophylactic vaccines are available for hepatitis A and B viruses.

There is no vaccine for hepatitis viruses C, D and E, although the hepatitis B vaccine may be given to help reduce the chance of hepatitis D infection. Treatment is supportive and the use of alcohol must be avoided. α-interferon is useful against hepatitis B and C. The antiviral drugs lamivudine and ribavirin can be used for hepatitis B and C respectively. All sexual and household contacts of the infected person with hepatitis B should be vaccinated, if possible.

## Liver abscess and non-viral liver infections

Liver abscesses are more common in developing parts of the world.

In the past, they were relatively common complications of appendicitis or perforation of the gastrointestinal tract, but improved management of these conditions has seen a decrease in the formation of abscesses.

They usually result from bacterial infection spread through the biliary tree (ascending cholangitis), carried from the gut in the portal system, from a penetrating injury to the liver, direct extension from a perinephric or other abscess, or infection carried in branches of the hepatic artery.

Amoebic abscesses must be considered in travellers, as *Entamoeba histolytica* causes abscesses as well as amoebic dysentery. Characteristically, the abscesses are filled with necrotic material which looks like anchovy paste.

Symptoms vary from general malaise to febrile jaundice with right upper quadrant pain and tender hepatomegaly.

Diagnosis is by ultrasonography, chest radiography, serological tests and analysis of the aspirated contents of the abscess.

Treatment of large abscesses is by radiologically controlled drainage and the administration of antibiotics. Complications include rupture and septicaemia.

Apart from viral hepatitis and bacterial infections, parasitic infections of the liver also occur, especially in the developing world. The two most important parasitic infections are those caused by helminths (worms) and protozoa.

Malaria (caused by the protozoon *Plasmodium* spp.) and visceral leishmaniasis (caused by *Leishmania donovani*) result in hepatomegaly apart from their other systemic symptoms.

Helminths which infect the liver include *Schistosoma* spp. and *Echinococcus granulosus*, apart from liver flukes. The first causes portal tract fibrosis leading to portal hypertension, while the second is the cause of hydatid cysts containing developing worms.

> Abscesses are collections of pus, caused by an inflammatory reaction, often as a result of bacterial infection. In general, 'if there is pus about, let it out'! Treatment of abscesses in accessible parts of the body is usually by surgical drainage or aspiration.

## Autoimmune hepatitis

This form of chronic hepatitis affects predominantly young and middle-aged women, and is associated with the HLA alleles HLA-B8, HLA-DR3 and HLA-DR4.

It is also associated with other autoimmune diseases, such as pernicious anaemia and thyroiditis. The patient may be asymptomatic, present with fatigue or present with acute hepatitis (25% of cases) displaying jaundice. On examination, the patient may have hepatosplenomegaly, bruises, cutaneous striae, acne, hirsutism and possibly ascites. Extrahepatic manifestations may be present, such as glomerulonephritis, fever or pleurisy.

The liver biochemistry shows elevated serum aminotransferases, alkaline phosphatases and bilirubin (to a lesser degree). Serum $\alpha$-globulins are usually twice the normal titre.

There are two types of autoimmune hepatitis, classified by the autoantibodies detected:

- Type I has antinuclear and anti-smooth muscle autoantibodies.
- Type II has anti-liver-kidney-microsomal (LKM) autoantibodies and anti-liver cytosolic autoantibodies.

Type I autoimmune hepatitis affects women, whereas type II mainly affects girls aged 5–20 years, and is generally less common.

Primary biliary cirrhosis (see below) is another form of autoimmune liver disease. Mitochondrial antibodies are found in the serum. Patients present with itching and jaundice, and slowly progress to cirrhosis.

Treatment for autoimmune hepatitis involves steroids (prednisolone) and immunosuppressants (azathioprine). The therapy is given indefinitely, and can bring remission to 90% of the cases. Liver transplantation is also an option if drug therapy fails.

## Diseases of the biliary tract associated with cirrhosis

### Primary biliary cirrhosis

Primary biliary cirrhosis (PBC) is an autoimmune disorder and, like other autoimmune diseases, affects women, especially those 40–50 years of age, more than men. It can occur in conjunction with other autoimmune diseases, e.g. Sjögren's syndrome, rheumatoid arthritis and scleroderma.

The epithelium of the bile ducts (especially that of the smaller intrahepatic ducts) is destroyed by an autoimmune reaction and the damaged areas become surrounded by lymphocytes. The surrounding hepatocytes undergo necrosis, in a pattern resembling piecemeal necrosis. Granulomas may also be present.

All patients with PBC have anti-mitochondrial autoantibodies and this, together with raised serum alkaline phosphatase, is diagnostic for the condition. The presence of anti-mitochondrial antibodies implies a connection with autoimmunity, although the exact pathogenetic mechanisms are unknown.

An attempt at regeneration then takes place in the form of proliferation of small bile ductules at the edges of the portal tracts, with consequent fibrosis disrupting the normal architecture of the liver.

Eventually, diffuse and irreversible cirrhosis occurs which may be complicated by liver failure, portal hypertension and, rarely, hepatocellular carcinoma.

Clinically, the patient will have pruritus, jaundice and xanthelasma (deposits of cholesterol-laden macrophages around the eyes, easily visible macroscopically).

The course and prognosis of the disease is slow (about 10 years) but variable and there is no effective medical treatment although ursodeoxycholate (a bile acid substitute) is of benefit in some patients, improving liver function and survival. Cholestyramine lessens pruritus.

Cholestasis results in malabsorption of the fat-soluble vitamins, therefore supplements are given. Treatment of PBC is difficult and often ineffective, so liver transplantation should be considered when the bilirubin levels rise above 100 µmol/L.

## Secondary biliary cirrhosis

Secondary biliary cirrhosis is caused by prolonged obstruction of extrahepatic bile ducts, often as a result of gallstones, biliary atresia, strictures caused by previous surgery or carcinoma of the head of the pancreas.

Bile remains in the obstructed ducts and inflammation and periportal fibrosis may result, eventually leading to cirrhosis.

Bile duct proliferation may occur and secondary bacterial infection (ascending cholangitis) may complicate biliary strictures and gallstones.

Diagnosis is by ultrasonography, endoscopic retrograde cholangiopancreatography (ERCP) or percutaneous transhepatic cholangiography.

## Primary sclerosing cholangitis

Primary sclerosing cholangitis (PSC) is a chronic inflammatory disease often associated with inflammatory bowel disease. Seventy per cent of cases occur in association with ulcerative colitis.

Male patients outnumber females by 2:1, and they usually present at around 39 years of age.

Intrahepatic, and sometimes extrahepatic, bile ducts become surrounded by a mantle of chronic inflammatory cells.

Eventually onion skin fibrosis occurs (concentric fibrosis around the ducts). The ducts are seen on ERCP as having a 'beaded' appearance. Small ducts near the portal tracts may be totally replaced by fibrous tissue ('vanishing bile ducts').

Patients vary from being asymptomatic to suffering from chronic liver disease, with pruritus, jaundice, fatigue and eventually portal hypertension.

Elevated serum alkaline phosphatase and myeloperoxidase ANCA antibodies in 80% of cases suggest a diagnosis of PSC. However, liver biopsy is the best diagnostic tool. Patients with PSC have a higher risk of developing cholangiocarcinoma.

# Alcohol-, drug- and toxin-associated disease

## Alcoholic liver disease

Alcohol produces a range of liver diseases, from fatty liver (steatosis) to cirrhosis. The pathogenesis of alcoholic liver disease is summarized in Fig. 4.28.

### Hepatic steatosis (fatty liver)

Fatty liver is seen in a number of disorders, including alcoholic liver disease and obesity with or without diabetes mellitus.

Normally, lipids from the diet or released from adipose tissue are transported to the liver where they are metabolized.

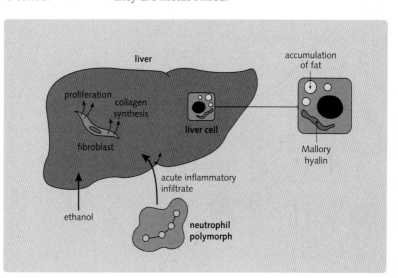

**Fig. 4.28** Pathogenesis of alcoholic liver disease.

Alcohol is toxic, and when it is drunk in excess its metabolism becomes a priority (Fig. 4.29). Cellular energy is diverted towards this and away from other essential metabolic pathways, including the metabolism of fat in the liver.

Fat then accumulates in the cytoplasm of liver cells, particularly in zone 3, the area adjacent to the central vein and furthest from the arterial supply.

In chronic ingestion of alcohol, the liver becomes a large greasy organ weighing as much as 5–6 kg.

If alcohol abuse continues, fibrosis and cirrhosis may occur but fatty change is reversible if alcohol intake is stopped.

### Alcoholic hepatitis

This is inflammation of the liver caused by alcohol ingestion.

Alcohol is directly cytotoxic at high concentrations and cells swell with granular cytoplasm. Intracytoplasmic aggregates of intermediate filaments (Mallory bodies) appear in the hepatocytes. There is aggregation of neutrophils around damaged liver cells (especially those with Mallory bodies), and lymphocytes and macrophages enter the lobule.

Focal necrosis is found in zone 3 (centrilobular zone) aided by damage caused by free radicals. These are produced by phagocytes in response to cytokines, and they are also generated by lipid peroxidation. Ballooning of hepatocytes can occur, due to the retention of proteins and water after injury to organelles.

Collagen deposition almost always ensues, especially with repeated bouts of high alcohol intake, and the risk of cirrhosis is greater than in purely fatty change.

Mallory bodies may also be seen in other conditions including primary biliary cirrhosis, Wilson's disease and hepatocellular carcinoma.

Patients with alcoholic hepatitis have elevated serum levels of alkaline phosphatase, alanine aminotransferase, aspartate aminotransferase, γ-glutamyl transpeptidase, bilirubin and an increased prothrombin time. Often a low serum albumin accompanies these findings.

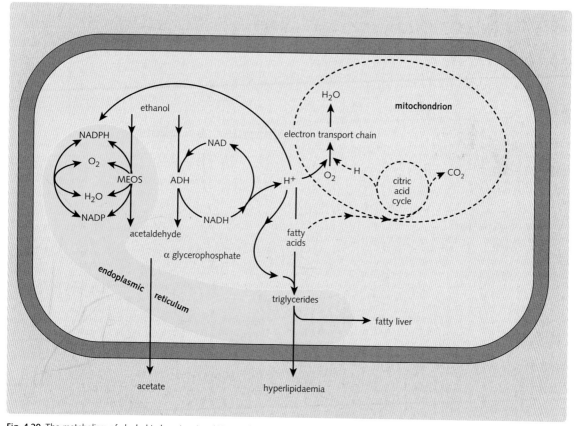

**Fig. 4.29** The metabolism of alcohol in hepatocytes. (ADH = alcohol dehydrogenase; MEOS = microsomal ethanol oxidizing system.) (From MacSween RNM, Whaley K. Muir's Textbook of Pathology, 13th edn. London: Edward Arnold, 1992. Reproduced by permission of Hodder/Arnold Publishers.)

If the patient stops drinking, the inflammation will resolve of its own accord.

## Alcoholic cirrhosis

Cirrhosis is the final and irreversible result of alcohol damage.

It usually develops over a number of years, but it may become apparent in as little as 2–3 years if associated with alcoholic hepatitis.

The underlying pathological mechanisms causing alcoholic cirrhosis are similar to those of cirrhosis due to other causes. The hepatocytes attempt to regenerate but the normal architecture is disturbed and nodules form, separated by fibrous septa. This disrupts the normal blood flow through the liver, and it becomes less efficient at performing its functions. In the early stages, the liver is usually large and fatty but later it shrinks to become small, brown and almost non-fatty.

Alcohol abuse usually causes a micronodular cirrhosis.

The nodular surface of the liver can vary in colour:

- Fatty changes give it a pale appearance.
- Cholestasis causes bile stains.
- Congestion causes the liver to look red, due to blood.

Remember the major complications of cirrhosis: liver failure, portal hypertension and hepatocellular carcinoma.

## Drugs and toxins

The liver is vital in the metabolism and excretion of drugs and toxins. At least 10% of all adverse reactions to drugs affect the liver.

Drug reactions may be predictable (occur in any individual if a sufficient dose is given) or unpredictable (idiosyncratic, or non-dose-related). Predictable drug reactions are also known as intrinsic reactions.

Drugs may cause damage to hepatocytes indistinguishable from viral hepatitis, cholestasis by affecting bile production or excretion, or other liver dysfunction.

The mechanisms of drug-induced damage include:

- Direct toxicity to cells.
- The conversion of the drug to a toxic metabolite.
- Drug-induced autoimmune reaction.

- Peroxidation of lipids.
- Denaturation of proteins.
- Mitochondrial dysfunction.
- Free radical generation.
- ATP depletion.
- Binding or blockage of transfer RNA (tRNA).
- Attachment to membrane receptors.
- Disruption of calcium homeostasis.
- Disruption of the cytoskeleton in hepatocytes.

Drug-induced autoimmunity usually occurs when the drug, or one of its metabolites, acts as a hapten (a small molecule that is not immunogenic on its own, but which can bind to another molecule and produce an immune response).

A careful drug history should be taken from anyone with signs or symptoms of liver disease, including drugs taken many months before, as there may be a long delay between the administration of the drug and signs of any injury becoming apparent. Injury may also be immediate, depending on the drug or toxin and the type of damage caused.

Diagnosis is made on the history and clinical signs, the fact that improvement should occur if the patient stops taking the offending drug, and by excluding other causes of liver damage.

A summary of hepatotoxins and their effects is given in Fig. 4.30.

## Vascular disorders

### Liver infarction

Liver infarction is rare because of the dual blood supply of the liver. It may occur if an intrahepatic branch of the hepatic artery is occluded, or the flow of blood through it is interrupted. This is seen in only five situations:

- Trauma to the artery.
- Embolization or ligation of the artery, e.g. for therapeutic reasons.
- Infective endocarditis.
- Eclampsia (seizures during pregnancy).
- Polyarteritis nodosa.

If the main hepatic artery is occluded, blood flow through the portal venous systems is usually sufficient to prevent necrosis, except in the case of a transplanted liver when occlusion usually leads to complete necrosis (in which case another transplant is needed).

**Fig. 4.30** Hepatotoxins and their effects on the liver. (From Friedman LS, Keefe E. Handbook of Liver Disease. Edinburgh: Churchill Livingstone, 1997.)

| Disorder | Hepatotoxic agents |
| --- | --- |
| *Acute disorders* | |
| Hepatitis-like syndromes (acute necroinflammatory liver disease) | Dapsone, isoniazid, indometacin, phenytoin |
| Fulminant hepatic failure | Paracetamol, halothane, isoniazid, methyldopa, nicotinic acid, nitrofurantoin, propylthiouracil, valproic acid |
| Cholestatic syndromes | Amitriptyline, ampicilin, carbamazepine, chlorpromazine, prochlorperazine, cimetidine, ranitidine, captopril, oestrogens, trimethoprim-sulfamethoxazole |
| Mixed necroinflammatory | Carbimazole, naproxen, phenytoin, thioridazine |
| Granulomatous hepatitis | Allopurinol, benzylpenicillin, dapsone, diazepam, diltiazem, phenytoin |
| Macrovesicular seatosis | Alcohol, glucocorticoids, methotrexate, minocycline, nifedipine, total parenteral nutrition |
| Microvesicular steatosis | Alcohol, amiodarone, aspirin, zidovudine (AZT), piroxicam, sodium valproate, tetracyclines |
| Budd–Chiari syndrome | Oral oestrogens |
| Ischaemic necrosis | Cocaine, methylenedioxymethamfetamine |
| *Chronic active* | |
| Chronic active hepatitis | $\alpha$-methyldopa, isoniazid, nitrofurantoin |
| Fibrosis/cirrhosis | Alcohol, $\alpha$-methyldopa, isoniazid, methotrexate |
| Peliosis hepatis | Anabolic/androgenic steroids, azathioprine, hydroxyurea, oral contraceptives, tamoxifen |
| Phospholipidosis | Amiodarone, diltiazem, nifedipine |
| Primary biliary cirrhosis | Chlorpromazine, haloperidol, prochlorperazine |
| Sclerosing cholangitis | Floxuridine FUDR via hepatic artery infusion |
| Steatohepatitis | Amiodarone, total parenteral nutrition |
| Veno-occlusive disease | Azathioprine, busulfan, cyclophosphamide, daunorubicin, tioguanine, X-irradiation |
| *Oncogenic effects* | |
| Cholangiocarcinoma | Thorotrast |
| Focal nodular hyperplasia | Oestrogens, oral contraceptives |
| Hepatic adenoma | Oestrogens, oral contraceptives |
| Hepatoma | Alcohol, anabolic/androgenic steroids |
| Hepatoblastoma | Oestrogens |
| Angiosarcoma | Arsenic, vinyl chloride, Thorotrast |

Occlusion of an intrahepatic branch of the portal vein causes an infarct of Zahn (or 'red infarct'). This is a well-demarcated area that looks red–blue because of stasis of blood in the sinusoids, which become distended. Despite its name, an infarct of Zahn is not a true infarct as necrosis does not occur, but hepatocellular atrophy may occur secondary to it.

## Portal vein obstruction and thrombosis

Portal vein obstruction may occur outside the liver (extrahepatic) or inside (intrahepatic). Extrahepatic obstruction is by thrombosis. Intrahepatic obstruction is most commonly caused by cirrhosis, but it can also be caused by congenital hepatic fibrosis and metastases, or primary carcinoma of the liver.

It may lead to portal hypertension (see earlier), with abdominal pain, ascites and oesophageal varices.

## Passive congestion and centrilobular necrosis

Passive congestion may be acute or chronic, and it is usually due to right-sided ('backward') heart failure (Fig. 4.31). It causes the classical 'nutmeg appearance' when looking at the cut surface of the liver. Centrilobular necrosis is usually due to left-sided ('forward') heart failure or shock causing hypoperfusion of the liver. As might be expected, zone 3 of the acini (being furthest from the portal triad) is most badly affected.

Where both hypoperfusion and congestion occur together, centrilobular haemorrhagic necrosis may occur.

## Hepatic vein thrombosis (Budd–Chiari syndrome)

Budd–Chiari syndrome is a rare condition in which occlusion (due to thrombosis) of the hepatic vein results in blockage of the flow of venous blood out of the liver.

It may be acute or chronic. Acute presentation is usually with sudden onset of abdominal tenderness, epigastric pain, nausea (and vomiting) and shock.

Chronic thrombosis results in hepatomegaly, portal hypertension (and its associated signs and symptoms), jaundice and cirrhosis. Ascites can be found in both acute and chronic forms of the disease.

It may be caused by any condition that predisposes to the formation of thrombi, most notably:

- Polycythaemia.
- Pregnancy.
- Postpartum states.
- Oral contraceptive.
- Hepatocellular carcinoma.
- Other intra-abdominal cancers.

Surgical treatment, with the creation of a portosystemic anastomosis is required. However, liver transplantation is often the treatment of choice. Mortality is higher in acute cases, with untreated cases resulting in death, but even in its chronic form, 5-year survival is only about 50%.

## Veno-occlusive disease

Veno-occlusive disease is similar to Budd–Chiari syndrome in its presentation. It is believed to be caused where damage to the endothelium of the sinusoids allows red blood cells into the space of Disse, which activates the coagulation cascade. The products of coagulation are then swept into the central vein, occluding it.

The incidence is higher in those receiving marrow transplants (25% in allogenic recipients), probably because chemotherapy and radiotherapy, given as part of transplant therapy, damage the endothelium.

Treatment of this disease is aimed at controlling hepatocellular failure and ascites formation.

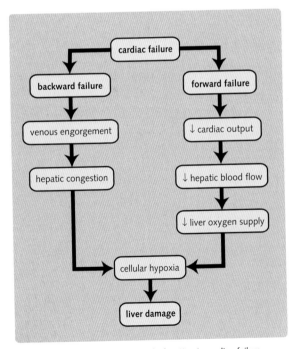

**Fig. 4.31** Pathophysiology of liver dysfunction in cardiac failure. (Redrawn with permission from Friedman LS, Keefe E. Handbook of Liver Disease. Edinburgh: Churchill Livingstone, 1997.)

It is also caused by ingestion of toxic plant alkaloids, which may be present in certain herbal teas and remedies.

# Neoplastic disease

## Hepatocellular carcinoma

Hepatocellular carcinoma (HCC) can develop following hepatitis B and C infections, alcoholic cirrhosis and haemochromatosis. Aflatoxin (a fungal metabolite), androgens and the contraceptive pill are all associated with HCC.

It affects men more than women, and usually presents before 50 years of age. The signs and symptoms include:

- Fever.
- Pain in the right hypochondrium.
- Hepatomegaly.
- Weight loss.
- Anorexia.
- Ascites.
- Elevated serum $\alpha$-fetoprotein.

Treatment usually involves surgical resection or transplantation. The prognosis is not good (survival is usually less than 6 months) but in a few cases surgical resection is possible, with palliation by percutaneous ethanol injection.

# The pancreas and biliary tract

## Learning objectives

After reading this chapter, you should be able to:

- Describe the anatomy of the pancreas, with regard to its macroscopic structure, relations, arterial supply, venous and lymphatic drainage, and nerve supply.
- Outline the embryological development of the pancreas.
- Outline the histological structure of the pancreas.
- Reproduce the structure of the pancreatic acinus.
- List the enzymes secreted by the pancreas and their functions.
- Describe the control of pancreatic secretion.
- Outline the following pancreatic disorders: pancreatitis, pseudocysts, pancreatic insufficiency, carcinoma and congenital abnormalities.
- Describe the anatomy of the gallbladder, with regard to its structure, relations, arterial supply, venous and lymphatic drainage, and nerve supply.
- Understand the role of cholecystokinin in gallbladder contraction.
- Outline the histological structure of the biliary tract.
- Outline the following disorders of the biliary system: gallstones, primary and secondary biliary cirrhosis, primary sclerosing cholangitis, malignant neoplasms and congenital abnormalities.

## THE PANCREAS

The pancreas is both an endocrine and an exocrine gland.

Most of the pancreas consists of exocrine tissue, in which are embedded islands of endocrine cells (islets of Langerhans). The exocrine cells produce enzymes that play an important role in digestion. The hormones produced by the islets are essential for the regulation of blood glucose.

## Anatomy

The pancreas is a soft, elongated digestive gland which is grey–pink and 'feather-like' in appearance. It is approximately 15 cm in length, lobular and weighs about 80 g.

It is retroperitoneal and extends transversely across the posterior abdominal wall from the curve of the duodenum to the hilum of the spleen.

The right side lies across the vertebral bodies of L1–L3. It is posterior to the stomach and the transverse mesocolon is attached to its anterior margin. It is located in the left hypochondriac and epigastric regions.

The pancreas has four parts: a head with an uncinate process (from the Latin meaning 'hook'), a neck, a body and a tail (Fig. 5.1):

- The *head* is the expanded right portion. It nestles in the curve of the duodenum, anterior to the inferior vena cava and the left renal vein. In a groove on the posterior surface of the head lies the common bile duct.
- The *uncinate process* is a small portion of the head extending superiorly and to the left, 'hooked' around the superior mesenteric vessels.
- The *neck* joins the body to the head, overlying the superior mesenteric vessels and the portal vein. The anterior surface of the neck is covered with peritoneum and is adjacent to the pylorus.
- The *body* is triangular in cross-section and extends as far as the hilum of the left kidney. It overlies the aorta, the left renal vein, the splenic vessels and the termination of the inferior mesenteric vein. It is crossed anteriorly by the attachment of the transverse mesocolon. Note that where the body crosses the aorta, superior mesenteric artery, left adrenal gland and left kidney, its posterior surface is not covered by peritoneum.

- The *tail* lies in the lienorenal ligament and ends at the hilum of the spleen.

The main pancreatic duct traverses the gland from left to right, i.e. from the tail to the head and together with the bile duct, opens into the second part of the duodenum at the hepatopancreatic ampulla (of Vater). This opens into the duodenum at the major duodenal papilla. There are two important sphincters in this region: the pancreatic duct sphincter at the termination of the pancreatic duct, and the hepatopancreatic sphincter (of Oddi) at the ampulla of Vater. They control the flow of pancreatic juice (as well as bile, in the case of the latter) into the duodenum.

An accessory duct, if present, may drain the inferior part of the head as well as the uncinate process. It has a separate opening into the duodenum at the minor duodenal papilla above the ampulla of Vater.

## Blood supply and venous drainage

Because the pancreas has an endocrine function, it has a rich blood supply.

The arteries supplying the pancreas arise from the splenic and pancreaticoduodenal arteries. The anterior and posterior superior and inferior pancreaticoduodenal arteries supply the head, while up to 10 branches of the splenic artery supply the remainder of the pancreas (Fig. 5.2).

Venous drainage is to the portal, splenic and superior mesenteric veins, with most going into the splenic vein.

## Lymphatic drainage and innervation

The course of lymphatic vessels draining the pancreas follows that of the blood vessels. Lymphatic drainage is to pancreaticosplenic or suprapancreatic nodes alongside the splenic artery and to preaortic nodes around the coeliac and superior mesenteric arteries. Some vessels also terminate in nodes near the gastric pylorus.

The innervation of the pancreas is from the splanchnic nerves and the vagi through the coeliac and superior mesenteric plexuses.

# Embryology and development

The pancreas develops between the mesenteric layers from two buds (the dorsal and ventral pancreatic buds) that originate from the endodermal lining of

Fig. 5.1 The relations of the pancreas.

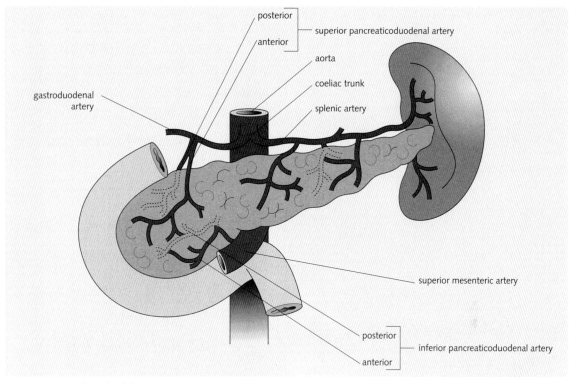

**Fig. 5.2** The arterial supply of the pancreas.

the caudal foregut (which goes on to form the proximal duodenum) in weeks 4–6 (Fig. 5.3). Most of the pancreas is formed from the dorsal bud, which is larger and appears before the ventral bud.

As the duodenum rotates to form a C-shape, the ventral pancreatic bud, which originates near the ampulla of Vater, migrates 270° around the back of the duodenum to lie below and behind the dorsal

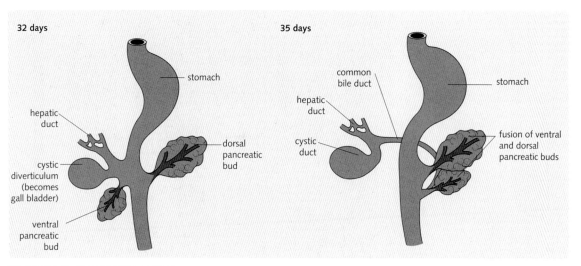

**Fig. 5.3** The development of the pancreas.

pancreatic bud, trapping the mesenteric vessels between them. This allows fusion of the ventral and dorsal pancreatic buds. Ultimately, part of the head as well as the uncinate process is derived from the ventral bud.

The distal part of the dorsal pancreatic duct normally joins with the duct of the ventral pancreatic bud, to become the main pancreatic duct. The proximal part of the dorsal pancreatic duct either regresses and disappears, or becomes an accessory pancreatic duct (of Santorini). The pancreatic islets of Langerhans develop from pancreatic parenchymal tissue in the 3rd month, and are scattered throughout the gland.

Insulin secretion begins during the 5th month of embryonic development and fetal levels of insulin are independent of those of the mother. Note that insulin does not cross the placenta.

## Histology

The pancreas is covered with a thin capsule of fibro-collagenous connective tissue, from which septa extend into the gland, dividing it into lobules. Nerves and larger blood vessels travel within the septa.

## The exocrine pancreas

The exocrine cells secrete digestive enzymes into a network of ducts that meet to form the main pancreatic duct, which joins the common bile duct and opens into the duodenum at the ampulla of Vater (see Fig. 6.2).

The basic unit of the exocrine pancreas is the acinus. The acini are tubuloacinar glands similar to salivary glands in their organization. They are called 'acinar' (Latin for 'berry-like') because the secretory portion is similar to a grape, with the duct resembling a stalk (Fig. 5.4). The acini consist principally of pyramidal epithelial cells, which produce the digestive enzymes of the pancreas. The apices of the cells surround a central lumen, which marks the termination of the duct system.

From the lumen, the intercalated ducts begin within the acini where the duct cells are called

**Fig. 5.4** A pancreatic acinus. The secretion of alkaline fluid and proenzymes is regulated separately, and pancreatic fluid rich in one or the other can be produced depending on the stimulus. Secretin initiates production of alkaline-rich fluid while cholecystokinin initiates production of an enzyme-rich fluid.

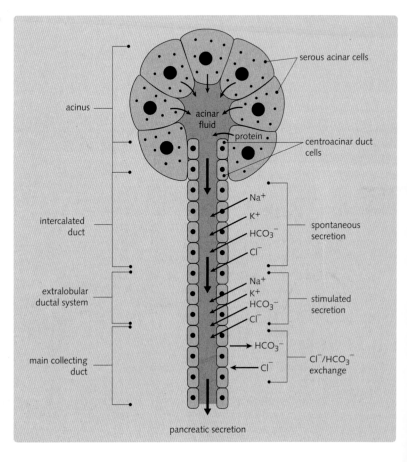

centroacinar cells. Intercalated ducts are the smallest members of the pancreatic duct system. The nuclei of the acinar cells are characteristically found at the cell base along with a large quantity of rough endoplasmic reticulum (RER). The abundance of RER is the reason the cell cytoplasm is basophilic. The apical portion has zymogen granules containing enzyme precursors, which are numerous in the resting gland. Microvilli extend from the apical surface into the lumen of the acini.

The intercalated ducts are lined with squamous epithelium. They drain into intralobular ducts lined with cuboidal or low columnar epithelium.

In turn, the intralobular ducts lead into larger interlobular ducts in the fibro-collagenous interlobular connective tissue. These are lined by columnar epithelium and also contain goblet and enteroendocrine (amine precursor uptake and decarboxylation, APUD) cells. As the size of the ducts increases, the supporting connective tissue becomes denser, with the wall of the main pancreatic duct containing a layer of smooth muscle.

## The endocrine pancreas

The islets of Langerhans form the primary component of the endocrine pancreas. These clusters of endocrine cells (Fig. 5.5) can be found throughout the pancreas but are most prevalent in the tail.

Pancreatic islet cells can be differentiated from the exocrine cells as they are smaller and paler. There is an extensive network of blood vessels surrounding the islets – each islet has its own capillary network which is in contact with every cell in that islet – into which the hormones insulin, glucagon and somatostatin are secreted.

- *Insulin* is produced by pancreatic β (or B) cells, which constitute 70% of pancreatic endocrine cells. It acts on all cells in the body to increase the uptake of glucose from the blood into the cells.
- *Glucagon* is produced by pancreatic α (or A) cells (20%) and it acts mainly on the liver. It increases glycogenolysis and gluconeogenesis to raise the blood glucose concentration.
- *Somatostatin* is secreted from δ (or D) cells (5–10%). It acts locally as a paracrine agent, inhibiting the production of insulin and glucagon. It also inhibits the gut peptides secretin, cholecystokinin (CCK), gastrin and motilin.
- *Pancreatic polypeptide* is produced by PP or F cells (1–2%).

Other cell types include vasoactive intestinal polypeptide (VIP)-secreting cells and enterochromaffin cells, which secrete serotonin, motilin and substance P.

A more detailed account of the endocrine function of the pancreas can be found in *Crash Course: Endocrine and Reproductive Systems*.

## Pancreatic exocrine functions and physiology

The pancreas secretes about 1.5 L of fluid a day (over ten times its own weight). This fluid contains cations, anions, albumin, globulin and digestive enzymes.

The bulk of the fluid is the sodium- and bicarbonate-rich juice secreted by cells of the small ducts, which neutralizes acid entering the duodenum from the stomach.

The acinar cells secrete a small volume of fluid rich in digestive enzymes, which break down carbohydrates, fats, proteins and nucleic acids.

Most of these enzymes are secreted in an inactive form to protect the pancreas from autodigestion, and are activated in the duodenum (see later).

**Fig. 5.5** High-power micrograph showing the α and β cells in the islets of Langerhans (in the endocrine pancreas). α cells produce glucagon and β cells produce insulin. Note that each cell is in contact with the capillary network. (Reproduced with permission from Stevens A, Lowe J. Human Histology, 2nd edn. Edinburgh: Mosby, 1997.)

## Alkaline secretion

The pancreas secretes a fluid rich in bicarbonate, which, together with secretions from the gallbladder and the intestinal juices, neutralizes gastric acid in the duodenum, raising the pH to 6 or 7.

Secretion in the pancreas takes place in a similar way to that in the salivary glands. The acini secrete a slightly hypertonic fluid, rich in bicarbonate, which is modified as it travels through the ducts (Fig. 5.4). Chloride is actively exchanged for bicarbonate by the epithelial cells of the extralobular ducts as the fluid travels through the ducts (Fig. 5.6) and concentrations of bicarbonate and chloride are reciprocal.

When the pancreas is stimulated to increase its rate of secretion, there is less time for chloride and bicarbonate to be exchanged and the fluid is richer in bicarbonate (Fig. 5.7). When the rate of secretion is low, the fluid is produced mainly by the intralobular ducts. However, when secretin stimulates an increased rate of production, most of the additional fluid is produced by the extralobular ducts.

The bicarbonate in pancreatic juice is derived from the blood and its concentration in the juice and the rate of production of juice are both proportional to the concentration of bicarbonate in the blood.

**Fig. 5.6** The mechanism by which bicarbonate is taken up by the epithelial cells of the pancreas. (Redrawn with permission from Johnson LR. Physiology of the Gastrointestinal Tract, 4th edn. New York: Raven Press, 2000.)

**Fig. 5.7** The variation in composition of pancreatic juice with rate of flow. (Redrawn with permission from Mangos JA, McSherry NR. Am J Physiol 1971 221:496.)

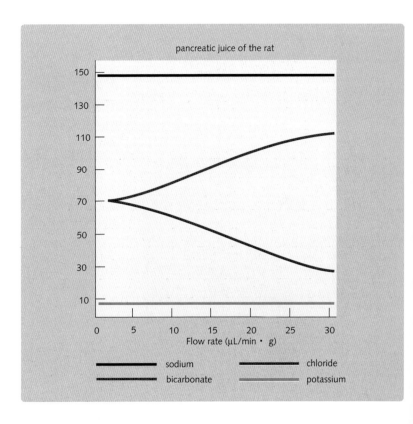

H+ ions, which are pumped out of the duct cells in exchange for $K^+$ and $Na^+$, neutralize bicarbonate in the blood by forming carbonic acid. This dissociates to form $CO_2$ and $H_2O$.

The dissociation is catalysed by carbonic anhydrase and is a similar reaction to that occurring in the kidney.

The carbon dioxide diffuses across the basolateral membrane into the duct epithelial cell. Here, it is combined with water by carbonic anhydrase, to make carbonic acid ($H_2CO_3$), which then dissociates to form $H^+$ and $HCO_3^-$ (bicarbonate) ions. The $H^+$ ions are actively eliminated at the basolateral membrane (which helps drive the reaction to produce more $CO_2$ in the blood and, therefore, $HCO_3^-$ ions).

$Na^+$ ions are thought to move through a paracellular junction from the interstitial fluid into the fluid in the duct.

## Enzyme secretion

There are three major types of enzymes secreted by the pancreas: proteolytic enzymes (trypsin, chymotrypsin and carboxypeptidase), amylase and lipase. Additionally, the pancreas also secretes ribonuclease and deoxyribonuclease. These are summarized in Fig. 5.8.

### Proteolytic enzymes

The proteolytic enzymes play an important role in protein digestion. It follows that these enzymes are capable of damaging the tissues of the pancreas and so they are secreted as proenzymes, which are activated by substances in the duodenum.

*Enterokinase* (enteropeptidase) in the brush border of the duodenum secreted in response to cholecystokinin, converts trypsinogen to trypsin. Trypsinogen is therefore not activated until it reaches the duodenum where it is needed.

*Trypsin* then activates the other proteolytic proenzymes, including its own proenzyme trypsinogen, resulting in an autocatalytic chain reaction.

To protect the pancreas from the chain reaction and autodigestion (that would result from even a small amount of trypsin in the pancreas), the pancreas contains a trypsin inhibitor called the kazal inhibitor. This forms a complex with trypsin and prevents it acting.

Other mechanisms are involved to prevent autodigestion of the pancreas by its enzymes. These include an enzyme called enzyme Y, which destroys zymogens (proenzymes) before they can be activated.

Also, the maintenance of an acid pH in the zymogen granules prevents the proenzymes being

**Fig. 5.8** The pancreatic enzymes.

| Enzyme | Activator | Substrate |
|---|---|---|
| Trypsin | Secreted as trypsinogen, activated by enteropeptidase (and by trypsin) | Proteins and polypeptides |
| Pancreatic lipase | | Triglycerides |
| Pancreatic α-amylase | Activated by $Cl^-$ | Starch |
| Ribonuclease | | RNA |
| Deoxyribonuclease | | DNA |
| Elastase | Activated by trypsin | Elastin and some other proteins |
| Phospholipase $A_2$ | Activated by trypsin | Phospholipids |
| Chymotrypsins | Secreted as chymotrypsinogen, activated by trypsin | Proteins and polypeptides |
| Carboxypeptidase A and B | Activated by trypsin | Proteins and polypeptides |
| Colipase | Activated by trypsin | Fat droplets |

exposed to their optimal pH. In acute pancreatitis, phospholipase $A_2$ is activated by trypsin in the pancreatic duct. It then acts on lecithin (a normal constituent of bile) to form lysolecithin, which damages cell membranes and causes disruption of pancreatic tissue and necrosis of surrounding fat. Circulating levels of pancreatic $\alpha$-amylase also increase in acute pancreatitis and measurement of levels in the blood is used as a diagnostic tool.

## Amylase

Like salivary amylase, pancreatic amylase hydrolyses polysaccharides into disaccharides, and therefore is involved in carbohydrate digestion in the duodenum. It is secreted in its active form as it does not damage pancreatic tissue.

## Lipase

This is the most important enzyme in terms of fat digestion, gastric lipase having a very minor role and only when pancreatic lipase is deficient. It hydrolyses triglycerides into glycerol and fatty acids, therefore in pancreatic insufficiency where enzyme secretion is deficient, fats cannot be digested and a malabsorption syndrome occurs (see section on 'Pancreatic insufficiency').

### The fate of pancreatic enzymes in the duodenum

The digestive enzymes survive for differing periods of time once they enter the intestines.

Measurements have shown that around 75% of amylase and 20% of trypsin were present in the distal ileum, but only 1% of lipase secreted actually reached this part of the small intestines. Different mechanisms are thought to be involved, and the small intestine is thought to be permeable to several digestive enzymes.

It has been found that chymotrypsinogen and amylase are capable of crossing the basolateral membranes of pancreatic cells.

Some foods contain inhibitors of the digestive enzymes. For example, soybeans contain the Bowman–Birk inhibitor, which stops trypsin and chymotrypsin activities.

## Control of pancreatic secretion

Pancreatic exocrine secretion is controlled by neuro-endocrine signals, which are hormones and substances released from nerve terminals (Fig. 5.9).

*Vagal* (*parasympathetic*) stimulation enhances the rate of secretion of both enzyme and aqueous components of pancreatic juice.

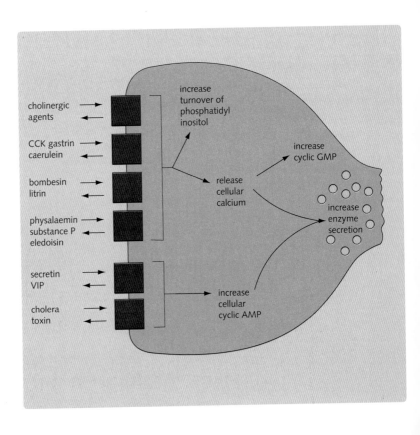

**Fig. 5.9** Summary diagram of all the stimulating substances of pancreatic secretion. (CCK = cholecystokinin; VIP = vasoactive intestinal peptide; AMP = adenosine monophosphate; GMP = guanosine monophosphate.)

*Sympathetic* stimulation inhibits secretion, probably by decreasing blood flow.

*Secretin* and *cholecystokinin* (released from the duodenal mucosa) stimulate secretion of the aqueous component of pancreatic fluid.

Separate control of the aqueous and enzymatic components explains the variation in composition of pancreatic juice (see Fig. 5.7).

The control of secretion can be split up into the *cephalic*, *gastric* and *intestinal* (*duodenal*) phases, like the control of gastric secretions.

### Cephalic phase

This is very minor in humans. Gastrin is released from the mucosa of the antrum in response to vagal stimulation (via acetylcholine and VIP). This causes the release of a small amount of pancreatic juice with a high protein content.

### Gastric phase

*Gastrin* is released in response to gastric distension (via the vago-vagal reflex) and the presence of amino acids and peptides in the antrum. This continues to stimulate release of pancreatic juice.

*Vago-vagal reflexes* elicited by distension of the fundus or antrum also cause the release of small amounts of pancreatic juice with a high enzyme content (by acting on receptors on the acinar cells in the pancreas).

### Intestinal phase

This is the longest and most important phase. It involves the secretion of two hormones, secretin and cholecystokinin. Chyme in the duodenum and upper jejunum stimulates pancreatic secretion.

*Secretin* is released from the duodenal and upper jejunal mucosal cells in response to acid in the lumen. Secretin acts on the pancreatic ducts to stimulate the secretion of a large volume of $HCO_3^-$-rich fluid (but with low levels of pancreatic enzymes). It also stimulates bile production in the liver.

*Cholecystokinin* (CCK, also called pancreozymin) is secreted from duodenal and upper jejunal mucosal cells in response to peptides, amino acids and fatty acids in the lumen. It has two actions:

- It acts on pancreatic acinar cells to stimulate enzyme synthesis and release.
- It acts on the gallbladder by stimulating its contraction and the relaxation of the sphincter of Oddi. This allows release of bile into the duodenum.

Therefore, CCK induces the secretion of a pancreatic juice that is rich in enzymes and which is accompanied by concentrated bile for fat absorption. The substances that stimulate pancreatic secretion are summarized in Fig. 5.9.

CCK has little direct effect on ductular epithelium but potentiates the effect of secretin, which is a weak agonist of acinar cells.

Vagal stimulation is important and vagotomy reduces the response to chyme in the duodenum by 50%.

Somatostatin has the opposite effect and by inhibiting adenylate cyclase and decreasing cyclic AMP, it inhibits the secretion of acinar and duct cells.

Insulin, insulin-like growth factors and epidermal growth factor potentiate enzyme synthesis and secretion, through the activation of receptor-associated tyrosine kinase.

## DISORDERS OF THE EXOCRINE PANCREAS

## Congenital abnormalities

### Agenesis and hypoplasia

Congenital abnormalities of the pancreas are rare. However, as with other organs, the pancreas may fail to develop at all (agenesis) or develop incompletely (hypoplasia).

### Annular pancreas and pancreas divisum

In normal development, the duodenum rotates and the ventral pancreatic bud migrates around the back of the duodenum to lie caudal and dorsal to the dorsal bud. This allows fusion of the ventral and dorsal pancreatic buds (Fig. 5.3).

Sometimes, migration of the ventral bud is incomplete, or it migrates in both directions, so that a ring of pancreatic tissue surrounds the duodenum. This is called an annular pancreas, and it may cause constriction or complete obstruction of the duodenum.

Pancreas divisum, either partial or complete, may occur where fusion of the two pancreatic buds does not take place. It is found in 5% of patients.

### Ectopic pancreatic tissue

Heterotopic pancreatic tissue is sometimes found in the mucosa of the stomach, the duodenum and in

Meckel's diverticula. More rarely, it may be found between the distal end of the oesophagus and any point proximal to the remnant of the attachment of the vitelline duct (the position at which Meckel's diverticulum would be found, if present). The pancreatic tissue is normal (although in an abnormal place), and so may produce substances normally made by the pancreas.

# Pancreatitis

Pancreatitis (inflammation of the pancreas) is classified as acute or chronic, but it is sometimes difficult to separate the two.

## Acute pancreatitis

Acute pancreatitis can be severe and complicated with a mortality of 5–10% but mild and moderate forms present with variable degrees of pain. The Glasgow or Ranson criteria (Fig. 5.10) are used to assess severity, although it is difficult to differentiate mild from severe pancreatitis in the first 24 hours. The presence of three or more items on either scoring system implies severe pancreatitis; if more than seven (out of 11) of Ranson's prognostic signs are present, mortality approaches 100%.

### Aetiology

The main cause in the UK, accounting for 50% of cases, is gallstones. The majority of non-gallstone pancreatitis is due to alcohol. Other causes include infection, trauma, drugs, e.g. azathioprine, sodium valproate and diuretics, hypothermia, hypercalcaemia, hyperlipidaemia, post-ERCP (endoscopic retrograde cholangiopancreatography) and post-operative states.

**Fig. 5.10** Ranson's prognostic signs: the Ranson criteria for assessment of the severity of pancreatitis. Three or more signs indicate a severe presentation.

Age > 5 years
Blood glucose > 10 mmol/L with no history of diabetes
White cell count > 15 × 109/L
Lactate degydrogenase (LDH) > 600 iu/L
Aspartate transaminase (AST) > 200 u/L
Corrected calcium < 2.0 mmol/L
Blood urea > 16 mmol/L and no improvement with
    intravenous fluids
Decreasing haematocrit
Arterial $pO_2$ < 8 kPa (60 mmHg)
Metabolic acidosis
Serum albumin < 32 g/L

Carcinoma of the pancreas may also cause acute pancreatitis. Rarely, it is hereditary (see below).

It is easy to remember the causes of acute pancreatitis using the mnemonic 'GET SMASHHHED': Gallstones, Ethanol, Trauma, Steroids, Mumps, Autoimmune, Scorpion bites, Hyperlipidaemia, Hyperthyroidism, Hypothermia, ERCP (or Emboli) and Drugs (especially azathioprine and diuretics).

### Pathology and clinical features

Different agents cause acute pancreatitis by different mechanisms. Fig. 5.11 summarizes the pathogenetic mechanisms of the major causes. Whatever the cause, they all lead to the release of lytic enzymes, which are then activated and cause damage. Pancreatic enzymes, in particular trypsin, lipase and phospholipase $A_2$, digest pancreatic tissue, in particular causing fat necrosis. Blood vessel walls are also damaged causing extravasation of blood or ecchymoses, which may be extensive enough to discolour the skin of the flanks (Grey Turner's sign) or around the umbilicus (Cullen's sign).

There are three general patterns of necrosis:

- *Periductal*: the acinar cells adjacent to the ducts undergo necrosis. This is seen in conditions caused by duct obstruction, which results in defective exocytosis of pancreatic enzymes.
- *Perilobular*: acinar cells in the periphery of the lobule undergo necrosis. This pattern is caused by impaired perfusion and so is seen in hypothermia and shocked states.
- *Panlobular*: the entire pancreatic lobule undergoes necrosis. The causes are those which damage the acini directly, e.g. drugs, hypercalcaemia, hyperlipidaemia and mumps. Alternatively, periductal and perilobular necrosis may become more widespread, affecting the whole lobule.

Calcium ions bind to the released fatty acid to form white precipitates. In severe cases this causes hypocalcaemia and tetany. Proteolytic enzymes may destroy the islets of Langerhans so that insulin and other hormones are not produced, leading to hyperglycaemia.

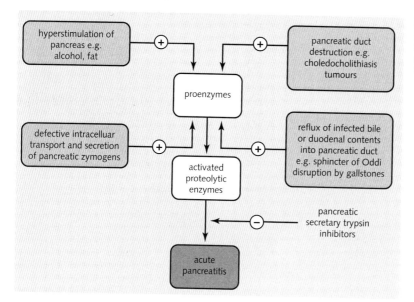

**Fig. 5.11** Pathogenesis of acute pancreatitis. (Reproduced with permission from Haslett C et al. Davidson's Principles and Practice of Medicine, 19th edn. Edinburgh: Churchill Livingstone, 2002.)

The typical presentation is with severe abdominal pain of sudden onset that may radiate into the back, together with nausea and vomiting. The upper abdomen is usually tender to palpation.

### Diagnosis

Diagnosis is by measurement of serum amylase. It is normally greatly elevated (five times or more) in acute pancreatitis. It is important to be aware that many other conditions, e.g. perforated peptic ulcer, intestinal obstruction and trauma can cause moderate increases in serum amylase, and only a marked elevation is characteristic of pancreatitis.

> Remember that not every patient with an elevated serum amylase has pancreatitis—there are numerous causes for a raised serum amylase. Only when levels are elevated fivefold or more should pancreatitis be diagnosed. Even then, be sure to correlate the findings on investigation with your clinical findings!

Radiography shows characteristic findings in the abdomen. The psoas shadow can be absent because of retroperitoneal fluid and an air-filled dilatation of the proximal jejunum will be seen, i.e. a 'sentinel' loop.

### Treatment

Patients with acute pancreatitis should be 'nil by mouth', and be given intravenous water and electrolyte replacement with opiate analgesia (not morphine). This allows the pancreas to 'rest' by removing secretory stimuli. Mild pancreatitis responds well to this supportive treatment. Complications of acute pancreatitis include formation of an abscess or a pseudocyst (see later), renal failure due to shock, relapses and diabetes mellitus if the inflammation is severe and necrosis ensues.

If the pancreatitis is severe, the patient must receive intravenous nutrition. Patients with cholangitis or jaundice and biliary pancreatitis may benefit from gallstone removal via ERCP from the bile duct.

Severe pancreatitis occasionally results in significant necrosis and surgical or laparoscopic necrosectomy may be required.

## Chronic pancreatitis

### Aetiology

Chronic pancreatitis is an on-going inflammation of the pancreas accompanied by irreversible architectural changes. It causes a great deal of pain and often permanent loss of pancreatic function, and may or may not be preceded by acute pancreatitis.

Alcohol consumption causes more than 85% of cases, and is the most common cause of pancreatitis in developed countries. High-fat and -protein diets amplify the damage done by alcohol.

Other causes include:

- Idiopathic chronic pancreatitis: this condition occurs in older people and is associated with peripheral vascular disease.
- Trauma and scar formation, leading to the obstruction of the main pancreatic duct.
- Previous episodes of acute pancreatitis predispose to others although they may often be subclinical.
- Hypercalcaemia causing the formation of calcified plugs, which obstruct the pancreatic duct.
- Cystic fibrosis resulting in protein plugs in the duct system.
- Hereditary forms of pancreatitis.

Unlike acute pancreatitis, gallstones do not play an important role in the aetiology of chronic pancreatitis.

Hereditary pancreatitis accounts for 5–15% of causes overall. It should be suspected in an individual with acute or chronic pancreatitis when detailed history either indicates a positive family history or the patient's history began in childhood or early adulthood. It can be confirmed by detection of an increasing number of identifiable genetic mutations, most commonly in the trypsinogen gene, the trypsin inactivator cascade or the cystic fibrosis genes. Treatment is the same as for other causes.

### Pathology

Chronic pancreatitis has four key pathological features:

- Continuous chronic inflammation.
- Fibrous scarring.
- Loss of pancreatic tissue.
- Duct strictures with formation of calculi.

### Clinical features

Patients normally present with a history of:

- Prolonged ill-health.
- Steatorrhoea (lipase deficiency prevents complete breakdown and absorption of fat in the diet).

- Weight loss from malabsorption.
- Recurrent abdominal pain.
- Diabetes mellitus (as a result of destruction of pancreatic islets).
- Some patients may be asymptomatic; if this is the case the diagnosis is made solely on the basis of radiography.
- Deficiency of the fat-soluble vitamins A, D, E and K also occurs.

### Diagnosis

Serum amylase will be normal, in contrast to acute pancreatitis. Diagnosis is by CT scan complemented by endoscopic ultrasound (EUS) or magnetic resonance imaging (MRI); plain abdominal radiography can show speckled calcification of the pancreas (caused by the binding of calcium ions to necrosed fat). Diabetes mellitus should be excluded.

### Treatment

Treatment involves avoiding alcohol and judicious use of analgesia. Surgery is an option in some cases, but only in those who are committed to stop drinking. Pancreatic supplements and a low-fat diet help the steatorrhoea, and diabetes mellitus is treated with insulin or diet control and oral hypoglycaemic agents.

## Pseudocysts

Pseudocysts are a complication of both acute and chronic pancreatitis. They are localized collections of serosanguinous fluid found 6 weeks after the onset of an acute attack of pancreatitis.

They are usually solitary, 5–10 cm in diameter and lie in the lesser sac. Typically, they are characterized by chronic pain and persistently raised serum amylase levels.

Pseudocysts may produce abdominal pain and, more rarely, haemorrhage, infection and peritonitis. As they usually present as an epigastric mass, they may be mistaken for a tumour in the pancreas.

They differ from true cysts in that true cysts have an epithelial lining and are often congenital, while pseudocysts are surrounded by granulation tissue. Those smaller than 6 cm may resolve of their own accord.

## Pancreatic insufficiency

In pancreatic insufficiency, pancreatic enzymes are absent or secreted in lower amounts than normal. Consequently, fat malabsorption occurs, with associated steatorrhoea. A deficiency in the fat-soluble vitamins A, D, E and K may also be found. The patient may be malnourished.

Cystic fibrosis is a major cause of pancreatic insufficiency. It is an autosomal recessive disorder (with a carrier rate of 1 in 25 among Caucasians but the disease incidence is 1:2500 live births), and its other major clinical feature is a tendency to chronic lung infections. The underlying defect is an abnormality in the chloride ion transporter.

Pancreatic insufficiency also occurs in chronic pancreatitis.

Treatment is with high-dose oral pancreatic enzymes. Additionally, a proton-pump inhibitor may help as it produces a pH in the duodenum which is optimal for fat digestion.

## Carcinoma of the pancreas

### Aetiology

About 6500 new cases of carcinoma of the pancreas occur in England and Wales every year, and it accounts for about 5% of all cancer deaths in the USA and the UK.

It is particularly common in diabetic females, being most common over the age of 60 years. It is associated with smoking. Of all pancreatic carcinomas, 60% occur in the head, 15–20% in the body and 5–10% in the tail. Twenty percent of cases involve the pancreas diffusely.

### Clinical features

Those arising in the head are likely to produce symptoms earlier than those arising elsewhere. They may obstruct the ampulla of Vater or common bile duct causing obstructive jaundice; in fact the classical presentation is with painless progressive jaundice. Other presenting symptoms include pain (50% of cases), intermittent jaundice, diabetes mellitus and the general features of malignancy, e.g. weight loss.

The gallbladder may be dilated and easily palpable (Courvoisier's sign).

Carcinomas arising in other parts of the pancreas are less likely to produce symptoms and so are discovered late. Consequently, they have a worse prognosis, often having metastasized before diagnosis.

Most are adenocarcinomas and almost all begin in the ductal epithelium. Less than 1% begin in the acinar cells.

Carcinoma of the head of the pancreas causes jaundice which develops over a few weeks. The jaundice is of the obstructive type, as the tumour compresses the common bile duct at the ampulla of Vater. The obstruction results in accumulation of bile in the proximal biliary tree, and so the gallbladder becomes enlarged and palpable. As inflammation is not usually involved, the jaundice is painless. Interestingly, even though the jaundice is due to a conjugated hyperbilirubinaemia, itching is uncommon; also, the jaundice of pancreatic carcinoma is more profound and progressive, unlike that due to other causes.

Weight loss usually occurs and some individuals develop thrombophlebitis migrans (flitting venous thromboses).

The carcinoma may be felt as a firm lump during surgery, similar to a pseudocyst.

### Treatment

The optimal treatment for carcinoma of the pancreas is surgical, but less than 30% of patients are suitable. Survival of up to 30% at 5 years with a surgical mortality of <5% can be achieved in some groups.

The operation is called Whipple's procedure. It is a major operation consisting of a partial gastrectomy, duodenectomy and a partial pancreatectomy. It may or may not include the removal of the gallbladder and distal common bile duct. For small tumours, a modified Whipple's prodecure preserves the duodenum and bile duct. Palliative surgical or endoscopic procedures can be used to relieve jaundice or gastric outlet obstruction.

## THE BILIARY SYSTEM

The biliary system comprises the gallbladder and bile ducts. It serves to remove waste products from the liver and carries bile salts to the intestine where they aid digestion. The biliary system is closely related both anatomically and functionally to the liver and pancreas.

## The gallbladder

The gallbladder is a pear-shaped sac that concentrates and stores bile secreted from the liver. It can hold between 30 and 60 mL of bile and, when stimulated, it releases its contents into the duodenum, through the cystic and biliary ducts.

It lies on the right edge of the hepatic quadrate lobe, in the gallbladder fossa on the visceral surface, partly covered by peritoneum on its posterior and inferior surfaces. The anterior surface contacts the hepatic visceral surface.

The gallbladder comprises three parts: the fundus, body and neck (Fig. 5.12), which tapers and makes an S-shaped bend to join with the cystic duct. The cystic duct is 2–4 cm long and joins the common hepatic duct to form the bile duct. This travels anterior to the portal vein and courses through the head of pancreas to open into the second part of the duodenum through the sphincter of Oddi (hepato-pancreatic sphincter) at the ampulla of Vater (duodenal papilla).

The neck, as well as the cystic duct, has a spiral folding of its mucus membrane, forming a spiral valve (of Heister). This keeps the cystic duct open constantly for two purposes:

- To allow bile to pass into the gallbladder from the liver when the bile duct is closed (by the sphincter of Oddi and the choledochal sphincter).
- To allow bile to be secreted into the duodenum when the gallbladder contracts.

## Blood supply

The blood supply to the gallbladder is from the cystic artery (a branch of the right hepatic artery). Variations in the cystic artery are common.

Venous drainage occurs via the cystic vein which drains the neck and ducts, and the veins draining the fundus and body. These terminate in three ways:

- Draining directly into the hepatic visceral surface.
- Joining the portal vein.
- Joining the gastric, duodenal and pancreatic veins (which then join the portal vein).

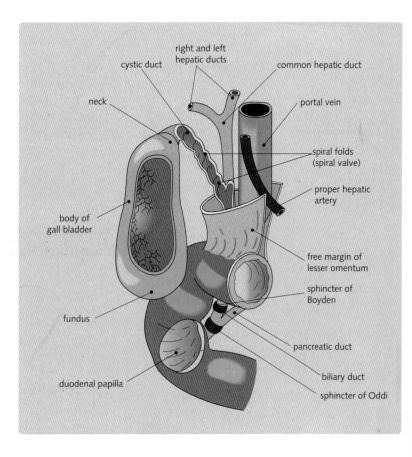

**Fig. 5.12** The gall bladder and biliary tract. (Redrawn with permission from Hall-Craggs ECB. Anatomy as a Basis for Clinical Medicine. London: Waverly Europe, 1995.)

## Lymphatic drainage

Lymph from the gallbladder passes to the hepatic nodes via the cystic nodes, near the neck of the gallbladder. These drain to the coeliac lymph nodes.

## Nerve supply

The innervation to the gallbladder is from the coeliac plexus (sympathetic), the vagus nerve (parasympathetic), the right phrenic nerve (sensory) and the hepatic plexus. The nerves follow the cystic artery.

## The biliary tract

The biliary tract, comprising the bile ducts, conveys bile from the liver to the duodenum. The left and right hepatic ducts join to form the common hepatic duct, which descends in the free edge of the lesser omentum and joins the cystic duct to form the common bile duct.

The common bile duct descends in the free edge of the lesser omentum with the hepatic artery and portal vein. It continues its descent behind the superior part of the duodenum and head of the pancreas.

The termination of the bile duct, together with that of the pancreatic duct forms the ampulla of Vater (hepatopancreatic ampulla) in the superior part of the duodenum.

There are two sphincters involved in the movement of bile:

- The *choledochal sphincter* at the distal end of the common bile duct. Contraction of this prevents bile entering the ampulla and duodenum, thus causing its storage in the gallbladder.
- The *sphincter of Oddi*—around the ampulla of Vater—which controls the secretion of both bile and pancreatic juice into the duodenum.

## Embryology and development

The embryology of the biliary system is intimately connected with that of the liver, hence it is worth reading this section together with that of its counterpart in Chapter 4. See also Fig. 5.3.

Important to the development of the biliary tract is the liver bud. The connection between this and the foregut (duodenum) narrows and forms the bile duct.

A small ventral outgrowth from the bile duct gives rise to the gallbladder and cystic duct.

When bile begins to be produced around the 12th week, the biliary tract and gallbladder are fully formed. This allows the bile to enter the duodenum.

## Histology of the gallbladder

The wall of the gallbladder consists of a mucous membrane, muscular layer, adventitia and a serous membrane.

The *mucous membrane* is made up of simple columnar epithelium and a lamina propria of loose connective tissue. The columnar epithelial cells have a brush border of many microvilli on their apical surfaces. The mucosa is thrown into folds when the gallbladder is empty. This allows it to distend when needed.

The *muscular layer* consists of smooth muscle oriented longitudinally, transversely and obliquely with associated collagenous elastic fibres.

The *adventitia* is made up of collagen and elastic fibres, and contains a rich blood vessel and lymphatic network.

The intrahepatic bile ducts are lined by cuboidal or low columnar epithelial cells. Increasing amounts of fibroelastic connective tissue surround the epithelium as the ducts become larger near the porta hepatis. The largest ducts have smooth muscle in their walls.

## Gallbladder functions and physiology

The primary functions of the gallbladder are the concentration and storage of bile.

In the fasting state, the sphincter of Oddi (Fig. 5.12) is contracted. However, in response to stimulation during and after meals to aid digestion (Fig. 5.13) it relaxes, allowing the gallbladder to release its contents. Nevertheless, it is not essential for life.

Cholecystectomy is a common operation, following which bile is discharged into the duodenum at a constant, slow rate which allows the digestion of moderate amounts of fat in the diet.

### Concentration of bile

The gallbladder stores bile secreted by the liver and has a capacity of about 35 mL (range 15–60 mL).

Stored bile is 5–20 times more concentrated than that secreted by the liver, principally because of the active transport of $Na^+$ from the gallbladder epithelium into the lateral intracellular spaces (Fig. 5.14). Water passively follows the active transport of $Na^+$ ions.

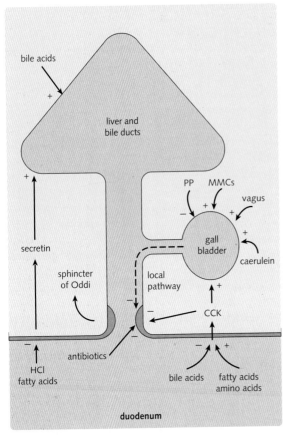

**Fig. 5.13** Mechanisms controlling the secretion of bile into the duodenum. (PP = pancreatic polypeptide; MMCs = migrating motor complexes; CCK = cholecystokinin.) (From Sanford PA. Digestive System Physiology, 2nd edn. London: Edward Arnold, 1992. Reproduced by permission of Hodder/Arnold Publishers.)

The gallbladder epithelial cells are highly specialized for absorption. They have a brush border of microvilli; they are rich in mitochondria; and they have numerous $Na^+/K^+$ ATPase transporters at their lateral surfaces.

## Gallbladder contraction

Gallbladder emptying begins several minutes after the start of a meal.

During the cephalic phase, the taste and smell of food and the presence of food in the mouth and pharynx cause impulses in branches of the vagus nerve that increase emptying of the gallbladder.

Distension of the stomach during the gastric phase also causes impulses in the vagus.

The highest rate of emptying of the gallbladder occurs during the intestinal phase, mostly in response to cholecystokinin released from the duodenal mucosa as a result of the presence of the products of fat digestion and essential amino acids in the duodenum.

Cholecystokinin enters the circulation and reaches the gallbladder, where it causes strong contractions of the smooth muscle of the wall and relaxation of the sphincter of Oddi.

**Fig. 5.14** The mechanism by which bile is concentrated in the gall bladder. The epithelial cells in the gall bladder mucosa have large lateral intercellular spaces near the basement membrane and tight junctions at the apices. $Na^+$ ions are coupled with $Cl^-$ ions and actively transported into the intercellular spaces. Water passively diffuses into the spaces as it follows the osmotic gradient set up by the active transport of ions.

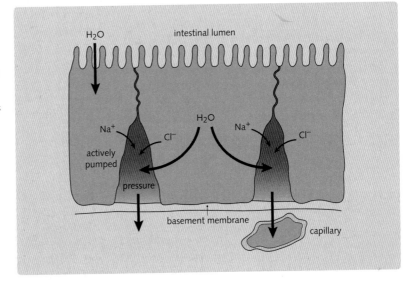

Gastrin, which has the same sequence of amino acid residues as cholecystokinin at its C-terminal, may also cause contractions of the gallbladder during the cephalic and gastric phases.

## DISORDERS OF THE GALLBLADDER AND BILIARY TRACT

### Congenital abnormalities

Anomalies of the biliary tree are characterized by changes in the architecture of the biliary tree within the liver.

In normal development, embryonic bile ducts involute (spiral and roll inwards at the edges). Anomalies of the biliary tree are thus thought to be caused by remnants that have not involuted completely.

Anomalies vary in severity. They may be clinically insignificant or be severe enough to cause hepato-splenomegaly and portal hypertension. They are often inherited.

### Gallstones

Gallstones (cholelithiasis) are a common complaint in the West. They affect the gallbladder and extra-hepatic bile ducts.

The incidence of gallstones is twice as high in women as in men overall. However, it increases with age in both sexes.

The commonly held belief that 'fair, fat females in their forties' have a higher risk of developing gallstones is merely an approximation to the truth. However, the incidence of gallstones is higher in overweight, middle-aged women; in the elderly, the sex ratio is about equal.

Obese people and those with diabetes mellitus are at higher risk. Gallstones are rare in children.

### Aetiology

Eighty percent of gallstones are composed predominantly of cholesterol. The rest are composed mainly of bile pigment and calcium (pigment stones). Most stones contain all three constituents.

A predisposition to cholesterol stones arises in two situations:

- Increased cholesterol in bile, e.g. due to obesity or diet.
- Decreased amount of bile acids in bile, e.g. due to malabsorption in cystic fibrosis patients.

Typically, cholesterol stones are large and can be either single or multiple. In cross-section, cholesterol crystals are seen radiating from the centre.

Pigment stones are seen when levels of unconjugated bilirubin are abnormally high, e.g. in haemolytic anaemias such as hereditary spherocytosis or when enterohepatic recycling of bile is impaired, e.g. in patients who have undergone ileal resections. Another risk factor is chronic infections of the biliary tract, as the bacteria act as foci for the formation of pigment stones. Pigment stones are usually small, black and fragile.

### Clinical features

Of all gallstones, 80% are asymptomatic. These remain in the gallbladder, but stones which impact in the neck of the cystic duct can cause biliary pain and acute cholecystitis.

If gallstones impact in the common bile duct, this can lead to obstruction of bile and cause pain and cholestatic jaundice. This sometimes gives rise to bacterial infections resulting in cholangitis.

If they impact in the gallbladder, either at the neck or in the cystic duct, the bile which is unable to escape becomes concentrated and produces a chemical cholecystitis. The bile may also become infected, resulting in acute cholecystitis. However, if the gallbladder is empty, it will secrete mucus, so that a mucocele results.

The clinical presentations and complications are summarized in Figs 5.15 and 5.16.

### Treatment

Treatment varies according to the location of the gallstones and how they present, e.g. whether inflammation or a bacterial infection (cholecystitis or ascending cholangitis) is present.

Cholecystectomy (surgical removal of the gallbladder) is often performed laparoscopically, with good effect. If gallstones are only present in the common bile duct then they can be removed via ERCP.

The cardinal feature of acute cholecystitis is pain in the right upper quadrant, but pain may also be felt at the epigastric or interscapular regions. This is because of the innervation of the gallbladder, which is derived from T5–T9, hence the referral to the corresponding dermatomes. Additionally, visceral pain from the gallbladder may also be referred to the right shoulder tip via C3–C5 if the inflammation irritates the diaphragm.

**Fig. 5.16** Complications of gallstones.

Acute cholecystitis

Pancreatitis

Gallstone ileus

Biliary enteric fistula

Ileum obstruction

Carcinoma of the gall bladder

Cholesterol stones may be dissolved or disrupted by giving bile acids to increase their solubility in bile. Dissolution of gallstones can take up to 2 years and 50% of the stones recur. This treatment is not suitable for calcified stones.

Antibiotics are administered if cholecystitis or cholangitis occur.

## Disorders associated with biliary cirrhosis

There are three main diseases in this category: primary and secondary biliary cirrhosis, and primary sclerosing cholangitis. These are disorders affecting the intrahepatic bile ducts which lead to cirrhosis of the liver. They are normally considered as hepatic diseases and so are covered in Chapter 4, but their aetiology should be borne in mind.

**Fig. 5.15** Causes and clinical presentation of gallstones.

| Clinical presentations | Causes |
| --- | --- |
| Biliary pain (in epigastrium and right hypochondrium) | Impacted in the cystic duct |
| Biliary pain, cholestatic jaundice and cholangitis | Impacted in the common bile duct |
| Asymptomatic | Located in the gall bladder |

# Neoplastic disease
## Cholangiocarcinoma

Cholangiocarcinomas (carcinomas of the bile ducts) are classified as intrahepatic or extrahepatic. These mucus-secreting adenocarcinomas cause jaundice and are not associated with the hepatitis B or C viruses, or cirrhosis. They are, however, associated with inflammatory bowel disease, especially if primary sclerosing cholangitis is present as well.

The prognosis is poor. There is usually no curative treatment but palliation can be effective for a couple of years.

## Primary adenocarcinoma of the gallbladder

This occurs mostly in women and in those over 70 years of age. It presents with right hypochondrial pain and nausea, and it is usually palpable. Obstructive jaundice occurs as the disease progresses.

Cholecystectomy is a possible treatment, but again, prognosis is poor.

In contrast, carcinoma of the ampulla has a 5-year survival rate of 40% after surgical resection because it presents earlier with jaundice.

# The small intestine

**6**

## Learning objectives

After reading this chapter, you should be able to:

- Describe the anatomy of the small intestine, with regard to its macroscopic structure, relations, arterial supply, venous and lymphatic drainage, and nerve supply.
- Outline the embryological development of the small intestine.
- Describe the histological structure of the small intestine and relate structure to function.
- Outline the functions of the small intestine.
- Describe the mechanisms controlling small intestinal motility.
- Describe the process of digestion and absorption in the small intestine, and understand the importance of villi.
- Outline the following types of small intestinal disorders: congenital abnormalities, malabsorption and neoplastic disease.

## OVERVIEW

The small intestine extends from the stomach to the ileocaecal valve where it joins the colon. It is about 6–7 m in length and is the site of most of the digestive and absorptive processes.

## ANATOMY

The small intestine consists of three parts: the duodenum, jejunum and ileum (Fig. 6.1).

### Duodenum

The duodenum is about 25 cm in length and extends from the pylorus to the duodenojejunal flexure. It is C-shaped and snakes around the head of the pancreas beginning 2–3 cm on the right side of the median plane and ending an equal distance from the median plane, but to the left. It lies in the umbilical region and, except for the first 2.5 cm, it is retroperitoneal and hence is the most fixed part of the small intestine.

It is divided into four parts for descriptive purposes:

- The first (superior) part (D1) is short (5 cm) and starts at the pylorus.

- The second (descending) part (D2) is 8 cm in length and descends to the right side of L3.
- The third (horizontal) part (D3) is 10 cm in length and passes to the left anterior to L3, before turning upwards to become the fourth part.
- The fourth (ascending) part (D4) is 3 cm in length and ascends to the duodenojejunal flexure to the left of L2. The duodenum becomes the jejunum at the ligament of Treitz, a fibromuscular band, which is also called the suspensory muscle of the duodenum.

The first 2 cm of D1 is called the duodenal cap. Only the proximal half has mesentery, which allows mobility. The greater omentum and hepatoduodenal ligament are attached proximally. The rest of D1, like the remainder of the duodenum, has no mesentery and so is not mobile.

The following structures are related to the first part:

- Anteriorly: the peritoneum, gall bladder and quadrate lobe of the liver.
- Posteriorly: the gastroduodenal artery, inferior vena cava, portal vein and bile duct.
- Inferiorly: the neck of the pancreas.

D2 is retroperitoneal. The common bile duct and pancreatic duct open into the posteromedial wall, coming together to form the ampulla of Vater

**Fig. 6.1** The position of the small and large intestines.

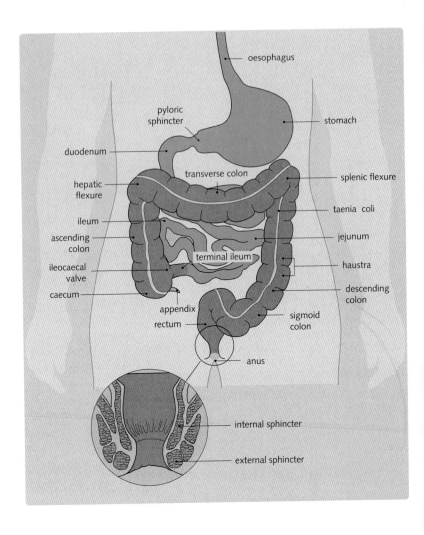

(hepatopancreatic ampulla) about two thirds along its length (Fig. 6.2). This opens at the major duodenal papilla.

The relations of the second part are:

- Anteriorly: the transverse colon, mesocolon and coils of the small intestine.
- Posteriorly: the hilum of the right kidney, its renal vessels, the right ureter and the psoas major muscle.
- Medially: the head of the pancreas and the bile and pancreatic ducts.

D3 also lies retroperitoneally. It is adherent to the posterior abdominal wall.

Its relations are:

- Posteriorly: the right psoas major muscle, right ureter, the abdominal aorta and inferior vena cava.
- Anteriorly: the coils of the small intestine and the superior mesenteric artery.
- Superiorly: the superior mesenteric vessels and the head of the pancreas.

The following are related to D4:

- Anteriorly: the coils of jejunum and the beginning of the root of the mesentery.

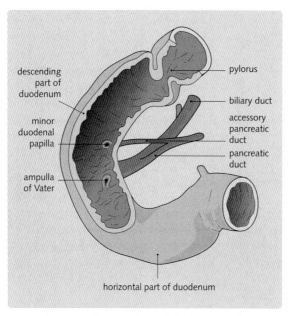

**Fig. 6.2** The second (descending) part of the duodenum, showing the periampullar structures.

- Posteriorly: the left psoas major muscle and the left margin of the aorta.
- The head and body of the pancreas lie medially and superiorly to D4, respectively.

An accessory pancreatic duct is sometimes present, formed by the proximal end of the dorsal pancreatic duct, which normally disappears. It opens into the minor duodenal papilla.

## Jejunum

The jejunum begins at the duodenojejunal flexure and makes up about two fifths of the small intestine. It is about 2.5 m long.

It lies mostly in the umbilical region. The jejunum has large and well-developed mucosal plicae circulares (circular folds) and these can be felt in a living person. It has no prominent Peyer's patches, but diffuse lymphoid tissue.

## Ileum

The ileum, which is about 3.5 m long, constitutes the rest of the small intestine. There is no clear demarcation between it and the jejunum, but the ileum is paler and less vascular than the jejunum. These differences, especially the fact that it is less vascular, are important surgically.

It is situated in the hypogastric and inguinal regions. Its terminal part lies in the pelvis major, ascending over the right psoas muscle and the right iliac vessels to join with the caecum at the ileocolic junction.

The plicae circulares are small in the superior part of the ileum and absent in the terminal end. The ileum is thinner walled and has more Peyer's patches than the jejunum.

## Mesentery

The small intestine has a fan-shaped mesentery, which suspends it from the posterior abdominal wall and allows the jejunum and ileum to be mobile. The root of the mesentery is about 15 cm long and this moves from left to right in an oblique and inferior direction.

It begins on the left side of L2 and crosses:

- The horizontal part (D3) of the duodenum.
- The aorta.
- The inferior vena cava.
- The right psoas major muscle.
- The right ureter.
- The right testicular (or ovarian) vessels.

The root of the mesentery ends at the right sacroiliac joint.

## Blood supply

The proximal half of the duodenum is a foregut structure and so is supplied by the coeliac trunk through the gastroduodenal artery and its branch, the superior pancreaticoduodenal artery. The distal half of the duodenum is a midgut structure. It is supplied by the inferior pancreaticoduodenal artery, which is a branch of the superior mesenteric artery.

The superior and inferior pancreaticoduodenal arteries form anastomoses called the anterior and posterior arcades. These lie in between the duodenum and the pancreas.

As they are midgut structures, the jejunum and ileum are supplied by the superior mesenteric artery, which arises from the abdominal aorta at the level of L1. Some 15–18 jejunal and ileal branches arise from the left side of the superior mesenteric artery and pass between the two layers of the mesentery, forming arches or loops called arcades.

Straight arteries called vasa recta branch off from the arcades and do not anastomose in the mesentery. Many blood vessel anastomoses are found within the walls of the intestines.

As mentioned earlier, the jejunum is more vascular than the ileum. It has longer arterial arcades, with straighter and less complex vasa recta. The arterial supplies of the jejunum and ileum are compared in Fig. 6.3.

The last ileal branch from the superior mesenteric artery anastomoses with a branch of the ileocolic artery.

**Fig. 6.3** (A) The arterial supplies of proximal jejunum and distal ileum. Note that the arterial arcades in the ileum are more complex and the vasa recta are shorter than in the jejunum. (B) Arteries of the gastrointestinal tract.

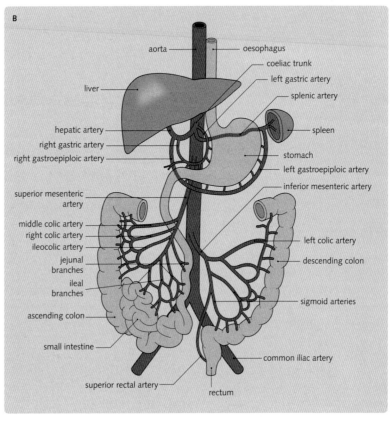

## Venous drainage

The venous drainage follows the arterial supply of the small intestine. From the duodenum, blood drains into the portal venous system, via the superior mesenteric vein.

Drainage to these occurs in three ways:

- Direct drainage to the portal vein.
- Indirect drainage, via small veins, to the pancreaticoduodenal veins.
- Indirect drainage, via the prepyloric veins, to the right gastric vein.

In the jejunum and ileum, all the tributaries of the superior mesenteric vein run alongside the branches of the superior mesenteric artery.

## Lymphatic drainage

In the duodenum, the anterior and posterior surface lymphatics anastomose. The anterior vessels drain to the pyloric and pancreaticoduodenal lymph nodes, which then drain to the coeliac lymph nodes. The posterior vessels drain to the superior mesenteric nodes.

In the jejunum and ileum, the lymphatics are present in the villi as lacteals. The lymph vessels drain into the mesenteric lymph nodes close to the intestinal wall, along the arterial arcades and along the proximal section of the superior mesenteric artery.

The terminal ileal lymph vessels drain to the ileocolic lymph nodes, which run with the ileal branch of the ileocolic artery.

## Innervation

Duodenal innervation comes from the vagus and sympathetic nerves via nerve plexuses on the pancreaticoduodenal arteries.

The jejunum and ileum are also supplied by the vagus and splanchnic nerves. These travel through the coeliac ganglion and form plexuses around the superior mesenteric artery.

The superior mesenteric nerve plexus, supplying the small intestine, receives sympathetic and parasympathetic supplies from the superior mesenteric ganglion and coeliac division of the vagal trunk, respectively.

## EMBRYOLOGY AND DEVELOPMENT

The proximal portion of the small intestine (from the pylorus to the duodenal papilla) develops from the foregut. The remainder of the intestine develops from the midgut and hindgut. Rapid elongation of the midgut, to form the primary intestinal loop, occurs from 5 weeks of embryonic life.

The midgut gives rise to the remainder of the duodenum (that part distal to the duodenal papilla) and to the proximal two thirds of the transverse colon.

The duodenum is, therefore, supplied by branches of the artery of the foregut (the coeliac artery) and the superior mesenteric artery (which supplies the midgut).

The midgut is suspended from the dorsal abdominal wall by a mesentery. It communicates with the yolk sac through the vitelline duct.

A small portion of the vitelline duct persists in 2% of individuals and forms an outpouching of the ileum known as *Meckel's diverticulum*.

During development, the liver and primitive gut grow so rapidly that there is not enough room in the fetal abdominal cavity, and the midgut herniates outside the abdominal cavity at about the 6th week. It develops in the umbilical cord until the end of the 3rd month, when it begins to return to the abdominal cavity.

While outside the abdomen, the primary intestinal loop rotates approximately 270° around the superior mesenteric artery. Viewed from the front, the rotation is anticlockwise (Fig. 6.4).

The jejunum and ileum form a number of coiled loops but the large intestine remains uncoiled. The jejunum is the first portion of gut to return to the abdominal cavity.

## HISTOLOGY

The tissue layers of the small intestine are essentially the same as those found elsewhere in the gastro-intestinal tract (see Fig. 1.2), consisting of a mucosa, submucosa, muscularis externa and serosa.

## The mucosa

The mucosa consists of an epithelial layer, the lamina propria and the muscularis mucosae. It is the main

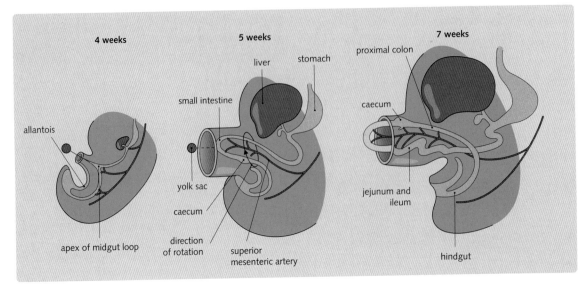

**Fig. 6.4** Rotation and herniation of the developing gut.

site of absorption for digestion products, such as amino acids, fats and sugars and so it, as well as the submucosa, is specialized to allow maximum absorption.

The mucosa has a much greater surface area than other parts of the gastrointestinal tract due to:

- The length of the small intestine.
- Plicae circulares.
- Numerous villi.
- A striated border of microvilli.

These factors together produce a 600-fold increase in the absorptive area of the small intestine. Plicae circulares are folds in the mucosa and submucosa, arranged on a circular fashion around the lumen of the small intestine. They are most prominent in the jejunum, but absent in the distal part of the small intestine.

Intestinal glands (crypts of Lieberkühn) are found throughout the length of the small intestine. They are simple tubular glands extending through the thickness of the mucous membrane and opening into the intestinal lumen at the base of the villi (Fig. 6.5).

## Villi

The villi change in shape along the length of the small intestine. In the duodenum they are broad, but they become leaf-like further down the tract. In the terminal ileum, villi are finger-like projections.

They consist of an epithelial cover and a lamina propria with a centrally placed lymphatic capillary (lacteal) that drains into the large lymphatic vessels in the submucosa (Fig. 6.6). Lacteals dilate after a meal, but they are collapsed in the fasting state.

Villi are projections consisting of a series of epithelial cells; microvilli are smaller protrusions from individual epithelial cells.

## Types of mucosal cell

### Enterocytes

Enterocytes are the most numerous cells and have an absorptive function. They are found chiefly on the villi and surface of the small intestine and, in smaller numbers, in the intestinal glands. They are tall columnar cells with striated microvilli and irregular outlines (Fig. 6.7).

The cells absorb water from the lumen of the gut, and the paracellular spaces contain ATPases (membrane pumps) which transport sodium from the cell into the spaces, drawing the water absorbed from the lumen from the cell by osmosis.

The ultrastructure of these cells is indicative of their absorptive role. They contain large quantities of rough endoplasmic reticulum (RER), mitochondria and Golgi bodies. Many ribosomes are present.

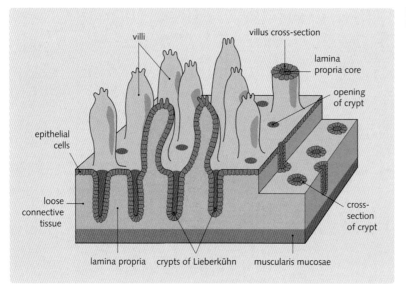

**Fig. 6.5** The villi and crypts of Lieberkühn.

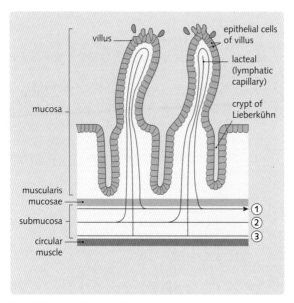

**Fig. 6.6** Cross-section of small intestinal villi. Drainage is to the hepatic portal vein (1), branches of superior mesenteric artery (2) and the lymphatic system (3).

The microvilli are covered by a protein coat, the glycocalyx. This contains many enzymes (e.g. lactase, alkaline phosphatase, lipases), which are involved in digestion and transport.

Microvilli are destroyed by the flagellate parasite *Giardia lamblia,* but they regenerate if the organism is eradicated.

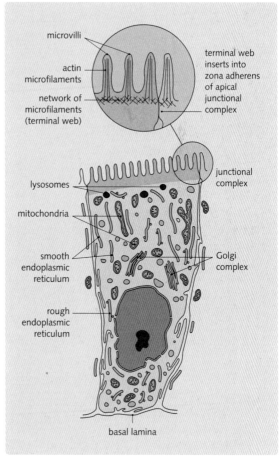

**Fig. 6.7** An enterocyte.

## Goblet cells

Goblet cells (Fig. 6.8) in the intestine produce mucus, as they do in other epithelia. They are packed with mucin and their cytoplasm has abundant RER, reflecting their secretory role.

They are interspersed between the enterocytes and are most numerous on the villi and in the superior two thirds of the crypts.

Goblet cells are least numerous in the duodenum, but they increase in frequency along the length of the small intestine. They are most numerous in the terminal ileum.

## Paneth cells

Paneth cells are found in the deepest part of the intestinal glands. They synthezise and secrete large amounts of protein, and thus have cytoplasm rich in RER. The secreted proteins are defensins which protect against infection by regulating the gut flora.

They are also phagocytic and contain granules of lysozyme, an enzyme that digests the walls of certain bacteria.

## Stem cells

Stem (undifferentiated) cells are located in the lower third of the crypts of Lieberkühn. They replenish all the other cells of the small intestine.

Approximately 1.7 billion enterocytes are shed from the adult intestine each day, being replaced by undifferentiated cells migrating up from the bases of the crypts. The turnover of enterocytes takes about 5 days.

As can be deduced from their role, the number of stem cells is increased in diseases where there is increased cell loss, e.g. coeliac disease.

## Enteroendocrine cells

The enteroendocrine (amine precursor uptake and decarboxylation, APUD) cells situated in the crypts of the small intestine are very similar to those found in the stomach. They are triangular-shaped with the luminal apex displaying microvilli, and contain neuroendocrine granules.

They secrete hormones and neuropeptides, including somatostatin, 5-hydroxytryptamine (serotonin), secretin, gastrin, motilin and vasoactive intestinal polypeptide.

## Peyer's patches

Peyer's patches are present in the mucosa of the ileum, extending into the submucosa, and are characteristically found opposite the attachment of the mesentery. They consist of aggregations of lymphoid nodules and form part of the mucosa-associated lymphoid (MALT) tissue system.

The Peyer's patches contain three types of cell:

- Membranous microfold 'M' cells, which allow antigen to enter.
- Dome cells, which are rich in MHC class II and present antigen to lymphocytes.
- Lymphocytes (B and T) found in the follicular zone.

The cell types of the small intestinal mucosa are summarized in Fig. 6.9.

Fig. 6.8 A goblet cell.

**Fig. 6.9** Cells of the small intestinal mucosa and their functions.

| Cell type | Function |
| --- | --- |
| Enterocytes | Intestinal absorptive cell. These tall columnar cells have microvilli and absorb water and nutrients from the lumen of the gut. |
| Goblet cells | These produce mucus and are found on the villi. They are least numerous in the duodenum and most numerous in the terminal ileum. |
| Paneth cells | These are phagocytic cells and contain lysozyme granules. They are found deep in the intestinal glands. |
| Membranous microfold 'M' cells | Epithelial cells, which overlie Peyer's patches and allow for entry of antigen. |
| Undifferentiated (stem) cells | These give rise to enterocytes, goblet cells and enteroendocrine cells. They are located in the lower thirds of the crypts. |
| Enteroendocrine (APUD) cells | These cells secrete hormones and neuropeptides, such as somatostatin, 5-HT, secretin and gastrin. They are found in the crypts of the small intestine and have microvilli at their luminal apices. |

## Lamina propria

The lamina propria of the small intestine is made up of a glycosaminoglycan (GAG) matrix, fibroblasts, collagen, reticulin and smooth muscle fibres.

It also contains capillaries, lymphatics, nerves and diffuse lymphoid tissue.

## Submucosa

The submucosa contains the submucosal (Meissner's) plexus as well as a large quantity of mucosa-associated lymphoid tissue (MALT) and lymphatics. It is vascular and extends into the plicae circulares.

In the duodenum, compound tubular Brunner's glands are also present. They secrete mucus, bicarbonate and growth factors such as epidermal growth factor. The last of these promotes the growth and regeneration of tissues.

Brunner's glands also secrete urogastrone, an inhibitor of acid secretion.

## Muscularis externa

The muscularis externa, like that of the rest of the gastrointestinal tract, is made up of two smooth msucle layers: an inner circular layer and an outer longitudinal one. The myenteric (Auerbach's) plexus is located between the muscle layers.

The protein content of the cells lost from the gut each day is approximately 30 g. It accounts for a substantial amount of the daily protein loss from the body.

## PHYSIOLOGY

The small intestine has a very large surface area and is specially adapted to digest and absorb nutrients, salt and water. Enzymes and hormones produced in the small intestine complete the digestion that began in the mouth and stomach.

The small intestine has immunological defences against antigens that have been ingested consisting of solitary lymph nodules and Peyer's patches (aggregations of lymphatic nodules).

Gastrointestinal hormones produced in the small intestine play an important role in gastrointestinal secretion and motility.

Defence against antigens is both mechanical, by the production of mucus, and immunological, principally through gut-associated lymphoid tissue, described below.

## Epithelial cell turnover

Enterocytes have a high rate of turnover and are replaced by undifferentiated (stem) cells, which migrate up from the bases of the crypts of Lieberkühn. The cells become partially differentiated and they continue to divide as they migrate upwards from the bottom of the crypts (Fig. 6.10).

The average lifespan of an enterocyte is about 2–3 days, but this is reduced in coeliac disease (see later) and as a side effect of some drugs, e.g. prolonged anticancer therapy. The undifferentiated cells cannot keep up with the increased loss, resulting in a flattening of the villi and malabsorption.

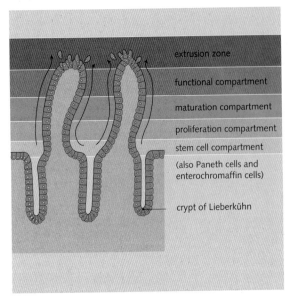

labels (top to bottom):
extrusion zone
functional compartment
maturation compartment
proliferation compartment
stem cell compartment
(also Paneth cells and enterochromaffin cells)
crypt of Lieberkühn

**Fig. 6.10** Cell turnover and migration of stem cells in the small intestine.

Radiotherapy may have a similar effect (radiation enteritis) depending on the dose and the site at which it is administered. Symptoms usually resolve within 6 weeks of the final dose of radiotherapy, but some patients experience chronic radiation enteritis (symptoms persisting for more than 3 months).

In coeliac disease, which is caused by an allergy to gluten in wheat, the surface of the jejunum is flattened and there is extensive loss of villi. This causes malabsorption, as the loss of villi results in a decrease in the available absorptive area.

This loss of villi also results in an increased enterocyte turnover and thus an increase in stem cell numbers, as the stem cells try to replenish the lost cells.

A gluten-free diet allows regeneration of villi and is curative for the disease.

## Secretions

The small intestine secretes mucus and gastrointestinal hormones.

- Mucus is produced by the goblet cells (Fig. 6.8), which are most numerous on the villi. The mucus lubricates the mucosal surface and protects it from trauma as particles of food pass through it.

- The gastrointestinal hormones which affect the small intestine are summarized in Fig. 6.11.

The epithelial cells secrete an aqueous solution during the course of digestion but, under normal conditions, they absorb slightly more than they secrete.

Under certain conditions, e.g. cholera (see Chapter 7), secretion greatly exceeds absorption and secretory diarrhoea occurs.

## Defence

The defences of the small intestine are in the most part due to lymphocytes of both T and B types.

T lymphocytes are made in the thymus gland, following which they migrate into encapsulated peripheral tissues such as those of the spleen and lymph nodes. T lymphocytes also migrate to non-encapsulated lymphoid tissue known as mucosa-associated lymphoid tissue (MALT). This gives protection against antigens entering the body through mucosal epithelial surfaces (Fig. 6.12).

The majority of MALT is present as gut-associated lymphoid tissue (GALT); smaller amounts are present in the bronchi, skin and genitourinary tract.

T cells are divided into:

- Helper (CD4) cells, which enhance the reaction of the immune system following the presentation of antigen to T helper cells by antigen-presenting cells, via MHC class II receptors.
- Cytotoxic (CD8) cells, which are capable of killing other cells, e.g. cancer cells and cells that have been infected with viruses, and can also downregulate the immune response. They are activated via an endogenous antigen–MHC class I complex.

CD4 and CD8 cells together make up approximately 75% of all lymphocytes.

B lymphocytes are made in the bone marrow and, in the fetus, in the liver. They also migrate to peripheral tissues, including MALT. B cells produce antibody and, once they have encountered a particular antigen, form memory cells, which can undergo clonal expansion (multiplication to form large numbers of identical B cells). They then differentiate to form plasma cells, which have a relatively short half-life but which produce large numbers of specific antibody to particular antigens. Scattered lymphoid cells are also found in the mucosa of the small intestine.

**Fig. 6.11** The main hormones acting on the small intestine and their functions.

| Hormone | Gastrointestinal source | Signal for release | Action |
|---|---|---|---|
| CCK | Enteroendocrine (APUD) cells in upper intestine | Peptides and amino acids and fats, elevated serum $Ca^{2+}$ in duodenum | Contracts gall bladder and relaxes sphincter of Oddi; causes secretion of alkaline enzymatic pancreatic juice, inhibits gastric emptying, exerts trophic effect on pancreas, acts as a satiety hormone, stimulates glucagon secretion and contracts the pyloric sphincter |
| Secretin | S cells in upper small intestine | Acid and products of fat digestion in duodenum | Increases secretion of $HCO_3^-$ by the pancreas and biliary tract, decreases acid secretion, contracts the pyloric sphincter and augments CCK's stimulation of pancreatic secretions |
| Gastrin | G cells in antrum | Peptides and amino acids, distension, vagal stimulation, blood-borne calcium and epinephrine | Acid and pepsinogen secretion, trophic to mucosa of stomach and small and large intestines, increases gastric motility, may close LOS, stimulates insulin and glucagon secretion after protein meal. Inhibits gastric emptying |
| Somatostatin | D cells of pancreatic islets, intestinal cells | Glucose, amino acids, free fatty acids, glucagon and β-adrenergic and cholinergic neurotransmitters | Inhibits secretion of insulin, glucagon, acid, pepsin, gastrin, secretin and intestinal juices, decreases gastric, duodenal and gall bladder motility |

The main type of antibody produced by intestinal B cells is IgA, the major immunoglobulin of external secretions. There are approximately $10^{10}$ plasma cells per metre of small intestine, the majority of which (70–90%) produce IgA. IgA dimers are transported across the glandular epithelium into the gut lumen by binding to a receptor on the epithelial surface. The IgA–receptor complex is endocytosed and transported across the cell into the lumen. Part of the receptor (the secretory component) remains attached to the IgA and protects IgA from proteolytic enzymes in the lumen.

IgA prevents microorganisms from entering as it binds and neutralizes them directly without the need for other effector systems. A much smaller amount of IgM is also secreted by the intestinal B cells.

Specialized M cells (so named because of the numerous microfolds on their luminal surface) overlie the Peyer's patches and they absorb, transport, process and present antigens to the lymphoid cells lying between them.

## Motility

Motility in the small intestine facilitates three main functions:

- Mixing of intestinal contents.
- Bringing the contents into contact with the absorptive surfaces of the small intestine.
- Forward propulsion of the contents.

Chyme takes between 2 and 3 hours to pass through the small intestine, which is the site at which most digestion and absorption of nutrients takes place. There are two main types of contraction seen in the fed state: segmentation and peristalsis.

Segmentation mixes the digested food and exposes it to the absorptive surfaces. It is a discontinuous, oscillating contraction resulting in alternating contracted and relaxed areas, the latter containing chyme. Although the movement is mainly in a forwards-and-backwards direction, there is a slow net movement towards the anus as the frequency of the contractions decreases down the length of the small intestine (Fig. 6.13).

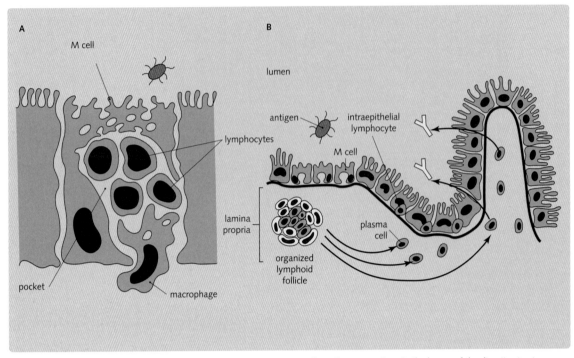

**Fig. 6.12** The mucosa-associated lymphoid tissue (MALT) of the gut. (A) M cells endocytose antigen in the lumen of the digestive tract, transport it across the cell and release it into the basolateral pocket. (B) Antigen activates B cells, which differentiate into IgA-producing plasma cells. (Redrawn with permission from Kuby J. Immunology, 3rd edn. New York: WH Freeman, 1997.)

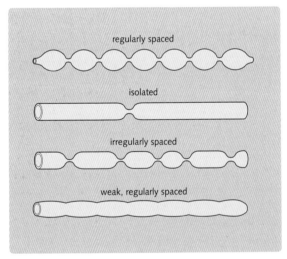

**Fig. 6.13** Segmentation in the small intestine.

Peristaltic contraction brings about rapid propulsion of the intestinal contents towards the anus, at a rate of 2–25 cm/s. It involves contraction of the longitudinal muscles and is a reflex initiated by local distension caused by the bolus of food. Peristalsis moves chyme more quickly towards the colon and does not mix it as efficiently as segmentation.

Motility in the fasting state is due to migrating motor complexes (MMC) which occur every 90–120 min. The MMC involves high-frequency bursts of powerful contractions, beginning in the stomach and moving towards the terminal ileum. The pyloric sphincter is open wide during the MMC.

The MMC has a number of functions:

- It moves indigestible food, e.g. tomato skins, nuts, sweetcorn into the lower bowel.
- It allows for the removal of dead epithelial cells.
- It prevents bacterial overgrowth.
- It prevents colonic bacteria entering the small intestine.

## Control of intestinal motility

The motility of the small intestine is controlled by nervous, hormonal and local factors which coordinate the various intestinal reflexes (Fig. 6.14). Of importance is the gastroileal reflex, which causes ileal segmentation in response to gastrin secreted due to the presence of chyme in the stomach.

When the ileocaecal valve opens, small amounts of chyme enter the colon at the rate at which the colon is able to reabsorb most of the salts and water contained in the chyme.

## The intestinal circulation

The intestinal circulation is part of the splanchnic circulation, which supplies the lower oesophagus, stomach, liver, gall bladder, pancreas, spleen and intestines.

At rest, approximately 10–30% of the cardiac output flows to the digestive organs and three quarters of this is required by the mucosa and submucosa for facilitation of absorption and transport. The remaining quarter is utilized by the smooth muscle layer of the bowels.

The splanchnic circulation has a major role as a large reservoir that can be mobilised easily when required, such as during exercise.

Another function of this circulation, is the intestinal counter-current system. In the mucosal villi, the blood vessels are arranged in a network of hairpin loops.

The arteriole enters at the base of the villus and divides into a capillary network at the tip of the villus, just deep to the epithelial lining of the villus. The arteriole and venule are only 20 mm apart and lipid-permeable molecules, such as oxygen, can pass from one vessel to the other.

The blood flows are opposite in direction (hence 'counter-current'). This facilitates some of the dissolved oxygen in the plasma to move along its diffusion gradient from the arteriole to the venule, without entering the capillary network.

When intestinal blood flow is low, this shunting of oxygen can cause death to the epithelial cells at the villus tip. Necrosis of enterocytes at the villus tip is a sign of severe intestinal ischaemia.

The most important function of the counter-current blood flow is to produce a region of hyperosmolarity in the villus tip by means of a multiplier system (Fig. 6.15).

Hyperosmolarity is achieved by the following mechanisms:

- $Na^+$ ions are pumped into the subepithelial extracellular fluid by the enterocytes and taken up in the capillary network. As blood flows down into the venule, $Na^+$ ions diffuse across to the capillary, which returns the $Na^+$ ions to the villus tip. This results in a hyperosmolar region at the tip, which draws in water molecules from the intestinal lumen.

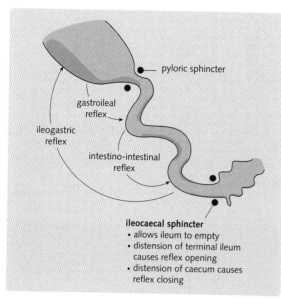

Fig. 6.14 Control of small intestine motility.

pyloric sphincter

gastroileal reflex

ileogastric reflex

intestino-intestinal reflex

**ileocaecal sphincter**
- allows ileum to empty
- distension of terminal ileum causes reflex opening
- distension of caecum causes reflex closing

Vagal stimulation is required to maintain the fed motor pattern. Segmentation is coordinated by the myenteric plexus, and circular muscle contraction is brought about by acetylcholine and substance P.

The peristaltic reflex occurs by the simultaneous oral (proximal) contraction and anal (distal) relaxation, either side of the bolus. The contraction is mediated by vagal excitatory contractions, via substance P and acetylcholine.

The relaxation is mediated by vagal inhibitory contractions, via nitric oxide (NO) and VIP. Movement of the bolus into the next section of the intestine triggers the next reflex.

In the fasting state, the MMC is coordinated by the enteric nervous system. It is initiated by vagal stimulation and motilin. During an MMC, plasma motilin concentrations increase, but they decrease on the arrival of food in the stomach.

### Control of the ileocaecal valve

The incompetent ileocaecal valve (see Chapter 7) separates the terminal ileum from the colon and is normally closed. However, it opens in response to:

- Distension of the terminal ileum (by a reflex mechanism).
- Short-range peristalsis in the terminal ileum.
- Gastroileal reflex (which enhances emptying of the ileum after a meal).

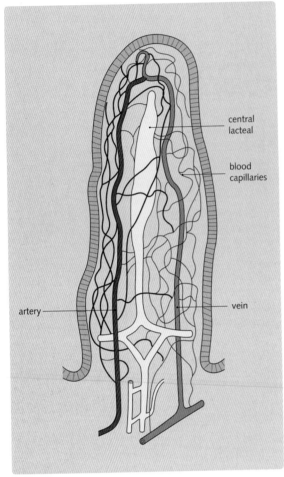

Fig. 6.15 The counter-current mechanism in the villi of the small intestine. This enables absorption of electrolytes and water.

- Water molecules may also be drawn into the descending capillaries from the arterial vessel, if there is an increased $Na^+$ concentration. This also results in the delivery of hyperosmolar blood to the villus tip.

The counter-current mechanism is very similar to that seen in the loop of Henle in the kidney.

## Control of the intestinal circulation

Nerves, hormones and local factors control the intestinal circulation.

A change in the cardiac output, arterial pressure or blood volume will have the same effect on this circulation as on the general systemic circulation. For example, massive haemorrhage will result in a decreased venous return to the heart, decreased cardiac output and a drop in arterial blood pressure.

This activates baroreceptors to bring about the sympathetic reflex of vasoconstriction in precapillary vessels. This is particularly marked in the intestinal circulation.

Autonomic nervous control regulates the blood flow by:

- Parasympathetic nerves, which are vasodilators, via acetylcholine and VIP.
- Sympathetic nerves, which are vasoconstrictors, via epinephrine and norepinephrine (acting on $\alpha_2$-adrenoreceptors).
- Enteric nerves, which are vasodilators, via acetylcholine and VIP.
- Primary sensory nerves (C fibres), which are vasodilators, via NO, substance P and calcitonin gene related peptide (CGRP).

Endocrine and paracrine controls can also regulate the intestinal circulation. These are summarized in Fig. 6.16.

Metabolites in the gut after a meal can act as vasodilators. Glucose and fatty acids cause postprandial hyperaemia, which is mediated by VIP release from the enteric nervous system.

Fig. 6.16 Control of the intestinal circulation by vasoactive hormones. (CCK = cholecystokinin; GI = gastrointestinal; JGA = juxtaglomerular apparatus.)

| Hormone | Source | Stimulus for release | Effect on GI circulation |
|---------|--------|----------------------|--------------------------|
| Catecholamines | Adrenal medulla | Oligaemic (hypovolaemic) shock | Vasoconstriction |
| Angiotensin II | Renal JGA | Heart failure | Vasoconstriction |
| Vasopressin | Posterior pituitary | Oligaemic shock | Vasoconstriction |
| Gastrin | GI mucosal G cells | Mealtimes | Vasodilatation |
| CCK | Intestinal mucosal I cells | Mealtimes | Vasodilatation |
| Secretin | Intestinal mucosal S cells | Mealtimes | Vasodilatation |

# DIGESTION AND ABSORPTION

Digestion begins in the mouth and continues in the stomach, but most digestion and absorption takes place in the small intestine.

## General concepts

For food to be absorbed, it must be broken down into small particles that can be transported across the epithelial cells of the gastrointestinal tract and into the bloodstream. Substances are then carried to the liver via the hepatic portal system.

As elsewhere in the body, molecules may be transported across the epithelial cells by simple diffusion, facilitated diffusion and primary or secondary active transport. The properties of these different types of transport are shown in Figs 6.17 and 6.18.

## Factors which control absorption by the small intestine

A number of factors control absorption by the small intestine:

- Adequate blood supply.
- Carrier molecule density and availability at the brush border.
- Cell maturation rate.
- Number of transporting cells.
- Passive permeability and the intracellular concentrations of molecules.
- The electrochemical gradient for $Na^+$.
- Sympathetic innervation and epinephrine in the plasma both increase the absorption of $Na^+$ and $Cl^-$ (and therefore water).

- Parasympathetic stimulation decreases the absorption of these substances.

## Digestion and absorption of different components of the diet

### Carbohydrates

Carbohydrates provide most of the calories in the average diet, the majority being in the form of starch (a polymer of glucose).

Starch contains $\alpha$-1,4 and $\alpha$-1,6 linkages: the former are hydrolysed by amylase in saliva (ptyalin) and in pancreatic secretions (pancreatic amylase).

This produces maltose and maltotriose (together known as malto-oligosaccharides), comprising 70% of the breakdown products, and $\alpha$-limit dextrans (the remaining 30%).

Starch is therefore partially digested in the mouth and its digestion continues in the duodenum, as salivary amylase is inactivated in the stomach by gastric acid.

Other enzymes exist in the brush border of the duodenum, and these complete the digestion of starch. These enzymes further break down starch into the monosaccharides glucose and galactose, which are actively taken up with sodium. Carbohydrates are only absorbed as monosaccharides through the gut mucosa.

Glucose and galactose then cross the basal membrane into the capillaries by facilitated transport and simple diffusion (Fig. 6.19). Another monosaccharide, fructose, is also produced and taken up by a sodium-independent mechanism.

A deficiency of enzymes in the digestive system can result in carbohydrate malabsorption. The most

Fig. 6.17 Cellular transport mechanisms. (Courtesy of Dr MA Rattray, UMDS, London.)

| Type of transport | Proteins required | Transport against or with concentration gradient | Energy required |
|---|---|---|---|
| Passive diffusion | No | With | No |
| Facilitated diffusion | Yes | With | No |
| Primary active transport | Yes | Against | Yes: hydrolysis of ATP |
| Secondary active transport | Yes | Against | Yes: electrochemical gradient |

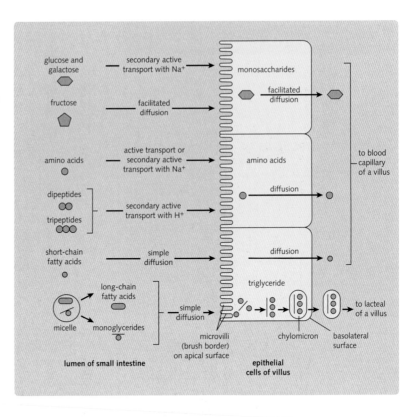

**Fig. 6.18** Absorption in the small intestine. For simplicity, all digested foods are shown in the lumen of the small intestine, even though some are digested by brush-border enzymes. (Redrawn with permission from Berne RM, Levy MN. Principles of Physiology, 3rd edn. St Louis: Mosby, 2000.)

common deficiency is lactase deficiency (see later). This is often acquired, and results in lactose intolerance in about 50% of adults worldwide. Congenital lactase deficiency is rare.

Lactase deficiency has a strong genetic component and its incidence varies in different races. Exclusion of milk and milk products relieves many of the symptoms.

The digestion of carbohydrates is summarized in Fig. 6.20.

## Protein

The protein requirement of a normal healthy adult is about 40 g/day (to replace the 5–7 g/day nitrogen lost as urea in the urine and so maintain nitrogen balance).

In the Western world, meat eaters usually exceed this, but in the developing world the amount of protein in the diet is less.

We do not have a store of protein in the body (unlike, for example, carbohydrate which is stored as glycogen). Every protein in the body performs a function and proteins are in a constant state of flux (1–2% of total body protein is turned over daily), being synthesized by ribosomes and then degraded in the body. We synthesize about 300 g/day.

Protein in the intestinal lumen comes from protein eaten in the diet and also from cell turnover, almost all of which are digested and absorbed.

Digestion of dietary protein begins in the stomach (pepsin hydrolyses about 15% of dietary protein to amino acids and small peptides). It continues in the duodenum and small intestine where pancreatic proteases continue the process of hydrolysis (Fig. 6.21).

### Absorption of the products of protein digestion

Small peptides, particularly dipeptides and tripeptides are absorbed more rapidly than amino acids. They are transported across the membrane by an active mechanism utilizing the electrochemical potential difference of $Na^+$.

There are a number of different amino acid carriers depending on the charge of the amino acid. Some of these require a $Na^+$ gradient for transport.

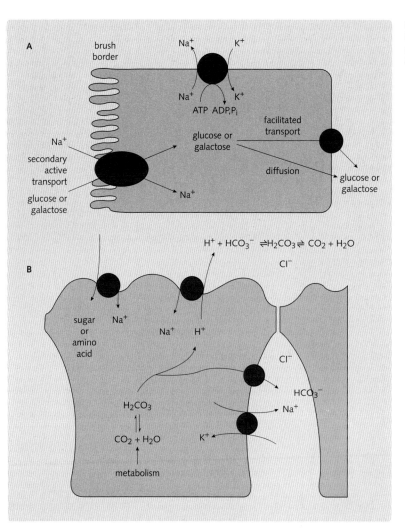

**Fig. 6.19** (A) Sugar and (B) ion transport in the small intestine. ([A] Redrawn with permission from Nature 330: 379; London: Macmillan Magazines Ltd, 1986.)

Amino acids enter the cells from the lumen and leave it to pass into the capillaries by three mechanisms: sodium-dependent transport, sodium-independent transport and simple diffusion.

Defects of amino acid absorption are rare.

## Fat

Fat is not water soluble and its digestion and absorption is more complex than that of other substances.

Fat in the diet is principally in the form of triglycerides (a complex of glycerol and fatty acids) and is only released from the stomach into the duodenum at the rate at which it can be digested. The presence of fat in the duodenum, therefore, inhibits gastric emptying.

Gastric lipase begins the hydrolysis of triglycerides, although it is not significant unless pancreatic lipase is deficient.

In the duodenum, bile acids, aided by lecithin, emulsify fat to form micelles by their detergent action. A minimum concentration of bile acids is needed to form micelles (the critical micelle concentration). Micelles consist of 20–30 molecules, arranged so that lipid (non-polar) molecules lie in the centre, surrounded by conjugated bile acids and water-soluble molecules. They increase the surface area for enzymatic digestion by pancreatic lipase. Other enzymes involved in fat digestion are cholesterol esterase and phospholipase 2, although the extent of their involvement is small.

**Fig. 6.20** Digestion of carbohydrates.

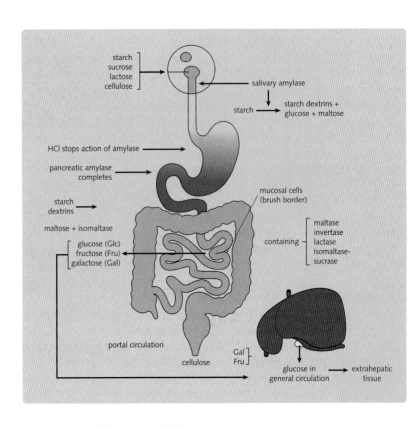

At the microscopic level, it is easy to tell the three sections of the small intestine apart. The duodenum has submucosal Brunner's glands. The jejunum has the most complex and numerous plicae circulares and villi while the ileum has the most developed Peyer's patches and GALT, which extend into the submucosa.

Pancreatic lipase is inactivated by acid and so is ineffective if excess acid is produced by the stomach. This occurs in the Zollinger–Ellison syndrome, where fat malabsorption occurs.

## Absorption of the products of fat digestion

The products of fat digestion, being lipids, diffuse across the lipid membrane of the brush border of the small intestine.

Different components are absorbed at different rates. Free fatty acids diffuse across rapidly, cholesterol more slowly. The micelles, therefore, become more concentrated in cholesterol as they move along the small intestine.

Under normal conditions, most dietary fat is absorbed before the contents reach the end of the jejunum and any fat in the stools (in the absence of steatorrhoea) is from desquamated epithelial cells and from bacterial flora in the gut.

Once inside the epithelial cells, lipid is taken into the smooth endoplasmic reticulum where much of it is re-esterified.

Some lipid is also synthesized in the epithelial cells. Dietary and synthesized lipids are then incorporated into chylomicrons and, provided β-lipoprotein is present, the chylomicrons are exocytosed into lateral intercellular spaces to enter the lacteals. Having reached the lymphatic system, they travel up the thoracic duct and enter the venous circulation.

Apolipoproteins are an important constituent of chylomicrons. They are made by hepatocytes and the epithelial cells of the intestine. Their absence leads to the accumulation of lipid in intestinal epithelial cells.

Chylomicrons consist mainly of triglyceride with a phospholipid coat studded with apolipoproteins

**Fig. 6.21** Digestion of protein.

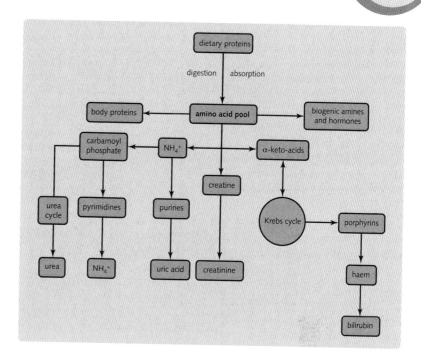

(Fig. 6.22). They contain small amounts of cholesterol and cholesterol esters in the centre, and their overall size depends on the amount of fat in the diet. Following a high fat intake, chylomicrons may have a diameter of up to 750 nm, in low-fat diets they may be as small as 60 nm.

Abetalipoproteinaemia is a rare inborn error of metabolism inherited as a recessive trait, characterized by failure of chylomicron formation and an accumulation of dietary fat within enterocytes.

A diagrammatic representation of the digestion and absorption of fat is shown in Fig. 6.23.

Remember that bile is not enzymatic; its acids emulsify fats via a detergent action and do not hydrolyse it.

## Vitamins

### Fat-soluble vitamins

Absorption of the fat-soluble vitamins A, D, E and K depends on the absorption of fat and any condition in which fat digestion and absorption is decreased will eventually lead to a deficiency of these vitamins.

### Water-soluble vitamins

At the concentrations present in a normal diet, most of these are taken up by specific transport mechanisms, many of which are sodium dependent.

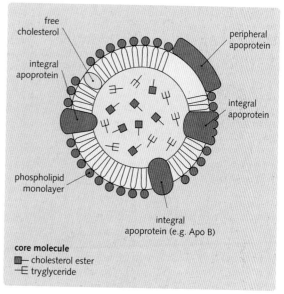

**core molecule**
■– cholesterol ester
–E tryglyceride

**Fig. 6.22** The structure of a chylomicron.

An important example of a water-soluble vitamin is vitamin $B_{12}$. On ingestion, it is bound to R protein found in saliva and in gastric secretions, which protects it from digestion in the stomach. Once vitamin $B_{12}$ has been separated from R protein in the duodenum by the action of pancreatic proteases, vitamin $B_{12}$ binds to intrinsic factor (IF) secreted by gastric parietal cells.

Receptors for the IF–$B_{12}$ dimer are present in the membranes of the epithelial cells of the terminal ileum, which bind the complex and allow uptake of vitamin $B_{12}$.

Vitamin $B_{12}$ is then transported across the basal membrane of the epithelial cells into the portal blood (Fig. 6.24). It is then bound to transcobalamin II and taken up by the liver, kidney, spleen, heart, placenta, reticulocytes and fibroblasts.

The presence of autoantibodies against IF causes malabsorption of vitamin $B_{12}$ and macrocytic anaemia. The resulting disease is called pernicious anaemia.

Diagnosis is by the Schilling test (see *Crash Course: Immunology and Haematology*), the demonstration of low-serum vitamin $B_{12}$ levels and the presence of anti-IF antibodies in the plasma.

Treatment of vitamin $B_{12}$ deficiency is by intramuscular injections of hydroxocobalamin (one of the forms of vitamin $B_{12}$) every 2-3 days until six injections have been given. If the cause of the deficiency remains uncorrected, injections should continue to be given at 3-monthly intervals.

## Water and electrolytes

The normal daily intake of water is about 1.5 L/day. However, up to 9 L water per day are absorbed from the gastrointestinal tract (through the reabsorption of secretions) under normal circumstances, most of it from the small intestine, especially the jejunum (Fig. 6.25).

### Sodium

Almost all of the $Na^+$ in the gastrointestinal tract is reabsorbed (about 99%), mostly from the jejunum in association with glucose, galactose and certain amino acids. $Na^+$ is transported across the epithelial cell membrane down its electrochemical gradient and pumped into the intercellular spaces in exchange for $K^+$.

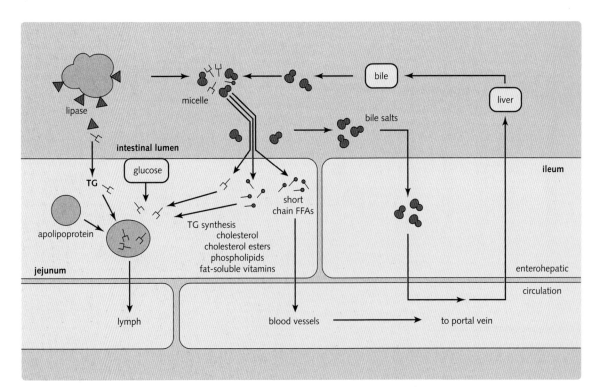

**Fig. 6.23** Cellular uptake of free fatty acids and chylomicrons. (TG = triglyceride; FFA = free fatty acid.)

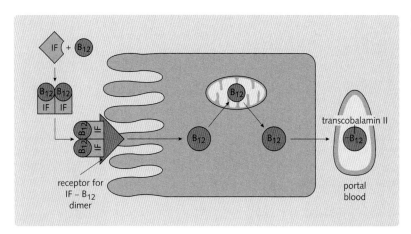

**Fig. 6.24** Vitamin $B_{12}$ absorption in the terminal ileum. (IF = intrinsic factor.)

$Na^+$ is absorbed against its electrochemical gradient in the ileum and the colon. Water follows the active pumping of $Na^+$ by $Na^+/K^+$ ATPases through a transcellular or paracellular (tight junctions) route.

### Potassium

$K^+$ is absorbed in the jejunum and ileum. It is secreted into the colon when $K^+$ concentrations in the lumen are less than 25 mmol/L.

### Calcium

This is absorbed throughout the small intestine (especially in the duodenum and jejunum) although absorption is disrupted in vitamin-D-deficient states.

The percentage of $Ca^{2+}$ absorbed on a low-$Ca^{2+}$ diet is higher than that absorbed from a high-$Ca^{2+}$ diet.

$Ca^{2+}$ passes across the luminal membrane and into the cytoplasm, where it is bound to a protein and then transported across the basolateral membrane, some of it in exchange for $Na^+$.

$Ca^{2+}$ deficiency is seen in vitamin D deficiency, for example in rickets. Vitamin D helps to regulate $Ca^{2+}$ absorption and metabolism in the body.

### Iron

Iron deficiency is relatively common, particularly in women of childbearing age.

The total amount of iron in the body is only about 3–4 g, of which about two-thirds is in haemoglobin.

An average Western diet contains about 20 mg of iron a day, of which only about 10% can be absorbed.

Both males and females lose almost 1 mg of iron a day in the urine and desquamated cells, and females lose about 50 mg of iron a month in the menstrual flow. Women of reproductive age therefore lose an average of 3 mg of iron a day and iron-deficiency anaemia is relatively common.

Absorption is increased in iron deficiency and by increased erythropoietic activity. Growing children, pregnant women and people who have bled are

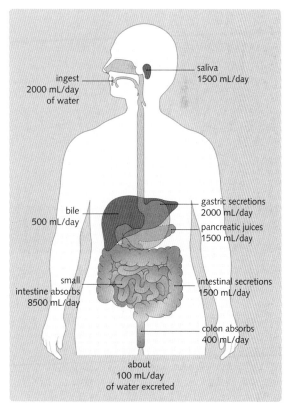

**Fig. 6.25** Fluid secretion and absorption in the gastrointestinal tract.

thus able to absorb increased amounts of iron to compensate for their greater need.

Most dietary iron is in the form $Fe^{3+}$, which is reduced to $Fe^{2+}$ by ascorbic acid in gastric secretions or ferrireductase in the mucosa and then absorbed. Anything that prevents this reduction decreases the absorption of iron, e.g. the production of an insoluble complex with other dietary compounds such as tannin (present in tea), phytate and certain fibres.

$Fe^{2+}$ is taken across the enterocyte membrane of the small intestinal villi by a divalent metal transporter. In the enterocyte, $Fe^{2+}$ is oxidized to $Fe^{3+}$ and then either released into the plasma where it binds to a transferrin molecule or stored in the epithelial cells, bound to ferritin.

The proportion of iron released depends on the body's requirement. A larger amount remains in the cell bound to ferritin when dietary intake exceeds the body's requirement. This iron is then shed when the epithelial cell is desquamated and prevents iron overload.

Excessive amounts of iron are absorbed in haemochromatosis (see Chapter 4), an autosomal recessive condition leading to deposition of iron in the liver, heart, pancreas and pituitary. This results in damage to those organs. The disease is more common in men because premenopausal women are protected by menstruation and childbirth.

Stem cells in the crypts of Lieberkühn can be programmed to absorb more iron, e.g. following haemorrhage. An increase in absorption may be seen 3–4 days after trauma and in response to other events causing blood loss (the time taken for stem cells to mature and reach the tips of the villi where most iron absorption takes place).

# THE FLORA OF THE SMALL INTESTINE

Bacteria may be commensal or pathogenic. Broadly, they may be classified as aerobic or anaerobic.

In health, most of these bacteria are commensal and many of them have important functions, particularly in protecting against colonization by pathogenic bacteria. However, flora which are harmless or even beneficial in one site may become pathogens in another part of the body.

A baby's gut is sterile at birth, but the baby picks up flora from its mother's rectum during delivery.

This colonizes the baby's gut over the next 12–18 hours.

Most of the gastrointestinal tract is heavily colonized with flora. Relatively sterile sites include the stomach (where the acid conditions are too hostile to support much flora), gall bladder and salivary glands.

The small intestine is also fairly sterile. The degree of colonization varies along its length. The duodenum has few microorganisms, mostly Gram-positive cocci and bacilli due to the acidic gastric juices and the alkaline biliary and pancreatic secretions.

The jejunum has more bacteria than the duodenum. *Enterococcus faecalis*, lactobacilli and diphtheroids are found here.

The ileum has a large flora of $10^4$–$10^8$ organisms per mL of fluid. The bacteria are obligate anaerobes and include *Bacteroides*, *Clostridium*, *Bifidobacterium* and Enterobactericeae.

# DISORDERS OF THE SMALL INTESTINE

Only those disorders affecting only or primarily the small intestine will be covered here. Disorders and diseases which involve both the small and large intestines are discussed in Chapter 7.

## Congenital abnormalities

### Meckel's diverticulum

Meckel's diverticulum is the remnant of the vitelline duct present in embryonic life. It connects the developing embryo with the yolk sac.

Meckel's diverticulum can be described with the 'rule of twos':

- It is present in 2% of the population.
- It is about 2 inches long.
- It is approximately 2 feet from the caecum.

In the embryo, the vitelline duct is found at the apex of the primary intestinal loop that forms when the midgut rapidly elongates (see Fig. 6.4). The long sides of the loop are known as the cephalic limb (which forms the duodenum, jejunum and part of the ileum) and the caudal limb (which forms the remainder of the ileum, the caecum, appendix, ascending colon and the proximal two thirds of the transverse colon).

Meckel's diverticulum, therefore, marks the junction of the cranial and caudal limbs of what was the embryonic midgut.

Heterotopic gastric epithelium (normal tissue present in the wrong place) may sometimes be found in the diverticulum, including HCl-secreting oxyntic cells, resulting in peptic ulceration. Rarely, ulcers may perforate or bleed. Heterotopic pancreatic tissue may also be found there.

Acute inflammation of the diverticulum may occur, mimicking acute appendicitis. The mucosa at the mouth of the diverticulum may become inflamed and lead to intussusception, or the diverticulum may perforate and cause peritonitis. In most cases, however, diverticula are asymptomatic.

If the vitelline duct remains patent throughout its length, a fistula may form onto the umbilicus.

The most important details of Meckel's diverticulum can be summed up by the 'rule of twos': it is present in about 2% of the population, is roughly 2 inches long and is found approximately 2 feet from the caecum.

## Atresia and stenosis

Atresia is a failure of canalization and results in complete obstruction. Stenosis is a narrowing of the lumen and results in partial obstruction.

Atresia and stenosis may occur anywhere along the length of the gastrointestinal tract, but they are found most often in the duodenum and least often in the colon.

The incidence is 1 in 5000 births. They are diagnosed quickly after birth. The causes of atresia and stenosis range from lack of recanalization (in the proximal duodenum) to malrotation and gastroschisis (in the distal duodenum), leading to the cessation of the blood supply.

The loss of a blood supply results in complete tissue necrosis to that part of the bowel. The anus may be imperforate, with the anal canal ending blindly at the anal membrane, or a fistula may form between the rectum and perineum.

Alternatively, the rectum may empty into the vagina forming a rectovaginal fistula or into the urethra, forming a urorectal fistula.

# Malabsorption syndromes

Malabsorption is the decreased absorption of nutrients and it may be caused by a number of conditions, including biochemical disorders (such as absent or defective digestive enzymes) and disease of the small intestine. A simple classification is given in Fig. 6.26.

## Causes and effects of malabsorption

The causes of decreased nutrient absorption include:

- Reduced small intestinal surface area.
- Infection leading to damage of the mucosa and bacterial removal of nutrients.
- Defective intraluminal hydrolysis or solubilization (due to lack of enzymes).
- Abnormalities of mucosal epithelial cells (involving loss of digestive enzymes or carriers).
- Drug-induced mechanisms.
- Lymphatic obstruction.
- Rapid transit though the small intestine.

**Fig. 6.26** Classification of malabsorption syndromes.

| Cause of malabsorption | Mechanism |
|---|---|
| Defective intraluminal hydrolysis | Lack of enzyme production<br>Dysfunctional enzymes |
| Primary mucosal cell abnormalities | Loss of enzymes in mucosa<br>Loss of carrier molecules<br>Damage to mucosa via drugs or inflammation |
| Decreased surface area of intestines | Inflammation<br>Drug-induced damage |
| Infection | Due to enterotoxic microorganisms in the food<br>Due to external injury to the bowel<br>Due to antibiotics |
| Iatrogenic | Antibiotics, leading to decreased commensals and increased opportunistic infection |
| Drug induced | Toxicity<br>Increased motility<br>Increased fluid secretion<br>Carrier inhibition<br>Decreased enzyme production<br>No uptake of fats from lacteals |
| Unexplained | Unknown |

- Failure of nutrients to reach the small intestine, e.g. because of a bypass fistula.
- After surgical resection of gut and/or radiation therapy.

Whatever the cause, the results of malabsorption are essentially the same.

Patients complain of frothy, greasy stools, which are difficult to flush away (steatorrhoea), diarrhoea, weight loss and abdominal distension.

Anaemia may be due to deficiency of iron, folate or vitamin $B_{12}$. Vitamin K deficiency can lead to bleeding disorders, purpura (extravasation of red cells into the skin, characterized by red skin lesions, which do not blanch on pressure) and petechiae (flat, red or purple spots about the size of a pinhead in the skin or mucous membranes).

Endocrine disorders may result from generalized malnutrition and deficiencies of vitamin A and $B_1$ may lead to peripheral neuropathy.

Deficient absorption of amino acids can result in hypoalbuminaemia and oedema. Dermatitis and hyperkeratosis may also be evident in the skin. The musculoskeletal system may also be affected with osteopenia and tetany. Fig. 6.27 summarizes the systemic effects of malabsorption.

## Coeliac disease

Coeliac disease is caused by an abnormal reaction to gluten, which is found in wheat.

It is most common in northern Europe, although it occurs worldwide. Many autoimmune diseases are associated with it, for instance dermatitis herpetiformis, type 1 diabetes mellitus and thyroid disease.

The disease causes damage to the enterocytes. The precise mechanism for this is unclear, although it is suggested that environmental factors allow gliadin, a protein found in gluten, to come into contact with tissue transglutaminase in the lamina propria. The gliadin is modified by TTG and is recognized as antigenic by $CD4^+$ T cells.

Stem cells are unable to keep up with the rate of loss of enterocytes. This results in villous atrophy and the presence of immature cells, which are unable to absorb nutrients normally on the flattened surface. This, in turn, causes malabsorption and an intolerance of lactose and other sugars because of a secondary disaccharide deficiency resulting from the loss of surface epithelial cells.

The production of gastrointestinal hormones may also be deficient. This has a knock-on effect on pancreatic secretion and bile flow. Malabsorption of fat therefore predominates.

Anaemia, due to iron deficiency is a common secondary complication, as the duodenum and proximal jejunum are affected more than the ileum.

The condition predisposes to T cell lymphomas in the small intestine (an unusual small bowel lymphoma among the non-coeliac population, in whom most small bowel lymphomas are B cells).

There is also a higher incidence of other gastrointestinal cancers such as cancer of the stomach and oesophagus. Splenic atrophy may occur and all or any of the other features of malabsorption can be present.

The gold standard for diagnosis is jejunal biopsy showing evidence of villous atrophy, although antigliadin and anti-TTG assays may also be used.

Treatment is a permanent gluten-free diet, the vast majority of patients showing a marked improvement on dietary change. Gluten is present in wheat, barley, oats and rye and these must all be excluded. It is not, however, present in rice or maize.

## Tropical sprue

Tropical sprue is a chronic, progressive malabsorption in patients from, or in, the tropics (mainly the West Indies and Asia) associated with abnormalities of small intestinal structure and function. It is thought to have an infective cause.

There is diarrhoea, abdominal distension, fatigue and weight loss. Megaloblastic anaemia caused by folate deficiency is common. Overgrowth of bacteria in the small intestine is commonly found.

Like coeliac disease, there is villous atrophy, although obviously a gluten-free diet is of no help.

Treatment is with broad-spectrum antibiotics, e.g. tetracycline.

## Whipple's disease

This is a rare bacterial infection usually occurring in middle-aged men. It is 10 times more common in men and is caused by the bacterium *Tropheryma whipplei* (a Gram-positive actinomycete).

Diagnosis is by jejunal biopsy, which shows intact villi where the normal cells of the lamina propria have been replaced by 'foamy' macrophages containing PAS-positive glycoprotein granules. Similar cells may be found in lymph nodes, spleen and liver.

Treatment is with tetracycline.

**Fig. 6.27** Systemic effects of malabsorption.

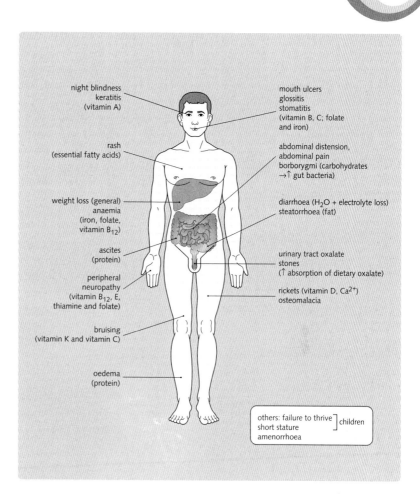

night blindness
keratitis
(vitamin A)

rash
(essential fatty acids)

weight loss (general)
anaemia
(iron, folate,
vitamin B$_{12}$)

ascites
(protein)

peripheral
neuropathy
(vitamin B$_{12}$, E,
thiamine and folate)

bruising
(vitamin K and vitamin C)

oedema
(protein)

mouth ulcers
glossitis
stomatitis
(vitamin B, C; folate
and iron)

abdominal distension,
abdominal pain
borborygmi (carbohydrates
→↑ gut bacteria)

diarrhoea (H$_2$O + electrolyte loss)
steatorrhoea (fat)

urinary tract oxalate
stones
(↑ absorption of dietary oxalate)

rickets (vitamin D, Ca$^{2+}$)
osteomalacia

others: failure to thrive ⎤ children
short stature
amenorrhoea

## Bacterial overgrowth

The small intestine normally supports a large number of flora but these are kept in check by peristalsis, the acidity of chyme leaving the stomach and the secretion of immunoglobulins into the intestinal lumen by the mucosal cells.

Where one or more of these factors is reduced, e.g. if there is a structural abnormality, bacterial overgrowth may occur. It may also occur in the elderly for unknown causes.

Jejunal biopsy may show a normal mucosa. Diagnosis is with the hydrogen breath test—an early rise in breath hydrogen levels is diagnostic.

These organisms may inactivate bile acids in the lumen by dehydroxylation, leading to fat malabsorption. The gut flora may catabolize ingested protein, metabolize sugars and bind vitamin B$_{12}$, preventing its absorption. Vitamin K levels may, however, be raised as the bacteria may produce it.

Treatment is with antibiotics, such as tetracycline, metronidazole or ciprofloxacin.

## Giardiasis

Giardiasis, prevalent in the tropics, is an important cause of traveller's diarrhoea. It is caused by the flagellate protozoan *Giardia lamblia*, which lives in the duodenum and jejunum and is transmitted by the faecal–oral route. It is more common among male homosexuals, in the immunosuppressed and in those with achlorhydria. Cases may occur in Britain among people who have never been abroad.

Asymptomatic carriage may occur. Alternatively, symptoms may develop within 1 or 2 weeks of ingesting cysts.

*Giardia lamblia* exists as a trophozoite and a cyst, the cyst being the transmissible form. Intestinal damage varies from slight changes in villous architecture to partial villous atrophy with severe malabsorption.

Diagnosis is by examination of stool. Both cysts and kite-shaped trophozoites may be found, but their absence does not exclude the diagnosis: in some cases they are only excreted at intervals. The parasite may also be seen in duodenal aspirates and in a jejunal biopsy.

Blood tests may show IgM antibodies to *Giardia* in acute infection and, later, anti-*Giardia* IgG. Treatment is with metronidazole or tinidazole.

## Abetalipoproteinaemia

Abetalipoproteinaemia is a rare autosomal recessive disorder, in which there is a failure to synthesize apo B-100 in the liver and apo B-48 in interstitial cells.

Normally, lipids (principally triglyceride cholesterol and cholesterol esters) are surrounded by a stabilizing coat of phospholipid because they are insoluble. Apoproteins are embedded in the surface of the complex of lipids and phospholipids to form lipoproteins.

In abetalipoproteinaemia, lipoproteins containing B apoproteins (for example, chylomicrons) cannot be made.

An absence of chylomicrons leads to accumulation of triglycerides within the absorptive cells of the gut, as they are responsible for transporting fat digestion products to the liver and peripheral tissues. Lipid vacuolation can be seen in these cells on biopsy.

Complications include atypical retinitis pigmentosa and neurological abnormalities, both linked to the malabsorption of the fat-soluble vitamins A, D, E and K.

The disease is characterized by failure to thrive, diarrhoea and steatorrhoea in infancy.

## Disaccharide deficiency

Normally, disaccharides in the diet are hydrolysed by lactase or sucrase on the luminal surface of mucosal cells. Lactase activity is high at birth, but it declines during childhood and it is low in adults.

Disaccharide deficiency leads to diarrhoea, bloating and flatulence, particularly with a high-milk diet.

Diarrhoea in lactase deficiency is caused by a failure to digest and absorb lactose. Lactose is broken down by bowel bacteria into its constituents glucose and galactose, and then to lactic acid. This process causes osmotic diarrhoea.

Increased disaccharide residues in the lower small intestine and colon lead to increased gas production and flatulence.

Congenital lactase deficiency is rare. Acquired deficiency due to decreased activity of lactase is common, however, and seen in about 15% of Caucasians and 70–90% of other races.

Congenital disaccharide deficiency becomes apparent early in life because of milk intolerance, which leads to the production of explosive, watery, frothy stools and abdominal distension. The more common acquired lactase deficiency often becomes apparent during viral and bacterial enteric infection.

## Neoplastic disease

Small intestinal tumours are rare. Patients may present with obstruction, bleeding, intussusception or volvulus.

Benign tumours include:

- Lipomas.
- Leiomyomas.
- Adenomas (often benign).
- Hamartomas.

Malignant lesions include:

- Adenocarcinomas.
- Carcinoid (see Chapter 7 for a fuller description).
- Lymphomas.
- Metastases, from lung, or melanoma.

## OVERVIEW

The large intestine extends from the ileocaecal junction to the anus, and is about 1.5 m in length.

Its main role is to concentrate faeces by absorbing water, hence it also plays a role in water and electrolyte balance. It also has to move faeces through its length to the anus; secreted mucus helps to lubricate the passage of faeces.

## ANATOMY

The large intestine can be divided into seven sections (Fig. 7.1):

- The caecum and appendix.
- The ascending colon.
- The transverse colon.
- The descending colon.
- The sigmoid colon.
- The rectum.
- The anal canal.

The outer, longitudinal muscle forms three distinct bands visible at dissection called taenia coli. These bands are shorter than the circular muscle layer and gather the caecum and colon into a series of pouch-like folds called haustrations or sacculations.

The haustra are visible on radiographs when an opaque medium is introduced through the rectum.

The outer surface of the large intestine has appendices epiploicae projecting from it. These are sacs of omentum distended with fat.

> The large intestine is easily distinguished from the small intestine as its haustra do not extend across the entire width, unlike the small intestine which has plicae circulares (also called valves of Kerckring or valvulae conniventes) visible across the whole width on radiographs.

### Caecum

The caecum is a sac lying in the right iliac fossa. It is continuous with the ascending colon distally and the ileum proximally, with which it communicates through the ileocaecal valve (Fig. 7.2).

> The ileocaecal valve is incompetent. This is good, because it prevents the build-up of wind or stools in the colon and allows the easing of pressure across the valve.

**Fig. 7.1** The large intestine.

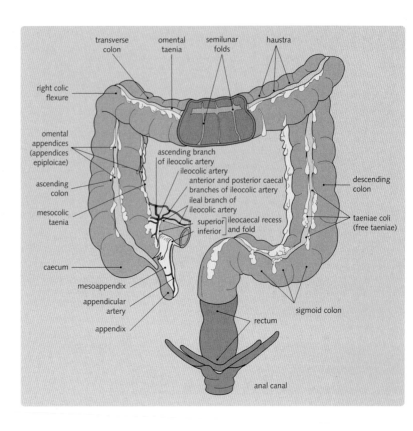

It is covered entirely in peritoneum, but has no mesentery. The caecum is often attached by peritoneal caecal folds to the iliac fossa to form the retrocaecal recess, a small peritoneal cavity in which the appendix lies.

The caecum is supplied by the ileocolic artery, a branch of the superior mesenteric artery. Venous blood from the caecum drains via the ileocolic vein into the superior mesenteric vein.

It is innervated via the superior mesenteric plexus.

## Appendix

The (vermiform) appendix is about 8 cm in length and protrudes from the posterolateral wall of the caecum (Fig. 7.1). It has aggregations of lymphatic tissue and the three taenia coli of the caecum come together at the base of the appendix, forming an outer longitudinal muscle coat.

It is a blind-ending sac and so may become inflamed (appendicitis) if obstructed, e.g. by faecoliths, which are small, hard masses of faeces. This requires

surgical removal of the appendix to prevent rupture and peritonitis.

The appendix is mobile as it has a mesentery, the mesoappendix. Because of this and the way it develops (see later), its position is variable. It usually lies behind the caecum or in the pelvis.

## Blood supply and lymphatic drainage

The appendix is covered in peritoneum and supplied by the appendicular artery (a branch of the ileocolic artery), which lies in the mesentery (the mesoappendix) that connects the appendix to the terminal ileum.

The ileocolic vein drains the appendix.

The lymphatic drainage and innervation for the caecum and appendix is the same. The lymph drains into the ileocolic lymph nodes (which lie along the ileocolic artery) and the lymph nodes in the mesoappendix.

## Innervation

The innervation to the caecum and appendix comes from the coeliac and superior mesenteric plexuses.

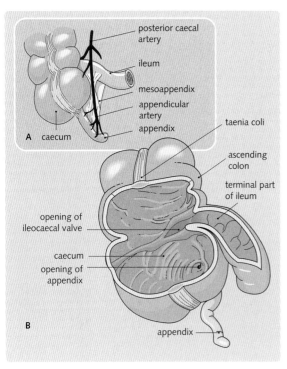

**Fig. 7.2** The ileocaecal valve (exterior view [A] and cutaway view [B]) and the appendix.

The base of the appendix is usually constant and can be located deep to McBurney's point. This is found at the junction of the lateral and middle thirds of the line between the anterior superior iliac spine and the umbilicus.

A gridiron incision can be made here to gain access to the appendix during appendicectomy.

## Ascending colon

The ascending colon arises from the ileocaecal valve to the inferior surface of the liver, where it turns to the left forming the hepatic (right colic) flexure (Fig. 7.1).

It has no mesentery and lies retroperitoneally. However, it has peritoneum covering the lateral and anterior surfaces, which attaches it to the posterior abdominal wall. The peritoneum on the medial and lateral sides of the ascending colon forms the right paracolic gutter.

Anterior to the ascending colon lie the coils of the small intestine and the greater omentum. These separate it from the anterior abdominal wall.

Posteriorly are the iliacus, transversus abdominis and quadratus lumborum muscles, and the right kidney.

## Blood supply and lymphatic drainage

The ascending colon, being a midgut structure, is supplied by the right colic artery and ileocolic artery, which are branches of the superior mesenteric artery.

Its venous drainage is via the right colic and ileo-colic veins, which drain into the superior mesenteric vein.

Lymph from this region drains to the paracolic and epicolic lymph nodes. These drain into the superior mesenteric lymph nodes.

## Innervation

Innervation to the ascending colon comes from the coeliac and superior mesenteric plexuses, like that of the caecum and appendix.

## Transverse colon

The transverse colon is not actually transverse, but extends from the hepatic (right colic) flexure to the splenic (left colic) flexure. It is the largest part of the large intestine and is about 45–50 cm in length.

The transverse colon is mobile due to its length and the presence of a mesentery (the mesocolon). This double layer of peritoneum is attached to the inferior border of the pancreas and greater omentum and allows the transverse colon to hang from the posterior abdominal wall, usually to the level of the umbilicus.

The splenic flexure is slightly more superior than the hepatic flexure, due to the spleen being smaller than the liver. The splenic flexure is attached to the diaphragm by the phrenicocolic ligament, a fold of peritoneum.

## Blood supply and lymphatic drainage

The arterial blood supply is from the middle, right and left colic arteries (Fig. 6.3B). The middle colic artery is the major arterial supply. It is a branch of the superior mesenteric artery, along with the right colic artery. These supply the proximal two-thirds of the transverse colon which is derived from the midgut.

The left colic artery is a branch of the inferior mesenteric artery supplying its distal, hindgut-derived third.

The superior mesenteric vein drains the transverse colon, and its lymph drains to the lymph nodes along the middle colic artery. These then drain into the superior mesenteric lymph nodes.

## Innervation

Innervation to the transverse colon comes from the superior mesenteric plexus, which follows the path of the middle and right colic arteries.

The nerves from the inferior mesenteric plexus follow the path of the left colic artery. Both sympathetic and parasympathetic (vagal) nerves supply the transverse colon.

# Descending colon

The descending colon is about 30 cm in length and is the narrowest part of the colon.

It extends from the splenic flexure to the left iliac fossa at the pelvic brim, where it becomes the sigmoid colon.

The descending colon has no mesentery and lies retroperitoneally, attached to the posterior abdominal wall. Like the ascending colon, it has paracolic gutters medially and laterally.

The lateral border of the left kidney, the transversus abdominis and quadratus lumborum muscles lie posterior to the descending colon.

## Blood supply and lymphatic drainage

The left colic and superior sigmoid arteries supply the descending colon. Both are branches of the inferior mesenteric artery.

Venous drainage is via the inferior mesenteric vein. The lymph drains to the intermediate colic lymph nodes, which lie along the left colic artery.

## Innervation

Parasympathetic innervation comes from the pelvic splanchnic nerves and sympathetic innervation is derived from the lumbar part of the sympathetic trunk and the superior hypogastric plexus.

# Sigmoid colon

The sigmoid colon is S-shaped and lies in the left iliac fossa. It extends from the pelvic brim to join the rectum at the level of S3.

The sigmoid colon has a long mesentery called the sigmoid mesocolon, which has a V-shaped root attachment. Therefore, it is very mobile.

It lies anterior to the left external iliac vessels, the left sacral plexus and the left piriformis muscle. Parts of it can also be found in the rectouterine pouch (of Douglas) in females or the rectovesical pouch in males.

Long appendices epiploicae hang from the external wall of the sigmoid colon. The position, size and shape of the sigmoid colon depend on how full of faeces it is. This is the main storage site of faeces, prior to defecation.

> The sigmoid colon is the part of the colon most prone to volvulus due to its length and high mobility. It is also the part most susceptible to perforation as it has the highest pressure in the colon and its walls are the weakest.

## Blood supply and lymphatic drainage

The sigmoid colon is supplied by two or three sigmoid arteries. These descend to the left and divide into ascending and descending branches. The descending branch of the left colic artery anastomoses with the most superior sigmoid artery.

The inferior mesenteric vein drains blood from the sigmoid colon, while the lymph drains to the intermediate colic lymph nodes, as in the descending colon.

## Innervation

The innervation is the same as that to the descending colon.

# Rectum

The rectum is continuous with the sigmoid colon proximally and the anus distally.

It starts at the level of S3, in the posterior part of the pelvis and curves along the sacrum and coccyx, in an S-shaped course before widening to form the rectal ampulla.

It has no mesentery and so is immobile.

Peritoneum covers the anterior and lateral surfaces in the superior third, and the anterior surface only in the middle third. The inferior third is not covered.

In males, it is reflected from the bladder to form the rectovesical pouch while in women it is reflected from the vagina to form the rectouterine pouch (of Douglas).

The rectum has three flexures, the most important being the anorectal flexure. This is produced by the puborectalis muscle encircling the rectum at the junction with the anal canal to form a 'sling' and a 90° anorectal angle.

At each flexure is a transverse fold formed by infoldings of the rectal wall. They are maintained by the taeniae coli and partly close the lumen.

The relations of the rectum are different in the male and female. In the male, the bladder, prostate, seminal vesicles and vasa deferentia lie in front of it; in the female it is related anteriorly to the uterus and vagina.

Posterior to the rectum lie:

- The three inferior sacral vertebrae.
- The coccyx.
- The anococcygeal ligament.
- The median sacral vessels.
- Branches of the superior rectal artery.
- The inferior ends of the sympathetic trunks and sacral plexuses.

The rectal ampulla stores faeces before defecation and is very distendable. It is supported by the levator ani muscles.

## Blood supply and lymphatic drainage

The arterial supply to the rectum comes from a number of sources:

- The median sacral arteries.
- The superior, middle and inferior rectal arteries. These supply the corresponding parts of the rectum.

The rectal arteries anastomose with each other. The superior rectal artery is a continuation of the inferior mesenteric artery while the middle and inferior rectal arteries are branches of the internal iliac arteries and the internal pudendal arteries, respectively.

The superior, middle and inferior rectal veins drain the rectum. They anastomose to form internal and external venous plexuses.

The external plexus is outside the muscular wall and the internal plexus is just deep to the mucosa. The internal venous plexus communicates with the uterovaginal venous plexus in the female and the vesical venous plexus in the male.

The different areas of the rectal venous plexus drain into different vessels:

- The superior part drains into the superior rectal vein, then into the inferior mesenteric vein.
- The middle part drains into the middle rectal vein, then into the internal iliac vein.
- The inferior part drains into the internal pudendal vein.

The superior rectal veins drain into the portal system and the inferior rectal veins drain into the systemic circulation. The rectum is thus a site of a porto-systemic anastomosis (see Chapter 4).

The superior part of the rectum drains lymph into the pararectal lymph nodes, which then drain to the sigmoid mesocolon lymph nodes and inferior mesenteric lymph nodes. The inferior part of the rectum drains lymph into the internal iliac lymph nodes.

## Innervation

The rectum receives sympathetic and parasympathetic innervation. Nerves from the inferior hypogastric plexus make up the middle rectal plexus.

Parasympathetic innervation is derived from S1, S3 and S4 nerves, which run with the pelvic splanchnic nerves, finally joining up with the inferior hypogastric plexus.

Sensory fibres follow the sympathetic fibres and are stimulated by rectal distension.

## Anus

The anal canal is continuous with the rectum and is about 3 cm long. It begins at the anorectal flexure and it is surrounded by the levator ani muscles, ending at the anus.

The anal canal descends between the perineal body and the anococcygeal ligament. The ischioanal fossae are two wedge-shaped spaces on either side of the anal canal.

The anus has an internal and an external sphincter (Fig. 7.3). The external sphincter surrounds the lower two thirds of the anal canal and is composed of striated muscle. It is thus under voluntary control, allowing delay of defecation.

The internal sphincter surrounds the upper two thirds of the anal canal and is made up of involuntary circular smooth muscle continuous with that

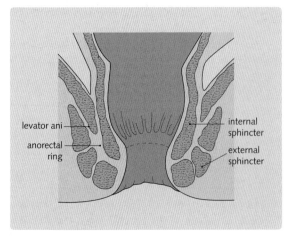

Fig. 7.3 The rectum and anal canal, showing the anal sphincters.

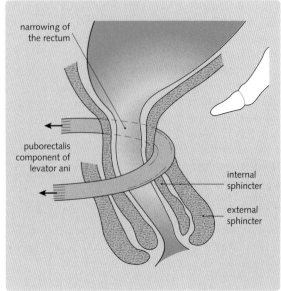

Fig. 7.4 The ano-rectal junction.

of the rectum. Both sphincters must relax for defecation to occur.

In the male, the anal canal lies behind the prostate and the bulb of the penis. The perineal body separates it from these structures, but a digital rectal examination can give important information about the prostate. In the female, the perineal body separates the anal canal from the vagina.

In the mucosa of the superior half are six to twelve longitudinal ridges called anal columns. They contain the terminal branches of the superior rectal artery and vein.

The superior ends of the anal columns mark the anorectal line or junction (Fig. 7.4). Folds of epithelium, called anal valves, connect the inferior ends of the anal columns.

Just superior to the anal valves are the anal sinuses, which release mucus to aid defecation.

The pectinate line is found between the superior and inferior parts of the anal canal. It is the boundary between the columnar epithelium of the superior part and the stratified squamous epithelium of the inferior part.

Anal canal structures above the pectinate line have developed from the endodermal hindgut. Structures below the pectinate line have developed from the ectodermal anal pit, or proctodeum. Therefore, the differences in blood, lymphatic and nerve supply above and below the pectinate line are due to embryological development.

## Blood supply and lymphatic drainage

The superior and both inferior rectal arteries drain the areas superior and inferior to the pectinate line respectively.

The terminal branches of the superior rectal artery anastomose in the anal valves. The middle rectal arteries anastomose with the superior and inferior rectal arteries.

Venous drainage occurs via the internal rectal venous plexus to the superior and inferior rectal veins respectively.

The veins in the wall of the anal canal provide a cushion for the passage of faeces and help to close the anus, but they can enlarge to form haemorrhoids.

In the superior part of the anal canal, the lymph drains to the internal iliac lymph nodes and then into the common iliac and lumbar lymph nodes. In the inferior part of the anal canal, lymph drainage is to the superficial inguinal nodes.

## Innervation

Superior to the pectinate line, the sympathetic nerve supply is derived from the inferior hypogastric plexus. The parasympathetic supply comes from the pelvic splanchnic nerves.

Inferior to the pectinate line, the nerve supply comes from the inferior rectal nerves, which are branches of the pudendal nerve. This region is sensitive to touch, temperature and pain.

The pelvic splanchnic nerves (parasympathetic) and the aortic and pelvic plexuses (sympathetic) innervate the internal anal sphincter.

The inferior rectal nerve, a branch of the pudendal nerve and the perineal branch of S4 innervate the external anal sphincter.

# EMBRYOLOGY AND DEVELOPMENT

This section focuses solely on the development of the large intestine. However, as it develops in tandem with the small intestine, it may be useful to read this section with its counterpart in Chapter 6.

The caecal bud appears on the caudal limb of the primitive gut tube at about week 6 and develops into the caecal swelling, which is the last part of the developing tube to re-enter the abdominal cavity.

The appendix develops from the distal end of the swelling during the descent of the colon and may come to lie in a variety of positions. However, it is usually found posterior to the large intestine.

Failure of the intestinal loops to return to the abdominal cavity results in exomphalos, the protrusion of abdominal contents through the abdominal wall at the site of insertion of the cord. The contents of this hernia are covered by amnion (which distinguishes them from gastroschisis—see later).

The distal third of the transverse colon and the upper part of the anal canal arise from the hindgut. They are supplied by the inferior mesenteric artery.

The distal part of the hindgut grows into the cloaca, an endodermal-lined cavity, which is in contact with the surface ectoderm.

During the 9th week of development, the anal membrane ruptures to open up the rectum to the external environment.

In the anal canal, the pectinate line indicates the junction between the endodermal and ectodermal parts. It is also the point at which the columnar epithelium in the upper part of the anal canal changes to stratified squamous epithelium in the lower part.

# HISTOLOGY

The tissue layers of the large intestine are essentially the same as those in the rest of the gastrointestinal tract (see Fig. 1.2).

However, the muscle walls are thicker in order to facilitate faecal movement, the lumen is larger and the outer longitudinal muscle layer forms taeniae coli visible on the outside of the intestine.

## Mucosa

The mucosa is thrown into folds when not distended. It consists of simple columnar epithelium and contains numerous straight tubular glands that extend throughout its thickness. Unlike the small intestine, there are no villi or plicae circulares.

The glands consist of two main types of cells: columnar absorptive cells and mucus-secreting goblet cells. The former are mainly found at the luminal surfaces, while goblet cells and stem cells which replenish the epithelium are found at the gland bases.

Paneth cells are present only when young. Isolated nodules of lymphatic tissue are found that extend into the submucosa.

The muscularis mucosae is prominent. Its contractions prevent clogging of the glands by aiding faecal movement.

## Anorectal junction

The rectum narrows towards its terminal end and it becomes the anal canal (Fig. 7.4).

The upper portion of the anal canal contains longitudinal folds (anal or rectal columns) separated by depressions (anal sinuses).

The sinuses contain straight, branched tubular glands (anal glands) which produce mucus and extend into the submucosa and sometimes into the muscularis externa.

The ducts of the anal glands open into crypts in the anal mucosa, and may thus become infected or blocked, forming a cyst.

The mucosa of the upper anal canal is similar to that of the large intestine but the lower portion consists of stratified squamous epithelium, continuous with the skin surrounding the anal canal. The middle portion contains stratified columnar epithelium.

Small folds of mucosa (anal valves) are present at the lower end of the anal canal. Above these, the mucosa is folded longitudinally forming the columns of Morgagni.

# THE FLORA OF THE LARGE INTESTINE

Most of the flora of the large intestine are anaerobes, e.g. *Bacteroides fragilis*. The large intestine also supports coliforms such as *Escherichia coli* and faecal streptococci, including *Enterococcus faecalis*.

There are at least 400 species of bacteria in the large bowel, with over $10^{10}$ organisms per gram of stool. Approximately one quarter of the weight of stool is bacteria.

Commensal bacteria keep pathogenic bacteria at bay by competing with them for space and nutrients. The significance of this becomes apparent during antibiotic administration. Antibiotics disrupt the normal flora and predispose to clostridial and other gut infections.

The intestinal flora convert conjugated bilirubin to urobilinogen, some of which is reabsorbed and excreted in the urine.

The flora also convert the remainder of the urobilinogen to stercobilinogen which is excreted in the faeces.

Many patients taking broad-spectrum antibiotics, e.g. cephalosporins and ampicillin develop diarrhoea which normally resolves on stopping the drug. However, in some patients an overgrowth of *Clostridium difficile* may ensue, causing pseudomembranous colitis (see later in the text).

Prophylactic antibiotics may be given during and after surgery when operating on a 'dirty site' like the large intestine.

The type and dose of antibiotic(s) given depend on the organisms likely to be encountered, and therefore the site of the operation. Commonly used antibiotics include cefuroxime and metronidazole.

Cefuroxime is effective against Gram-negatives e.g. *Neisseria* and coliforms, and metronidazole against Gram-negative and Gram-positive anaerobes. Most anaerobes are sensitive to metronidazole, but aerobes are not.

# FUNCTIONS AND PHYSIOLOGY

## Water absorption

Absorption of water in the colon is similar to the mechanism used to concentrate the contents of the gall bladder described in Chapter 5.

$Na^+$ and $Cl^-$ are pumped into the paracellular (lateral intercellular) spaces and water follows by osmosis. Water molecules, $Na^+$ and $Cl^-$ then flow through the lateral intercellular spaces away from the lumen, and across the basement membrane of the epithelial cells of the colon.

Some $Cl^-$ from the colonic lumen also crosses the tight junction into the intercellular space because of the potential difference. It travels in the opposite direction to $K^+$ and increases the concentration of $Cl^-$ in the intercellular space and, therefore, the passage of water.

The concentration of ions in that part of the intercellular space closest to the lumen is hypertonic, but the fluid at the basement membrane end is isotonic. It is the isotonic fluid that crosses the basement membrane and moves into the intestinal capillaries. Absorbed amino acids and sugars also increase the osmotic absorption of water.

Abnormalities in water absorption in the intestines can result in diarrhoea (see later).

## Transport of urea and electrolytes

The main function of the colon is absorption. It absorbs over 90% of the water from the contents passing through it, reducing the volume from 1–2 L to about 200 mL of semi-solid faecal matter.

By the time they reach the end of the gastro-intestinal tract, faeces are about 50–75% water. The remainder is solid material, which is partly composed of bacteria and desquamated mucosal cells. Desquamated cells largely account for the fact that a starving person continues to produce stools.

The ion transport processes of the colon are shown in Fig. 7.5. $Na^+$ in the lumen is exchanged for $H^+$ ($Na^+$ is pumped into the epithelial cells and $H^+$ pumped out of it). $HCO_3^-$ is exchanged for $Cl^-$ ($Cl^-$ is reabsorbed, bicarbonate pumped out).

In addition, paracellular spaces exist into which $Na^+$ and $Cl^-$ is pumped, and from which $K^+$ passes out into the lumen. $K^+$ is pumped into the cells in exchange for the $Na^+$ pumped out into the paracellular spaces.

The net result of this is the creation of a potential difference of about $-30$ mV across the colonic mucosa (a greater difference than that across the jejunal and ileal mucosa).

It is this potential difference that allows the passage of $K^+$ across the tight junctions from the paracellular space into the lumen and accounts for the potassium-rich secretions found in the colon.

Urea synthesis is greater than its excretion by about 20%. The excess is secreted into the colon for metabolism by bacteria. The products are then absorbed.

Metabolism occurs near the mucosa, rather than in the lumen. $NH_4^+$ and $HCO_3^-$ ions are produced and converted into $NH_3$, $CO_2$ and water. These freely diffuse across the mucosal epithelium into the circulation. The $NH_3$ is transported to the liver for synthesis of amino acids. Electrolyte movement in the colon is shown in Fig. 7.5.

## Secretion of mucus

The colonic mucosa has many goblet cells in its crypts and surface epithelium. They secrete mucus in response to mechanical irritation of the mucosa caused by substances passing through it, and as a result of cholinergic stimulation.

Conversely, secretion of mucus is inhibited by sympathetic stimulation.

Mucus lubricates the colon, preventing trauma from the contents passing through it, which become increasingly solid as water is reabsorbed on the way

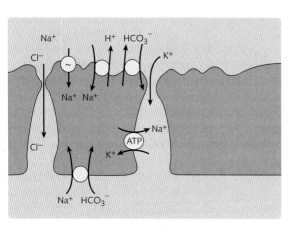

**Fig. 7.5** Electrolyte movement in the colon.

through. The ratio of mucous to aqueous secretion is greater in the colon than elsewhere in the gastrointestinal tract.

The aqueous component contains bicarbonate, which plays an important role in buffering, and is rich in potassium. Chloride is absorbed in exchange for bicarbonate.

## Motility of the large intestine

The movement of intestinal contents through the colon is slower than that seen in the rest of the gastrointestinal tract. This is partly due to the nature of the activity and partly due to its absorptive function of water and electrolytes.

The large intestine has three main modes of movement:

- Segmental (or haustral) contractions.
- Peristalsis.
- Mass movement.

### Segmental contractions

Segmental (or haustral) contractions are brought about by the contraction of the taeniae coli. These three bands of longitudinal muscles gather the colon into haustra. The haustra fill with intestinal contents and the distension stimulates contraction.

Contraction of adjacent haustra causes a mixing effect and allows the contents to be in contact with the mucosal surfaces, thus facilitating absorption.

Segmental contractions are initiated by acetylcholine and substance P release.

### Peristalsis

Peristalsis is slower in the large intestine than in the small intestine. It provides waves of propulsive contractions, slowly moving the intestinal contents towards the anus. As in the small intestine, distension initiates the contractions and vagal inhibitory and excitatory fibres control the movement.

### Mass movement

Mass movement describes the intense contraction that begins halfway along the transverse colon and pushes the intestinal contents towards the rectum. This type of contraction occurs only a few times a day and is responsible for colonic evacuation.

It occurs shortly after a meal and if faeces are present in the rectum, stimulates the urge to defecate. This is called the gastrocolic reflex. It is partly neuronal and partly hormonal (via the action of cholecystokinin). The gastrocolic reflex is particularly strong after breakfast.

## Control of colonic motility

As in other parts of the gastrointestinal tract, Auerbach's and Meissner's plexuses are present in the walls of the colon (see Fig. 1.2). Their activity is modulated by parasympathetic and sympathetic activity.

Parasympathetic stimulation is via branches of the vagus and pelvic nerves from the sacral spinal cord. It increases contraction of the proximal colon, allowing greater absorption of salts and water.

Sympathetic innervation is via the superior and inferior mesenteric and hypogastric plexuses. It decreases colonic movements.

Colo-colonic reflexes occur (mediated in part by the sympathetic system) causing one part of the colon to relax if an adjacent part is distended (Fig. 7.6).

## Defecation

### Control of defecation

The urge to defecate is felt because stretching of the rectum causes impulses in the cholinergic parasympathetic nerves of the pelvis. These are transmitted to a nerve centre in the sacral spinal cord. A pressure of about 18 mmHg in the rectum is needed.

Impulses are then conveyed to higher centres, allowing an individual to decide whether to defecate, i.e. whether to voluntarily relax the external sphincter, or not. In the latter case, the internal sphincter will recontract and the urge to defecate will subside.

As mentioned earlier, the external anal sphincter is made up of striated (voluntary) muscle while the internal sphincter is composed of involuntary smooth muscle. The latter relaxes as a reflex in response to distension of the distal rectum.

Intact Auerbach's and Meissner's plexuses are needed for this reflex relaxation to occur. Thus in Hirschsprung's disease (see later), the internal sphincter does not relax in response to colonic distension as there is a congenital absence of ganglion cells in these plexuses in the rectum and sometimes in the colon.

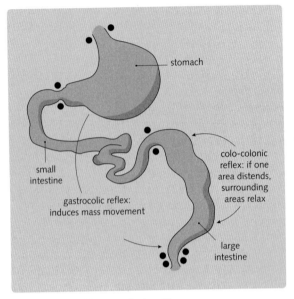

**Fig. 7.6** Control of large intestinal motility.

If there has been damage to the spinal nerves and therefore to the control of the external sphincter, it will relax when the pressure in the rectum reaches about 55 mmHg.

The anal canal is a remarkable structure. It can differentiate between air, liquid and solid contents, and allow the selective release of air as flatus.

Normally the rectum is distended as a result of mass movements filling it with faecal material. It may also be distended by a neoplasm or other mass, however, giving rise to tenesmus (the feeling of incomplete evacuation).

Patients complaining of tenesmus should be investigated promptly so that neoplasms are not missed.

## Mechanics of defecation

When a person decides to defecate, i.e. when the external sphincter is voluntarily relaxed, an increase in intra-abdominal pressure must be achieved to expel the faeces.

Thus, a breath is taken in and the glottis closes over the trachea. The respiratory muscles contract on lungs filled with air, which increases both the intrathoracic and intra-abdominal pressures.

The pelvic floor muscles relax and the floor 'drops', thus straightening the rectum and preventing rectal prolapse. The faeces are then expelled from the anus.

# PHARMACOLOGY OF INTESTINAL MOTILITY

Bowel motility is under autonomic control (see earlier). Two classes of drugs increase bowel movements: laxatives, which cause purgation and true motility stimulants, which do not. Antidiarrhoeals and antispasmodics decrease bowel movements. The modes of action of these drugs vary (Fig. 7.7).

## Drugs which increase movements

### Laxatives

Strictly speaking, laxatives (also known as purgatives) do not increase gastrointestinal motility. However, they do increase the speed with which food passes through the intestine, hence the purgation. There are four kinds of laxative: osmotic laxatives, bulk laxatives, stimulant laxatives and faecal softeners.

### Osmotic laxatives

Osmotic laxatives accelerate the transit of food by preserving the higher water contect of residue in the small intestine. An increased (hydrated) volume is thus delivered to the colon, distending it and causing purgation. They are poorly absorbed solutes, which accounts for their osmotic effect.

Two types of osmotic laxatives are in use: lactulose and the saline purgatives. Lactulose is a semi-synthetic disaccharide of fructose and galactose which is degraded to its component monosaccharides by gut bacteria. These are then fermented, producing lactate and acetate which draw water into the intestine by osmosis. Lactulose takes 2–3 days to have an effect.

The main saline purgatives are magnesium sulphate and magnesium hydroxide. As they are insoluble salts, they remain in the intestinal lumen and osmotically increase water content.

### Bulk laxatives

These are polysaccharides which cannot be digested. They act by retaining water and promoting peristalsis. However, they take several days to work but have no major side-effects. Examples include methylcellulose, bran and sterculia.

**Fig. 7.7** Sites and mechanisms of action of drugs which affect intestinal motility. (ACh = acetylcholine.)

### Stimulant laxatives

As their name suggests, they act possibly by stimulating enteric nerves causing increased mucosal water and electrolyte secretion. Senna is an important example of this class of drug. It is a glycoside of sugars with anthracene derivatives like emodin. In the colon, senna is hydrolysed, releasing free anthracene derivatives which then stimulate the myenteric plexus. As a result, smooth muscle activity is increased and defecation occurs.

Other examples are bisacodyl and sodium picosulphate (Picolax); the latter is commonly used when preparing the bowel for surgery ('bowel prep').

### Faecal softeners

An example of a faecal softener is docusate sodium, which acts via a detergent action in the intestine. It is also a weak stimulant laxative.

## Motility stimulants

There are two main drugs in this category: metoclopramide and domperidone. All increase motility but without causing purgation.

The anti-emetic function of metoclopramide has already been mentioned above. In addition to that, however, metoclopramide also acts locally in the stomach to stimulate acetylcholine release. Consequently, gastric motility is stimulated, with an increase in gastric emptying but without a corresponding increase in gastric acid secretion.

Domperidone is another dopamine-receptor antagonist. However, the mechanism by which it enhances gastrointestinal motility is unexplained, although it has been suggested that it acts to facilitate acetylcholine release from the myenteric plexus as well. Its effects are to increase gastric emptying (without increasing gastric acid secretion) and duodenal peristalsis, as well as increasing the pressure of the lower oesophageal sphincter.

## Drugs which decrease movements

### Antidiarrhoeal drugs

When treating diarrhoea (see later), the maintenance of normal fluid and electrolyte balance must be the first priority. Then, depending on the aetiology, either antimicrobial drugs or non-antimicrobial drugs may be necessary. Antimicrobial drugs are beyond the scope of this book; for more information on them

consult the relevant chapter in *Crash Course: Pharmacology*.

If fluid and electrolyte balance is deranged due to excessive loss, it can be restored by means of oral rehydration solutions. These are easy to use; the most common preparation is a powder mix of glucose and sodium chloride which can be dissolved in water. Glucose increases sodium, and thus water, absorption as it is absorbed by secondary active transport with sodium. The use of oral rehydration therapy may be sufficient in many cases; in fact, it is the treatment of choice for cholera.

The main non-antimicrobial antidiarrhoeal drugs are opioids. Opioids act on μ-receptors on myenteric neurons. The tone and contractions of the intestinal smooth muscle are increased, but opioids also reduce peristalsis, making a reduction in gastrointestinal motility their overall effect. Additionally, they also increase the tone of the pyloric, ileocolic and anal sphincters. For a more detailed account of the mechanism of action of opioids, see the relevant chapter in *Crash Course: Pharmacology*.

Loperamide, codeine and diphenoxylate are the main opiates used in the treatment of diarrhoea. Loperamide and codeine also have antisecretory effects besides inhibiting gastrointestinal motility. Note, however, that the opioids used to treat diarrhoea have side-effects such as constipation, drowsiness and abdominal cramps, and should not be used in young children.

You should be able to work out the major side-effects of drugs by understanding their mechanism of action, especially as many drugs are not selective for a particular organ or system. A good understanding of pharmacology is therefore essential.

## Antispasmodics

Antispasmodics are sometimes used in the treatment of irritable bowel syndrome and diverticular disease. Two types exist: muscarinic receptor antagonists and mebeverine. The former decrease muscle tone by inhibiting parasympathetic activity in the alimentary tract. Examples are dicyclomine and propantheline. As would be expected of parasympathetic blockade, side-effects include dry mouth, decreased sweating and blurred vision. Mebeverine acts directly on gastrointestinal smooth muscle causing it to relax.

# DISORDERS OF THE LARGE INTESTINE

The diseases and disorders covered in this section affect primarily the large intestine and/or both small and large intestines.

## Congenital abnormalities

### Hirschsprung's disease (congenital aganglionic megacolon)

Hirschsprung's disease is caused by an absence of ganglion cells in Auerbach's and Meissner's plexuses in the distal bowel as a result of the failure of neuroblasts to migrate during weeks 5–12 of gestation.

When these parasympathetic plexuses fail to develop, the circular muscle layer of the intestine goes into spasm, resulting in intestinal obstruction. As in other causes of obstruction, dilatation of the intestine occurs proximal to the area in spasm (Fig. 7.8).

Hirschsprung's disease usually affects the rectum and distal colon but, in severe cases, it may also affect the small intestine. The colon may become

distended with faeces resulting in megacolon and death from acute enterocolitis.

It is four times more likely to occur in males and severe cases may become apparent shortly after birth with symptoms of obstruction. Less severe cases may simply result in chronic constipation.

The incidence is 1 in 5000 live births; it is ten times as likely to occur in children with Down's syndrome (trisomy 21) and is often found in association with other congenital abnormalities.

Diagnosis is by barium enema and biopsy showing an absence of ganglion cells. Pressure studies show a failure of relaxation of the internal anal sphincter.

### Acquired megacolon

Megacolon may also be acquired, usually as a result of chronic constipation in childhood. It may also be seen in the elderly.

Causes of acquired megacolon include Chagas' disease, inflammatory bowel disease and bowel obstruction.

Acquired megacolon may be differentiated from Hirschsprung's disease by rectal examination. In patients with Hirschsprung's disease, a narrow empty segment of rectum can be felt, above which the colon is dilated and full of faeces. In patients with acquired megacolon, in contrast, no empty segment of rectum is felt and faeces are present in the distal rectum.

The definitive distinguishing test is a rectal biopsy. In acquired megacolon, ganglion cells are present in the rectal wall.

## Gastroschisis and exomphalos

Gastroschisis is a congenital herniation of bowel through the abdominal wall, usually just to the right of the umbilical cord.

The bowel is exposed to fetal urine *in utero* which causes inflammation and paralytic ileus, and so neonates cannot be fed orally until the bowel recovers. The condition is not associated with other abnormalities and overall mortality is about 5%.

Exomphalos occurs when the gut fails to return to the abdominal cavity after its physiological herniation and development outside the cavity during weeks 7–11 of gestation. Affected children are born with gut and sometimes liver protruding through the umbilicus, covered by amnion and hence protected from fetal urine. This is the key feature distinguishing it from gastroschisis, where the amnion does not cover the herniated intestine. The

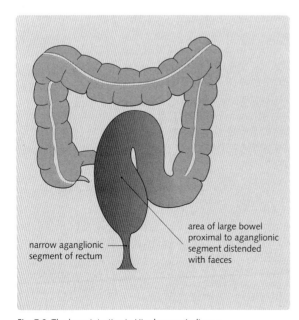

narrow aganglionic segment of rectum

area of large bowel proximal to aganglionic segment distended with faeces

**Fig. 7.8** The large intestine in Hirschsprung's disease.

condition is associated with other congenital abnormalities however, most commonly cardiac, renal or chromosomal. Overall mortality is 25–50%.

Treatment of both conditions is surgical.

# Infectious and inflammatory disease

## Diarrhoea

Diarrhoea is an increase in frequency of bowel opening associated with increased volume and fluidity of faeces. A more technical definition is passage of more than three unformed stools per 24 hours. It is important to note that a change in bowel habit, not the absolute frequency, is the key abnormality.

More water is reabsorbed in the intestine than is secreted. Clearly, if there is failure of absorption, the faeces will contain abnormal amounts of water and diarrhoea will result.

Dysentery is painful, bloody, but low-volume, diarrhoea.

Reduced absorption may be due to one or more of a number of factors including:

- An increase in the number of osmotic particles in the lumen, resulting in a flow of water into the lumen (osmotic diarrhoea).
- An increase in the rate of flow of intestinal contents, leaving less time for the absorption processes to take place (deranged motility diarrhoea).
- An abnormal increase in secretions of the gastrointestinal tract (secretory diarrhoea).

The main categories and causes of diarrhoea are summarized in Fig. 7.9.

### Osmotic diarrhoea

Both electrolytes and absorbed nutrients (such as sugar and amino acids) contribute to osmosis. If the absorption of either of these is reduced, e.g. in a protein-losing enteropathy, osmotic diarrhoea will occur.

### Secretory diarrhoea

Mature cells near the tips of the small intestinal villi are responsible for absorption. They are stimulated to increase their rate of secretion by a number of factors such as acetylcholine, substance P, 5-hydroxytryptamine (serotonin) and neurotensin, all of which increase intracellular calcium.

Potentially fatal secretory diarrhoea can also be caused by cholera. The causative organism, *Vibrio*

**Fig. 7.9** Types and causes of diarrhoea.

**Osmotic diarrhoea**
Disaccharidase deficiencies
Drug-induced
Galactose
Generalized malabsorption

**Secretory diarrhoea**
Infectious
Defects in intraluminal digestion and absorption
Excess laxative use

**Deranged motility**
Increased intestinal transit time
Decreased motility

**Malabsorption**

**Exudative diseases**
Infectious
Inflammatory bowel disease

*cholerae*, is endemic in certain parts of the developing world. Infection is spread by the faecal–oral route and pandemics are by no means unusual.

The organism can survive in the acid conditions of the stomach and multiplies in the small intestine where it produces an enterotoxin that binds to receptors on the immature cells in the crypts.

This causes an increase in adenylate cyclase, elevating cyclic AMP and increasing the secretion of $Na^+$, $Cl^-$ and water into the lumen. The main symptom is profuse 'rice water' stools.

Treatment with oral rehydration therapy to replace water and electrolytes is curative.

### Deranged motility (rapid transit) diarrhoea

Increased gut motility leads to lack of absorption (due to rapid transit), which can result in diarrhoea. Some agents may stimulate secretion as well as motility.

Gastrointestinal stasis may also cause diarrhoea by facilitating bacterial overgrowth.

## Parasitic causes of diarrhoea

The protozoan organisms *Entamoeba histolytica* and *Giardia lamblia* commonly cause diarrhoea. Both are transmitted by the faecal–oral route.

Infection with the former may be asymptomatic or cause amoebic dysentery (a notifiable disease), which may have a gradual onset accompanied by systemic symptoms, such as anorexia and headache.

Treatment of acute amoebic dysentery is with metronidazole. Diloxanide is given in chronic disease.

Giardiasis causes steatorrhoea and abdominal pain. It may also lead to malabsorption (see Chapter 6). Treatment is with metronidazole or tinidazole.

Inflammation, infection or neoplasms can cause bloody diarrhoea. If the diarrhoea is very bloody then it is due to chronic disease, such as a neoplasm or ulcerative colitis. Inflammatory bowel disease can cause chronic exudative diarrhoea.

# Infective enterocolitis

Enterocolitis is inflammation of the intestines. It may be caused by a variety of agents. In 40–50% of cases, no specific agent is isolated and an educated guess must be taken according to the age, circumstances and degree of immunocompetence of the patient.

Improved sanitation has led to a decreased prevalence of infective enterocolitis in the developed world, but it still accounts for more than 50% of all deaths before the age of 5 years worldwide and over 12 000 deaths each day among children in developing countries.

## Viral gastroenteritis

Gastroenteritis is the inflammation of the stomach and intestines. The illness includes vomiting, fever, abdominal pain and diarrhoea. The rapid loss of water and electrolytes can result in metabolic disturbances.

Causes, transmitted faecal–orally, include rotaviruses, enteric adenoviruses, caliciviruses, astroviruses and noroviruses (Fig. 7.10).

## Bacterial enterocolitis

The major causes of bacterial enterocolitis are summarized in Fig. 7.11. In the UK, *Campylobacter* infection, usually acquired by eating contaminated poultry, is the commonest cause.

The principal mechanisms by which bacterial infection may lead to gastroenteritis are:

- The ingestion of a bacterial organism that proliferates in the gut lumen and that is enterotoxic.
- Ingestion of a ready-made (preformed) toxin in contaminated food, which is heat stable, e.g. *Staphylococcus aureus*, *Vibrio cholerae* and *Clostridium perfringens*.
- The ingestion of an enteroinvasive bacterial organism, which proliferates in the gut and destroys the mucosal epithelial cells.

The incubation period can give clues as to whether the food poisoning was due to bacterial contamination or preformed toxins. Usually, the incubation period of bacterial contamination is longer, as time is required to establish an enterotoxic colony in the gut.

Treatment consists of fluid replacement therapy with antibiotics. Sometimes intravenous fluids must be given if vomiting is severe.

## Necrotizing enterocolitis

As the name suggests, this is a necrotizing inflammation of the small and large intestines (primarily the terminal ileum and ascending colon) and is the most common acquired gastrointestinal emergency in neonates.

**Fig. 7.10** Common causes of viral gastroenteritis.

| Virus | Host age | Transmission method |
| --- | --- | --- |
| Rotavirus (group A) | 6–24 months | Person-to-person, food, water |
| Astroviruses | Child | Person-to-person, water, raw shellfish |
| Norwalk-like viruses | School age, adult | Person-to-person, water, cold foods, raw shellfish |
| Enteric adenoviruses | Child under 2 years | Person-to-person |
| Caliciviruses | Child | Person-to-person, water, cold foods, raw shellfish |

**Fig. 7.11** Common causes of bacterial enterocolitis.

| Organism | Source of transmission |
|---|---|
| Campylobacter | Milk, poultry, animal contact |
| Clostridium difficile | Nosocomial environment |
| Clostridium perfringens | Meat, poultry, fish |
| Escherichia coli | Food, water, undercooked beef products, weaning foods, cheese, person-to-person |
| Mycobacterium tuberculosis | Contaminated milk, swallowing of coughed-up organisms |
| Salmonella | Milk, beef, eggs, poultry |
| Shigella | Person-to-person, low-inoculum |
| Vibrio cholerae, other vibrios | Water, shellfish, person-to-person |
| Yersinia enterocolitica | Milk, pork |

It is most common within the first few days of life (when infants start oral feeding), but it may occur at any time within the first 3 months, especially in premature or low-birth-weight babies being given formula milk rather than breast milk.

Symptoms vary from mild gastrointestinal upset to perforation of necrosed intestine leading to shock and, if untreated, death. Surgical resection of affected intestine may be necessary.

## Pseudomembranous colitis

Pseudomembranous colitis (PMC) is caused by an overgrowth of *Clostridium difficile* following antibiotic therapy, as this may suppress the normal gut flora.

There is loss of epithelial cells and the formation of a whitish pseudomembrane on the bowel surface composed of mucin, polymorphs and fibrin.

While PMC is associated mainly with broad-spectrum antibiotics, e.g. cephalosporins, almost any antibiotic may precipitate it. Elderly patients should not be put on cephalosporins for this reason.

Treatment is with vancomycin or metronidazole.

## Appendicitis

As mentioned above, acute appendicitis is usually caused when the appendix is obstructed, mostly by faecaliths. Rarely, it can occur when the appendix is not obstructed, e.g. when the lymphoid follicles are infected.

Typically, patients initially present with central abdominal pain, which then becomes localized after 6 hours or so to the right iliac fossa as the peritoneum adjacent to the appendix is affected. Movement exacerbates the pain. There may be vomiting, and fever and tachycardia are present.

Appendicectomy is curative. However, if the appendix has ruptured and there is generalized peritonitis, surgery should not be carried out and treatment should be conservative.

## Inflammatory bowel disease

There are two major non-specific inflammatory bowel diseases: Crohn's disease and ulcerative colitis.

### Crohn's disease

Crohn's disease may affect any part of the gastro-intestinal tract from the mouth to the anus (Fig. 7.12). It is most common in the terminal ileum and ascending colon.

Crohn's disease is more frequent in the Western world, particularly amongst Caucasians, where the incidence is approximately 5–7 per 100 000 and prevalence 50–60 per 100 000. It commonly presents in adolescence, but the peak onset is between 20 and 40 years of age. Both sexes are equally affected.

There is a high rate of concordance in monozygotic twins, which suggests both a genetic and environmental cause. However, the exact aetiology is unknown.

There is a 3–4-fold increase in risk with smoking and Crohn's patients generally eat a diet higher in refined sugars and lower in fibre than those without Crohn's.

**Crohn's disease**

ileum or ileocolonic disease only (40%)

small intestine only (30–40%)

colon only (about 20%)

perianal region only (less than 10%)

**Ulcerative colitis**

rectum or rectum and sigmoid colon only (40–50%)

left side of colon only, or extensive disease (30–40%)

entire colon (pancolitis, 20%)

**Fig. 7.12** Distribution patterns of inflammatory bowel disease.

Macroscopically, the bowel appears bright red and swollen. Later, small, discrete aphthoid ulcers with a haemorrhagic rim form, so named because they look similar to aphthous ulcers in the mouth.

These progress to deeper longitudinal ulcers, which may develop into deep fissures involving the full thickness of the wall of the gastrointestinal tract. Because of this, the mucosa is often described as cobble-stoned (Fig. 7.13).

Fibrosis may follow, with stricture formation visible as a narrow string-like area on contrast radiographs (the 'string sign').

Aggregations of inflammatory cells and lymphocytes infiltrate the bowel wall. Mesenteric lymph nodes may be enlarged due to reactive hyperplasia. Granulomas may be present in the lymph nodes.

Damage to the gastrointestinal tract in Crohn's disease is often patchy (skip lesions) with normal areas of tissue found in between the patches. Symptoms include diarrhoea, with or without malabsorption, abdominal cramps, fever, malaise and weight loss. The signs include:

- Abdominal tenderness.
- Perianal lesions.
- Anaemia.
- Aphthous ulcers in the mouth.
- Weight loss.

Diagnosis involves sigmoidoscopy, rectal biopsy and contrast radiography.

**Complications**

Complications depend on the site and extent of the lesions.

Malabsorption may occur where large areas of small intestine are affected (short bowel syndrome, following surgical resection). Fistulae may form because of deep fissuring. These may be internal (between loops of gut or from the gut to the bladder), perianal, or, following surgery, open onto the skin.

Crohn's disease may also cause stricture formation, which may lead to obstruction.

Acutely, perforation or haemorrhage may occur.

**Ulcerative colitis**

no areas of normal mucosa between inflamed areas

horizontal superficial ulcers

**Crohn's disease**

areas of normal gut mucosa between inflammatory lesions

deep fissure ulcer

aggregations of inflammatory cells

**Fig. 7.13** Histopathological features of ulcerative colitis and Crohn's disease. Unlike Crohn's disease, ulcerative colitis is continuous and areas of normal gut are not found between lesions.

A variety of lesions may be seen around the anus, most commonly skin tags, fissures and fistulae in 60% of patients.

### Treatment

All Crohn's disease patients require symptomatic relief and, for some, this is all the treatment they ever need. Diarrhoea is treated with anti-diarrhoeal drugs, such as loperamide and codeine phosphate.

Vitamin and nutrient supplements are given to overcome any deficiency from malabsorption. Other treatments include anti-inflammatory steroids, e.g. prednisolone and immunosuppressive drugs, e.g.

ciclosporin or azathioprine. Antibodies to TNF-α induce remission in 70–80% of patients unresponsive to corticosteroids.

Antibiotics, such as metronidazole and cotrimoxazole, are useful in severe perianal disease. However, 80% of patients will require surgery at some point in their life because of:

- Failure to thrive in children.
- Complications, e.g. perforation, obstruction, stricture or fistula formation.
- Failure or side effects of drug therapy.

Surgery is never curative. Remission is achievable, but most patients have significant relapses.

Granulomas are collections of epithelioid macrophages and giant cells surrounded by a cuff of lymphocytes. The non-caseating granulomas in Crohn's disease are different from those found in tuberculosis, which are tubercular granulomas characterized by central caseous (cheese-like) necrosis.

## Ulcerative colitis

Ulcerative colitis only affects the large intestine (Fig. 7.12). The incidence of ulcerative colitis is 10 per 100 000 and the prevalence is 80–120 per 100 000.

Ulcerative colitis affects women more than men and is most common between the ages of 20 and 40 years, although it can occur at any age.

It usually starts in the rectum and it may extend proximally, although never beyond the colon. Occasionally, inflammation of the terminal ileum is seen (backwash ileitis) but this is a result of an incompetent ileocaecal valve rather than ulcerative colitis itself. Its aetiology is unknown, although possible causative agents include genetics, infection and immunological factors.

Unlike Crohn's, which commonly shows skip lesions, ulcerative colitis is continuous. Areas of normal gut are not found between lesions.

The disease is a chronic relapsing inflammatory disorder. Inflammation is diffuse but superficial. The mucosa is granular and haemorrhagic (Fig. 7.13), rarely involving the muscle layer.

Both acute and chronic inflammatory cells are found infiltrating the mucosa, and aggregates of polymorphs are seen in the crypts (crypt abscesses). Healing of ulcers leads to periods of remission but, in areas of healing, the normal large bowel epithelium may be replaced by a simple layer of mucus-secreting cells without crypts.

The major symptom in ulcerative colitis is bloody exudative diarrhoea. Often lower abdominal pain, anorexia and malaise accompany this. If the disease is confined to the rectum, urgency and tenesmus accompany the bloody diarrhoea.

Diagnosis requires rectal examination, sigmoidoscopy and biopsy. A barium enema can show fine ulceration.

In the developed world, this is the most frequent cause of prolonged bloody diarrhoea and it should be suspected whenever bloody diarrhoea lasts for more than 7 days.

### Complications

The mucosa may haemorrhage, leading to blood loss and anaemia.

Toxic megacolon, where the colonic diameter is greater than 6 cm may occur in acute fulminating cases. It allows passage of bacterial toxins into the systemic circulation and predisposes to perforation.

Ulcerative colitis is premalignant and carcinoma of the colon may develop after 10 years in people with extensive disease.

Extraintestinal complications may also occur in both Crohn's disease and ulcerative colitis (Fig. 7.14). These include:

- Skin involvement: pyoderma gangrenosum and/or erythema nodosum.
- Primary sclerosing cholangitis.
- Fatty liver and/or liver abscesses.
- Iritis and/or episcleritis.
- Arthritis and spondylitis.

### Treatment

There are two types of treatment for ulcerative colitis, depending on whether acute management or the maintenance of remission is needed. Acute cases are treated with prednisolone. All ulcerative colitis patients are treated with 5-aminosalicylic acid (5-ASA, e.g. mesalazine) or sulfasalazine (a compound of 5-ASA and sulfapyridine) to maintain remission and reduce the risk of colon cancer.

Some patients receive prednisolone. Azathioprine can induce remission in some cases.

Surgery is curative in ulcerative colitis. Colectomy with an ileorectal or ileoanal anastomosis with an ileal reservoir, avoids the need for an ileostomy.

A colectomy also removes the risk of cancer in the diseased bowel, in patients with total or sub-total colitis, who have had the disease for more than 10 years.

Prognosis depends on the extent of the disease and it is better in proctitis (disease limited to the rectum) than in severe fulminant disease (which carries a 15–25% mortality).

It is important to distinguish between a diagnosis of Crohn's and ulcerative colitis as the management of each is different (Fig. 7.15).

## Irritable bowel syndrome

Irritable bowel syndrome (IBS) is a functional bowel disease. No single cause has been identified, and it is diagnosed on the basis of the presence of particular symptoms and, in patients over 40 presenting for the first time, the exclusion of organic diseases.

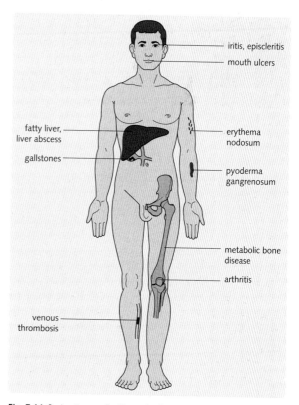

Fig. 7.14 Systemic complications of inflammatory bowel disease.

**Fig. 7.15** Comparison of ulcerative colitis and Crohn's disease.

| Crohn's disease | Ulcerative colitis |
|---|---|
| Affects anywhere from mouth to anus | Only affects large bowel (but backwash ileitis occurs in 10%) |
| Deep ulcers and fissures (rose-thorn ulcers) in mucosa | No fissures, horizontal undermining ulcers |
| Malignant change less common than ulcerative colitis | Malignant change relatively common |
| 10% have fistulae | Fistulae rare |
| 60% have anal involvement | 25% have anal involvement |
| Fibrous shortening and early strictures of intestine | Muscular shortening of colon but strictures rare and late |
| Skip lesions | No skip lesions |
| Fat and vitamin malabsorption (if small intestine affected) | No fat or vitamin malabsorption |
| Granulomas in 50% | No granulomas |
| Marked lymphoid reaction | Mild lymphoid reaction |
| Fibrosis | Mild fibrosis |
| Serositis | Mild serositis (if any) |
| No raised ANCA | Raised ANCA |
| Increased incidence in smokers | Decreased incidence in smokers |

IBS is very common, affecting 10–20% of the general population, and is more prevalent in young women. It comprises a cluster of symptoms, the most important being abdominal pain, altered bowel habit, abdominal distension, tenesmus and the presence of rectal mucus.

Diagnostic criteria for IBS are:

- Exclusion of structural or metabolic abnormalities, e.g. ulcers, inflammatory bowel disease, lactose intolerance.
- Abdominal pain for 12 weeks or more in a 12-month period.
- Presence of two or more accompanying symptoms:
  - Pain relieved by defecation.
  - Onset of pain associated with a change in frequency of the stools.
  - Onset of pain associated with a change in the form of the stools.

Irritable bowel syndrome is generally referred to as constipation-predominant or diarrhoea-predominant. The course of the disease is often relapsing and remitting. Stress can bring on attacks of IBS.

A management algorithm for IBS is given in Fig. 7.16. Reassurance and avoidance of unecessary investigation is very important.

# Bowel obstruction

Bowel obstruction may have mechanical or non-mechanical causes (pseudo-obstruction).

The signs and symptoms are similar, regardless of the cause, and depend primarily on the level of the obstruction.

Vomiting is a symptom of high obstruction, but it may be absent (or occur late) in low-level obstruction. Conversely, distension and colic are early symptoms of obstruction lower in the intestine.

Obstruction causes distension of the gut, with a build-up of gas and intestinal secretions above the level of the obstruction. There is progressive depletion of extracellular fluid and the multiplication of bacteria, especially coliforms, *Enterococcus faecalis*, *Clostridium perfringens* and *Bacteroides*.

Diagnosis requires a thorough history and erect and supine radiography. This shows distended, gas-filled loops of bowel with multiple horizontal fluid levels.

Treatment depends on the cause and level of the obstruction, and whether the bowel is strangulated. Strangulated bowel is an emergency and requires urgent surgery.

Simple obstruction, i.e. not due to strangulation may be treated conservatively initially. Conservative treatment consists of 'drip and suck': intravenous

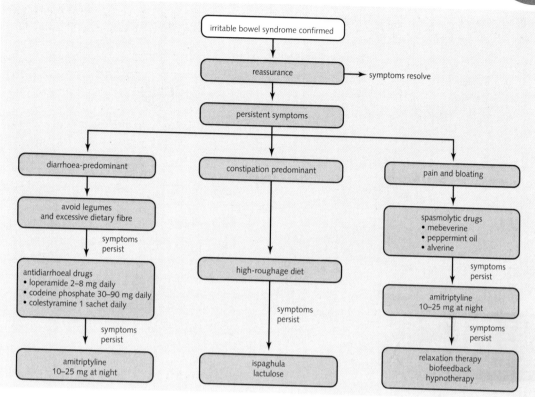

**Fig. 7.16** Management of irritable bowel syndrome (Reproduced with permission from Haslett C et al. Davidson's Principles and Practice of Medicine, 19th edn. Edinburgh: Churchill Livingstone, 2002.)

fluids and continuous aspiration by nasogastric tube.

In general, obstruction high in the gastrointestinal tract presents with vomiting. Obstruction lower down causes distension.

## Causes of bowel obstruction

Mechanical causes of obstruction of a tube like the intestine may be:

- In the wall, e.g. malignancy, inflammatory bowel disease, congenital strictures and diverticular disease.
- In the lumen, e.g. foreign material, faecaliths, polypoid tumours and meconium in cystic fibrosis.
- Outside the wall, e.g. intussusception, adhesions, hernias, volvulus and intra-abdominal tumours.

Pseudo-obstruction may be due to Hirschsprung's disease, paralytic ileus and bowel infarction.

Paralytc ileus is atony of the intestine resulting in lack of peristalsis. It occurs transiently after almost every laparotomy. Other major causes include interruption of the autonomic innervation of the gut, peritonitis (which may cause toxin-mediated paralysis of the intrinsic nerve plexuses of the gut) and potassium depletion.

### Hernias

A hernia is the protrusion of any organ or tissue through its coverings and outside its normal body cavity.

Hernias are common, occurring in about 1% of the population, and may be congenital or acquired (Fig. 7.17). Within these two groups, they may be reducible, irreducible or strangulated (Fig. 7.18).

Reducible hernias can be pushed back into the compartment from which they came, while irreducible ones cannot and may become strangulated if their blood supply is cut off by the neck of the sac.

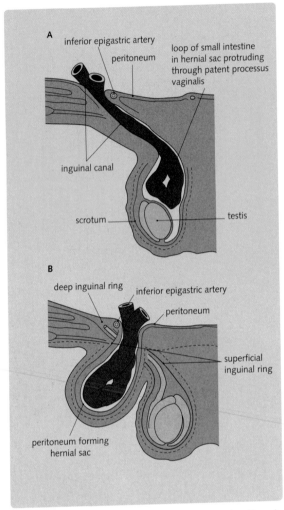

**Fig. 7.17** (A) Congenital indirect hernia passing into scrotum through patent processus vaginalis. (B) Acquired direct hernia passing through a defect in the abdominal wall. (Redrawn with permission from Hall-Craggs ECB. Anatomy as a Basis for Clinical Medicine. London: Waverly Europe, 1995.)

Strangulated hernias present with signs and symptoms of obstruction and if untreated, become gangrenous and necrotic. The most common sites of herniation through the abdominal wall are:

- Inguinal (about 90%).
- Femoral.
- Umbilical.
- Incisional.
- Ventral and epigastric.

Inguinal hernias may be:

- Direct (protruding through the posterior wall of the inguinal canal).
- Indirect (passing through the inguinal canal).

Direct inguinal hernias are less common (20% of inguinal hernias) and they lie medial to the inferior epigastric vessels. Indirect hernias are much more common, lie lateral to the inferior epigastric vessels and are more likely to strangulate, as the neck (the internal ring of the inguinal canal) is narrower. See also *Crash Course: Anatomy*.

Treatment depends on the type of hernia. Reducible hernias often require no treatment so long as they remain reducible. Strangulated hernias must be treated surgically.

Synthetic meshes are often used to reinforce closure of hernia orifices.

### Adhesions

Adhesions occur where two parts of the body that are normally separate are connected by bands of fibrous tissue.

Some are congenital, but most occur as a result of post-inflammatory scarring, e.g. after peritonitis, endometriosis, or scars that form as a result of surgery.

Adhesions may cause external constriction of the bowel, leading to obstruction or strangulation. Urgent surgery is required to relieve the strangulation.

If there are scars from past abdominal surgery, consider adhesions as a cause of the obstruction.

### Intussusception

Intussusception occurs when one segment of bowel (the intussusceptum) slides inside the adjacent segment (Fig. 7.19), like a telescope. It is most common in early childhood (95% of all cases) and occurs mainly at the ileocaecal valve (ileocolic intussusception), although it may also occur at other sites. The ratio of males to females affected is 2:1.

The aetiology is unclear, but it may be related to an adenovirus causing enlargement of lymphatic tissue in the intestinal wall. This protrudes into the lumen and is pushed into the adjacent section by peristalsis.

In some cases a polyp (such as Peutz–Jeghers polyps), Meckel's diverticulum or carcinoma may project into the lumen and be pushed along in a similar way.

Patients present aged 5–12 months of age, with periods of screaming, vomiting, blood in the faeces ('redcurrant jelly') and drawing up of the legs.

The child is pale and a sausage-shaped mass may be felt on palpation of the abdomen.

Peritonitis and gangrene may occur within 24 hours if untreated. A barium enema may resolve the

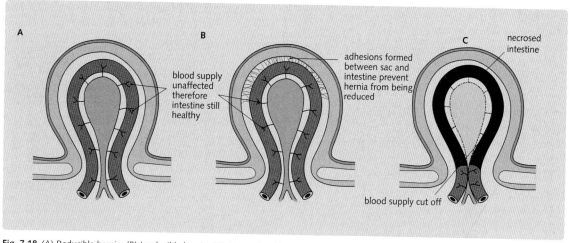

**Fig. 7.18** (A) Reducible hernia. (B) Irreducible hernia. (C) Strangulated hernia. Reducible hernias can be pushed back into the compartment from which they came, irreducible ones cannot. Strangulated hernias have had their blood supply cut off.

intussusception by forcing the invaginated segment back with hydrostatic pressure. Alternatively, surgery may be required.

### Volvulus

Volvulus occurs when a loop of bowel is twisted 180 degrees about its mesenteric axis. This usually occurs in the sigmoid colon, but it may be found in the caecum, small intestine, gall bladder or stomach. It is rare in the UK.

Risk factors include chronic constipation, adhesions and abnormally mobile loops of intestine.

Twisting of the bowel causes obstruction and occlusion of the vessels supplying the affected section.

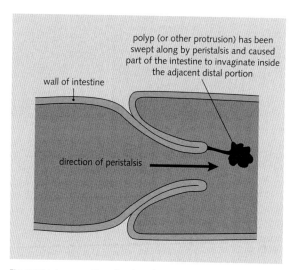

**Fig. 7.19** Intussusception. One bowel segment has slipped inside an adjacent one.

Potentially fatal gangrene and peritonitis may occur if the volvulus is not treated. Symptoms include the sudden onset of colicky pain in the right iliac fossa and rapid abdominal distension.

Diagnosis is by plain radiography, which shows a dilated section of bowel full of gas and forming a characteristic loop or inverted 'U' (the 'bent inner tube' sign). Treatment depends on the site of the volvulus: surgery is often necessary. Sigmoid volvulus is sometimes resolved by sigmoidoscopy and the passing of a flatus tube.

## Diverticulosis

Some important definitions:

- A diverticulum is an outpouching of the wall of the gut. They occur at weak points in the wall, usually due to increased pressure from within the gut or pulling from outside.
- Diverticulosis means that diverticula are present.
- Diverticular disease means that diverticula are causing symptoms, such as abdominal pain or change in bowel habit. However, the pain is due to muscle spasm, not inflammation.
- Diverticulitis means that one or more diverticula are inflamed. This is usually caused by an infection and leads to inflammatory abdominal pain and diarrhoea, or constipation.

### Diverticulosis

Diverticula may be congenital or acquired. They may occur in any part of the gut.

Congenital diverticula are outpouchings of the full thickness of the bowel wall. They are found most commonly in the duodenum and jejunum. They are usually asymptomatic, but they may lead to bacterial overgrowth, steatorrhoea and vitamin $B_{12}$ malabsorption. They may also perforate or bleed.

Acquired colonic diverticula increase in incidence with increasing age. They are predominantly a Western condition, present in about 50% of people aged over 50 years. There is no difference in distribution between the sexes. Low-fibre diets are a risk factor. They are more common in the left side of the colon than the right, and are usually found in the sigmoid and descending colon.

They form when the muscle layer of the wall thickens (hypertrophies) and high intraluminal pressures force a pouch of mucosa out through an area of weakness in the muscle layer. Areas of weakness often occur near blood vessels (Fig. 7.20).

Acquired diverticula do not consist of all three layers of the intestinal wall and this differentiates them from congenital ones.

Diagnosis of diverticula is often incidental during other investigations. As over 90% of cases are asymptomatic, in many cases no treatment is required.

Patients should, however, be advised to increase the amount of fibre and liquids in their diet (fibre has no beneficial effect unless there is sufficient liquid in the diet).

## Diverticulitis

Diverticulitis may occur if the neck of the diverticulum becomes obstructed by faeces. Patients with

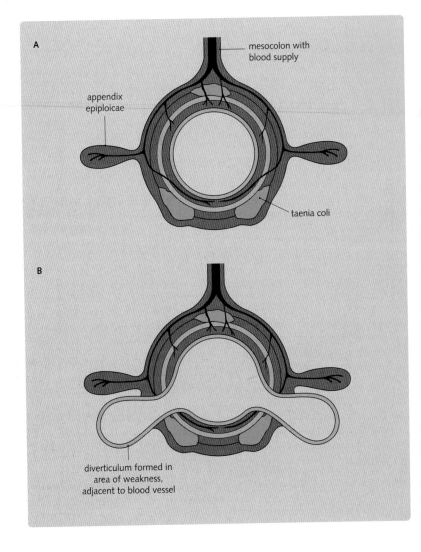

**Fig. 7.20** Colonic diverticulosis. High intraluminal pressure has forced pouches of mucosa through weak muscle areas. (Redrawn with permission from Ellis H, Calne R, Watson C. Lecture Notes on General Surgery, 10th edn. Oxford: Blackwell Science, 2002.)

A

mesocolon with blood supply

appendix epiploicae

taenia coli

B

diverticulum formed in area of weakness, adjacent to blood vessel acute diverticulitis often present in a similar way to those with appendicitis, except that the pain is usually in the left iliac fossa instead of the right. The most common site is the sigmoid colon.

Signs include tenderness and guarding on the left side of the abdomen, pyrexia and tachycardia. Radiographs should be taken to exclude air under the diaphragm (an indication of perforation).

Complications include:

- Haemorrhage if a vessel is eroded.
- Perforation, causing peritonitis if it occurs into the peritoneal cavity, abscess formation or fistulae if it occurs into the bladder or vagina.
- Chronic infection causing fibrosis and obstruction.

In the absence of complications, acute diverticulitis is treated conservatively with a liquid diet and appropriate antibiotic treatment.

## Vascular disorders

### Bowel ischaemia

Essentially, the causes of ischaemic bowel disease are the same as ischaemia in other parts of the body.

Common causes include:

- Stenosis.
- Thrombosis.
- Emboli.

Strangulation may also cause ischaemia as the blood supply is disrupted.

Ischaemic bowel disease may occur in the small intestine or the colon. The effect depends on the size of the ischaemic area and the length of time ischaemia has persisted.

It may be classified as mucosal, mural or transmural, the effects of which are summarized in Fig. 7.21.

The blood supply to the wall is 'from outside in' and mucosal or mural infarction often results from underperfusion. Transmural infarction is usually due to mechanical compromise of the artery.

The splenic flexure and an area of the rectum are particularly prone to ischaemic damage. These are the 'watershed' areas where the arterial supply switches from the superior to the inferior mesenteric artery, and from the inferior mesenteric and hypogastric arteries, respectively (Fig. 7.22).

Mucosal ischaemia causes release of proteolytic enzymes, which may cause deeper damage to the wall. However, complete regeneration is more common.

After mural ischaemia, ulcers form, the mucosa haemorrhages and granulation tissue forms. This is replaced by fibrotic tissue, which can form a stricture.

Transmural ischaemia leads to gangrene, perforation and, if untreated, death. It should be suspected in any elderly patient with atherosclerosis or atrial fibrillation with a tender abdomen and absent bowel sounds.

Symptoms in acute bowel ischaemia include:

- Acute severe abdominal pain.
- No abdominal signs, such as distension.
- Shock, due to hypovolaemia.
- Increased haemoglobin and white cell count.
- Persistent metabolic acidosis.
- Gasless abdomen on X-ray.

Fig. 7.21 The effects of acute intestinal infarction.

**Fig. 7.22** Areas of large bowel particularly prone to ischaemic injury.

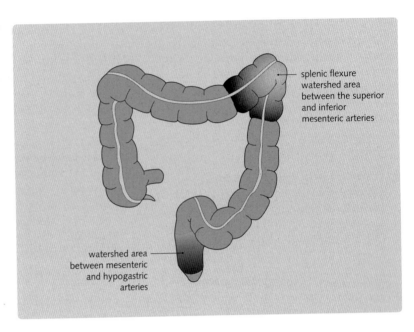

splenic flexure watershed area between the superior and inferior mesenteric arteries

watershed area between mesenteric and hypogastric arteries

Diagnosis relies on abdominal X-ray and endoscopy. A sigmoidoscopy shows a normal rectal mucosa, but it also shows blood and mucus coming from further along the bowel. A full colonoscopy is not performed, due to the risk of perforation.

Histological changes in chronic ischaemic bowel disease include fibrosis, haemorrhage, ulceration and granulation. On biopsy, the mucosa has a large infiltration of polymorphonuclear cells. Macrophages laden with haemosiderin are uncommon, but thought to be characteristic of ischaemic bowel disease.

The patient is treated with fluid replacement, heparin and antibiotics. Surgery is absolutely necessary to remove the dead segment of bowel. Revascularization may also be attempted, but note that reperfusion injury caused by free radicals commonly occurs following hypoperfusion.

The prognosis is poor in acute bowel ischaemia, with a less than 20% survival rate.

## Angiodysplasia

Angiodysplasia refers to small vascular anomalies, most commonly venous malformations in the mucosa or submucosa. They are usually asymptomatic and their only presentation is bleeding from the large bowel. They are more common in the elderly and can be diagnosed by angiography or colonoscopy. The right side of the colon is affected more commonly than the left.

Treatment is by diathermy coagulation or surgical removal.

## Haemorrhoids

Haemorrhoids are the enlargement of the normal spongy blood-filled cushions in the wall of the anus. They are the most common cause of rectal bleeding, and patients normally complain of blood on the toilet paper after defecation.

The anal cushions (and hence sites of haemorrhoids) are at 3, 7 and 11 o'clock when viewed in the lithotomy position and attached by elastic tissue and smooth muscle.

However, gravity, increased anal tone and straining on defecation all put stress on the cushions, making them protrude and bleed readily from the underlying capillaries. Pregnancy and portal hypertension (see Chapter 4) can also cause haemorrhoids.

Haemorrhoids are classified as:

- First degree (confined to the anal canal, and which bleed but do not prolapse).
- Second degree (which prolapse on defecation, but spontaneously reduce).
- Third degree (which prolapse on defecation, but require reduction with the fingers).

Patients present with bright red bleeding from the rectum, and they are often very anaemic.

Mucus discharge and pruritus ani (anal itching) accompany this. Often internal haemorrhoids are asymptomatic.

Diagnosis involves rectal examination, proctoscopy and exclusion of any abdominal malignancies, which may also cause bleeding.

Haemorrhoids can be treated by:

- Infra-red coagulation.
- Injection sclerotherapy.
- Banding (rubber band ligation).
- Cryotherapy.
- Haemorrhoidectomy.

The choice of treatment depends on the type of haemorrhoids, associated symptoms and history. All patients are advised to have a high-fibre diet, drink plenty of water and use a faecal-softening agent, if necessary.

## Neoplastic disease

### Hamartomatous polyps

Some 90% of colonic epithelial polyps are non-neoplastic and therefore benign. Hamartomatous polyps are an example. Thy are derived from over-growth of mature tissue and are usually large and pedunculated. They fall into two main categories: juvenile and Peutz–Jeghers polyps.

Hamartomas are malformations containing two or more types of mature cell which are normally present in the organ in which they arise. They are always benign.

### Juvenile polyps

Juvenile polyps are usually solitary focal hamar-tomatous malformations of mucosal tissue.

They occur in children and teenagers, but they are most common below the age of 5 years. About 80% of them occur in the rectum.

However, in juvenile polyposis, an autosomal dominant condition presenting with ten or more colonic polyps, the risk of colonic cancer is increased. Children with this must begin a screening programme to help spot cancer in its early stages.

### Peutz–Jeghers polyps

Peutz–Jeghers syndrome is a rare autosomal domi-nant syndrome characterized by multiple polyps scattered throughout the gastrointestinal tract. Abnormal pigmentation also occurs in the skin and oral mucosa.

The polyps may bleed and cause anaemia. Although the polyps themselves are not premalig-nant, being hamartomas, people with Peutz–Jeghers syndrome do have a slightly increased risk of develop-ing certain carcinomas, notably in the gastrointestinal tract and ovary.

## Neoplastic epithelial lesions

### Adenomas

Adenomas (a type of polyp) are derived from glan-dular epithelium, and they are the most important of the epithelial polyps. They are relatively common, especially in the elderly.

Of all adenomas, 75% are tubular, 10% villous and the remainder a mixture of the two (tubulovillous).

Tubular adenomas are smaller than villous adenomas (up to 1 cm in diameter) and they are usually pedunculated. They look a little like a blackberry on a stalk.

Villous adenomas, on the other hand, are usually sessile and larger (up to several centimetres in diameter) and, as the name suggests, have villi lined with dysplastic columnar epithelium protruding from their surface.

Villous adenomas have a greater tendency to malignant change (Fig. 7.23). They carry the addi-tional risk of electrolyte imbalance and, more rarely, acute renal failure resulting from their secretion of electrolyte-rich mucus.

### Familial adenomatous polyposis

People with familial adenomatous polyposis (FAP), a rare autosomal dominant disorder, almost always develop cancer of the intestine by the age of 35 years. FAP is characterized by the development of numerous adenomas in the large and, to a lesser extent, the small intestine during the teens and twenties.

The gene involved in FAP is called *APC* and is on the long arm of chromosome 5 (between q21 and q22). Non-steroidal anti-inflammatory drugs are thought to be protective.

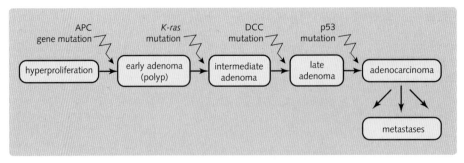

**Fig. 7.23** Development of colorectal carcinoma, showing the consecutive gene mutations involved.

## Hereditary non-polyposis colorectal cancer

Hereditary non-polyposis colorectal cancer (HNPCC) is similar to FAP in that it greatly predisposes to colorectal cancer and is an autosomal dominant condition, but is commoner. The carcinomas also tend to be more aggressive in nature, with a propensity to produce mucin.

Other associated carcinomas include those of the stomach, ovary and endometrium. The cause is a mutation, of which four have been identified, in DNA mismatch genes. The two most important mutations are those in hMSH2 (chromosome 2p) and hMLH1 (chromosome 3p).

## Colorectal cancer

Colorectal cancer is common in the developed world. It is the second biggest cause of cancer death in the UK, coming second only to lung cancer.

It is closely related to diet. Its incidence is low in Japan but, among second-generation Japanese living in the United States, the incidence is the same as that of the indigenous American population. FAP and HNPCC predispose to the condition, as mentioned above.

Diets carrying a greater risk of colorectal cancer are:

- Low in fibre.
- High in carbohydrate.
- High in fat—a typical modern Western diet!

Fibre increases the bulk of faeces as long as fluid intake is adequate, which reduces the time taken for the contents of the intestine to pass through and out of the rectum. In a low-fibre diet, faeces remain in the intestine for longer, altering the normal flora. This is thought to predispose to cancer.

Inadequate intake of the free radical scavengers, vitamins A, C and E, also leads to an increased risk of colorectal and some other cancers.

Survival after diagnosis of colorectal cancer depends on the stage. Dukes' classification is most widely used (Fig. 7.24) and is a common examination question. Dukes' stages are:

- Stage A: invaded submucosa and muscle layer of the bowel, but confined to the wall.
- Stage B: breached the muscle layer and bowel wall, but no involvement of lymph nodes.
- Stage C1: spread to immediately draining pericolic lymph nodes.
- Stage C2: spread to higher mesenteric lymph nodes.
- Stage D: distant visceral metastases.

## Other neoplasms

### Carcinoid tumours

These arise from neuroendocrine (APUD) cells (see Chapters 3 and 6) in the gut and elsewhere, e.g. pancreas, biliary tract and lung. They are slow growing and potentially malignant but their malignant potential depends on the site.

Larger tumours in the appendix and ileum tend to spread to regional lymph nodes and the liver. Small tumours (less than 2 cm diameter) near the tip of the appendix rarely do so.

Because of the cells in which they arise, tumours produce hormones that may have local or systemic effects:

- 5-HT produced by midgut carcinoid tumours causes diarrhoea and borborygmi as a result of local stimulation of the contractility of the intestine.

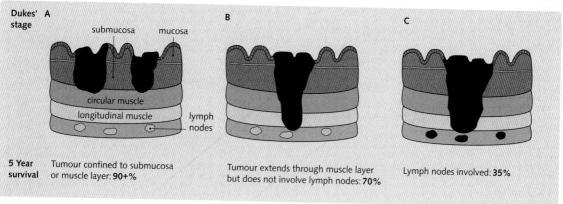

Fig. 7.24 Dukes' staging for colorectal carcinoma.

- 5-HT may also be produced from metastases in the liver and give rise to the carcinoid syndrome with facial flushing, cyanosis and pulmonary and tricuspid valve stenosis or incompetence.
- Adrenocorticotrophic hormone (ACTH) may be secreted and can result in Cushing's syndrome.

Palliative treatment is usually chosen. Survival can be anything from 3 years to 30 years, even if metastases are present.

### Intestinal lymphomas

Intestinal lymphoma is rare, but is the second most common extranodal origin of lymphoma (after gastric lymphoma). Lymphomas are more common in the small intestine than in the large, and may be of B cell or T cell lineage.

T cell lymphomas are associated with coeliac disease; B cell lymphomas are not and most occur sporadically.

# CLINICAL
# ASSESSMENT

## Learning objectives

After reading this chapter, you should be able to outline the following key manifestations of gastrointestinal disease:

- Dysphagia.
- Dyspepsia.
- Vomiting.
- Upper gastrointestinal bleeding.
- Lower gastrointestinal bleeding.
- Abdominal pain.
- Diarrhoea.
- Constipation.
- Weight loss.

## DYSPHAGIA

Dysphagia means having difficulty in swallowing. This is a symptom of a number of conditions, principally obstruction, stricture, neurological lesions or uncoordinated peristalsis as in achalasia, but it can also occur in the context of simple reflux oesophagitis (Fig. 8.1). Note that it is not the same as globus, where a 'lump in the throat' is felt in anxiety states, or odynophagia, which is pain on swallowing.

It is important to differentiate between these two types of dysphagia. Thus, when taking the history, ask whether it is difficult to make the swallowing movement. Is it difficult to swallow fluids as well as solids? Is it painful? Does the neck bulge or gurgle when drinking? Does swallowing precipitate coughing? Difficulty making the swallowing movement is likely to be caused by a neurological lesion, e.g. a cerebrovascular accident. The ability to drink liquids, but not to swallow food, suggests a stricture. However, failure to swallow food as well as fluid is seen in achalasia.

Constant, painful dysphagia with weight loss may be caused by a malignant stricture. Bulging or gurgling is a symptom of a pharyngeal pouch.

## DYSPEPSIA

This is a general term for symptoms which originate in the upper gastrointestinal tract. Heartburn, indigestion and peptic symptoms all come under this heading. Dyspepsia is therefore very common.

It is important to ask patients to clarify potentially ambiguous terms such as 'indigestion', as often your understanding of the word will be different from theirs.

Although most of the time no abnormality is found, if a patient has 'alarm symptoms' (Fig. 8.2)

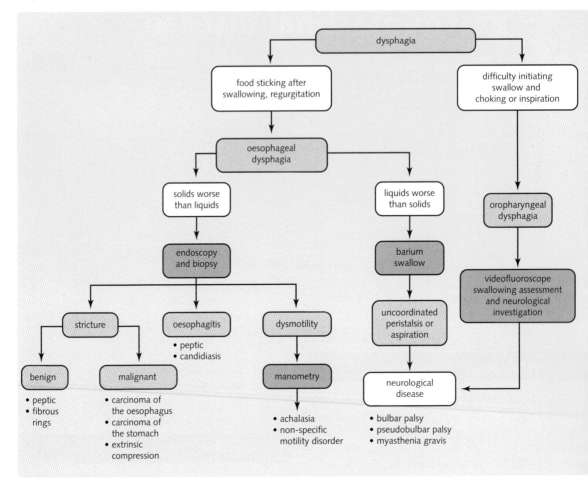

**Fig. 8.1** Investigation of dysphagia. (Reproduced with permission from Haslett C et al. Davidson's Principles and Practice of Medicine, 19th edn. Edinburgh: Churchill Livingstone, 2002.)

they should be investigated thoroughly to rule out serious gastrointestinal disease.

Heartburn is common, especially in developed countries. It is pain behind the sternum (retrosternal pain) that may radiate up towards the throat. It is worse on bending and lying flat. It can also be worse after drinking alcohol or eating something acidic or spicy (Fig. 8.3).

It is important to distinguish this from the retrosternal pain of a myocardial infarct (typically described as a central crushing pain, as if someone were tightening a band around the chest). Indigestion has different meanings to different people and is commonly used to mean any discomfort experienced after eating or drinking. It is important to establish exactly what the patient means by the word (Fig. 8.4).

**Fig. 8.2** Signs and symptoms ('alarm features') in dyspepsia which require prompt further investigation.

Weight loss
Dysphagia
Vomiting
Melaena and/or haematemesis
Anaemia (on full blood count)
A palpable mass in the abdomen

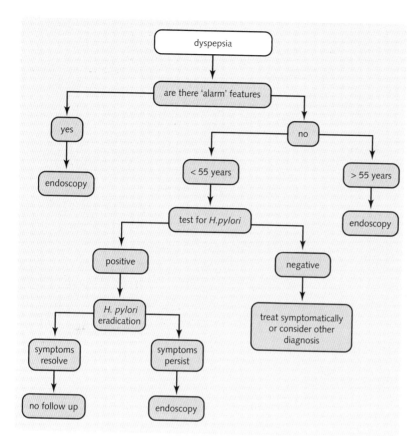

**Fig. 8.3** Investigation of dyspepsia. (Reproduced with permission from Haslett C et al. Davidson's Principles and Practice of Medicine, 19th edn. Edinburgh: Churchill Livingstone, 2002.)

# NAUSEA AND VOMITING

Nausea is a feeling that one is about to vomit. It is often accompanied by hypersalivation, which protects the mouth against the acid contents of the stomach. A differential diagnosis is given in Fig. 8.5.

Some patterns of vomiting are almost diagnostic, for example the projectile vomiting seen in pyloric stenosis in babies. Note that it is important to differentiate true vomiting from regurgitation of gastric contents.

The content of the vomit (especially blood or bile), the frequency and amount all give important

**Fig. 8.4** Differential diagnosis of indigestion. (From Greene HL et al. Clinical Medicine, 2nd edn. St Louis, USA: Mosby, 1995.)

Peptic disease
Gastro-oesophageal reflux
Oesophagitis
Gall bladder disease
Pancreatitis
Ischaemic heart disease
Malabsorptive diseases
Irritable bowel syndrome
Motility disorders
Inflammatory bowel disease
Abdominal angina

**Fig. 8.5** Differential diagnosis of nausea and vomiting. (From Greene HL et al. Clinical Medicine, 2nd edn. St. Louis, USA: Mosby, 1995.)

| Associated abdominal pain | Associated neurological signs | Predominant symptoms | |
|---|---|---|---|
| | | **Acute** | **Recurrent or chronic** |
| Viral gastroenteritis | Increased intracranial pressure | Digitalis toxicity | Psychogenic vomiting |
| Acute gastritis | Midline cerebellar haemorrhage | Ketoacidosis | Metabolic disturbances |
| Food poisoning | Vestibular disturbances | Opiate use | Gastric retention |
| Peptic ulcer disease | Migraine headaches | Cancer chemotherapeutic agents | Bile reflux after gastric surgery |
| Acute pancreatitis | | Early pregnancy | Pregnancy |
| Small bowel obstruction | | Inferior myocardial infarction | |
| Acute appendicitis | | Drug withdrawal | |
| Acute cholecystitis | | Binge drinking | |
| Acute cholangitis | | Hepatitis | |
| Acute pyelonephritis | | | |
| Inferior myocardial infarction | | | |

information. The presence of bile suggests that the lesion is below the ampulla of Vater.

Associated symptoms, including abdominal pain, onset relative to food consumption, headache, fever and weight loss, should be enquired about in the history. This is because nausea and vomiting are non-specific symptoms, hence the history is crucial in coming to a diagnosis.

Distension may have intraluminal, intramural or intraperitoneal causes. A diagnostic algorithm is given in Fig. 8.6.

As with other disorders, the rate of onset, i.e. the rate at which the abdomen distends is important. A neoplasm, for example, will not produce distension as quickly as gas.

Benign causes are also less likely to cause other symptoms. Aetiologies are given in Fig. 8.7.

## ABDOMINAL DISTENSION

Abdominal distension may be caused by one of the five Fs (flatus, fluid, fetus, fat or faeces).

Obstruction low in the gastrointestinal tract typically leads to distension. Obstruction higher up causes vomiting.

## ABDOMINAL PAIN

Because of the embryological development of the gut, pain in a structure that develops from the foregut may be referred to the epigastric region, that from midgut structures to the umbilical area and hindgut structures to the suprapubic area.

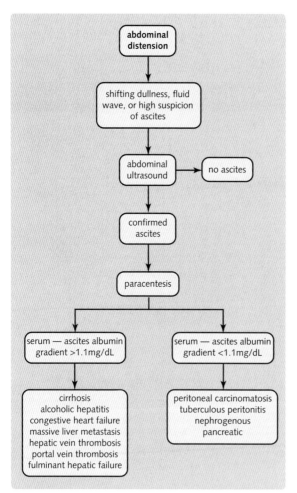

**Fig. 8.6** Investigation of abdominal distension. (From Greene HL et al. Clinical Medicine, 2nd edn. St Louis, USA: Mosby, 1995.)

**Fig. 8.7** Causes of abdominal distension. (From Greene HL et al. Clinical Medicine, 2nd edn. St Louis, USA: Mosby, 1995.)

**Gaseous causes**
Functional gas/bloat syndrome
Gastric outlet obstruction
Small bowel obstruction
Ileus
Intestinal pseudo-obstruction
Pneumatosis cystoides intestinalis
Perforated viscus

**Solid causes**
Organomegaly
    Liver
    Spleen
    Kidney
Tumour mass
Constipation with faecal retention
Pregnancy
Obesity

**Fluid causes**
Ascites
Perforated viscus
Abdominal haemorrhage
Cysts
Abscesses
Pancreatic pseudocysts
Gastric outlet obstruction
Small bowel obstruction
Ileus
Intestinal pseudo-obstruction
Bladder outlet obstruction

There are many possible causes of abdominal pain (Fig. 8.8), and it may be acute or chronic (Figs 8.9 and 8.10). Broadly, abdominal pain may be classified as one of the following types: visceral (from organs), parietal (from the parietal peritoneum), referred or psychogenic. Accompanying symptoms will give clues as to the mechanisms behind the pain.

## The acute abdomen

This accounts for about half of urgent general surgical admissions. Many of the causes (Fig. 8.11) are serious and require prompt treatment, although relatively simple conditions, e.g. constipation may also cause it.

Generally, the causes of an acute abdomen are:

- Inflammation – the pain develops gradually and is diffuse at first. Movement exacerbates it.

**Fig. 8.8** Mechanisms of abdominal pain. (From Greene HL et al. Clinical Medicine, 2nd edn. St Louis, USA: Mosby, 1995.)

| Obstruction | Metabolic disturbance |
|---|---|
| Gastric outlet | Diabetic ketoacidosis |
| Small bowel | Porphyria |
| Large bowel | Lead poisoning |
| Biliary tract | |
| Urinary tract | **Nerve injury** |
| | Herpes zoster |
| **Peritoneal irritation** | Root compression |
| Infection | |
| Chemical irritation (blood, | **Muscle wall disease** |
| bile, gastric acid) | Trauma |
| Systemic inflammatory | Myositis |
| process | Haematoma |
| Spread from a local | |
| inflammatory process | **Referred pain** |
| | Pneumonia (lower lobes) |
| **Vascular insufficiency** | Inferior myocardial infarction |
| Embolization | Pulmonary infarction |
| Atherosclerotic narrowing | |
| Hypotension | **Psychological stress** |
| Aortic aneurysm/dissection | Depression |
| | Situational stress |
| **Mucosal injury** | Intrapsychic conflict |
| Peptic ulcer disease | |
| Gastric cancer | |
| | |
| **Altered motility** | |
| Gastroenteritis | |
| Inflammatory bowel disease | |
| Irritable colon | |
| Diverticular disease | |

- Obstruction – the pain is colicky, as the bowel goes into spasm trying to move the obstruction.
- Perforation of a viscus – the pain comes on suddenly, is severe and if untreated leads to generalized peritonitis, with possible fatal consequences.

The most important factor to consider is whether the patient shows signs of peritonitis (see Chapter 7). If yes, it is an emergency: resuscitation is needed and prompt surgical treatment arranged with minimal further investigations.

# GASTROINTESTINAL BLEEDING

In general, bright red blood signifies fresh blood, and dark, black blood is from an old bleed.

## Upper gastrointestinal (GI) bleeding

Acute upper GI bleeding is by far the most common gastrointestinal emergency. Up to half of all cases are caused by bleeding from peptic ulcers. Other important causes are bleeding oesophageal varices, oesophagitis and gastric erosions.

The haematemesis is red with clots if the bleeding is severe; black, 'coffee grounds' haematemesis indicates a lesser severity. The stools may be tarry and black (melaena), as the blood will have been digested in the gut.

A patient suffering from an acute upper GI bleed may rapidly go into shock with fatal consequences if the bleeding is severe, hence assessment of circulatory status is a key part of management. Intravenous access is a priority and the patient should be resuscitated if necessary. Blood should be crossmatched in case surgical treatment is needed.

Investigations include a full blood count, urea and electrolytes and liver function tests (see Chapter 10).

Once the patient is sufficiently resuscitated, endoscopy may be carried out. This is diagnostic in about 80% of all cases.

## Lower GI bleeding

This is caused by bleeding from the anus or intestine and may be acute, subacute or chronic. Patients typically complain of blood on the toilet paper when they open their bowels.

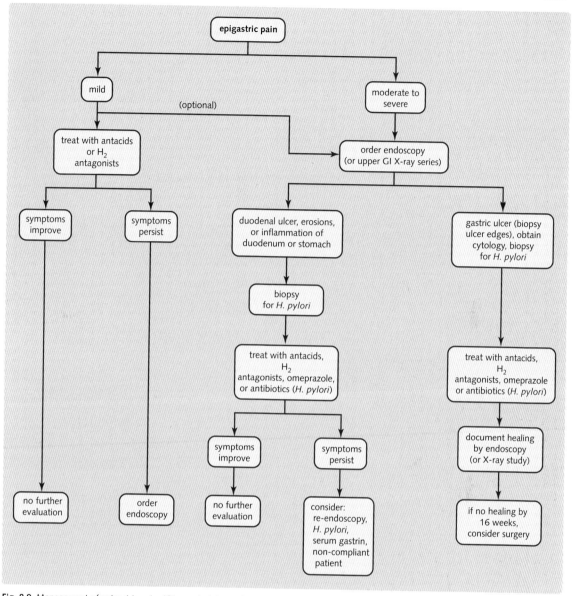

**Fig. 8.9** Management of epigastric pain. (GI = gastrointestinal.) (From Greene HL et al. Clinical Medicine, 2nd edn. St Louis, USA: Mosby, 1995.)

Severe acute lower GI bleeding is uncommon. Diverticular disease is the most likely cause.

Subacute or chronic bleeding is very common across all age groups. Usually it is due to haemorrhoids (the commonest cause of rectal bleeding) or anal fissures and this can be ascertained by proctoscopy. Nevertheless, in older patients (those over 50), colonoscopy should be performed to rule out colorectal carcinoma.

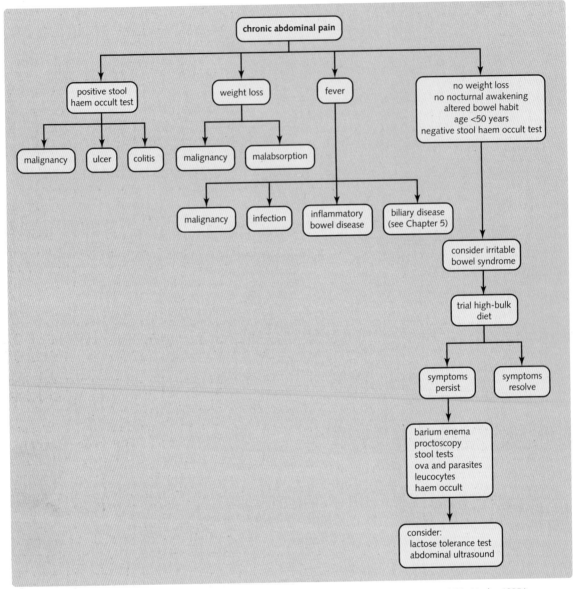

**Fig. 8.10** Management of chronic abdominal pain. (From Greene HL et al. Clinical Medicine, 2nd edn. St Louis, USA: Mosby, 1995.)

Fig. 8.12 gives an algorithm for the management of GI bleeding.

# WEIGHT LOSS

Any weight loss over 3 kg within a 6-month period is considered pathological until proven otherwise. It is an unspecific symptom, and may be due to gastrointestinal, systemic (e.g. malignancy, tuberculosis) or psychiatric causes (e.g. anorexia nervosa), apart from being associated with a number of diseases affecting particular organ systems, e.g. diabetes mellitus, hyperthyroidism.

Many gastrointestinal diseases have weight loss as a symptom, hence it is important to take a

**Fig. 8.11** Causes of the acute abdomen.

**Inflammation**
Acute appendicitis
Cholecystitis
Pancreatitis
Diverticulitis
Abscess
Pelvic inflammatory disease

**Perforation**
Peptic ulcer
Aortic aneurysm
Diverticula

**Obstruction**
Intestinal
Biliary

**Other causes**
Torted ovarian cyst
Ectopic pregnancy

detailed history and perform a thorough examination. Gastrointestinal tract malignancy must be excluded.

Other gastrointestinal causes include malabsorption, inflammatory bowel disease, dysphagia and obstruction.

# JAUNDICE

Jaundice is characterized by yellow skin and sclerae (observed in a good light), and is caused when plasma bilirubin levels exceed 45 μmol/L.

The mechanisms by which levels may become elevated are described in Chapter 4.

Jaundice is classified as prehepatic, hepatic or posthepatic. It may also be described as intrahepatic and extrahepatic—again, refer to Chapter 4.

# DIARRHOEA AND CONSTIPATION

Diarrhoea refers to excess frequency of bowel motions with stools being more liquid than usual.

Severe diarrhoea causes electrolyte disturbances and is a significant cause of mortality in children worldwide.

It may be classified as acute or chronic. Acute cases are usually due to dietary indiscretion or infections. Chronic diarrhoea often has more serious causes (Fig. 8.13). Fig. 8.14 shows an algorithm for the management of acute diarrhoea.

Constipation is a subjective complaint. Some people believe they must open their bowels at least once a day to remain healthy but in fact anything from once every three days to three times a day is well within the normal range. Therefore, when considering diarrhoea or constipation, an important question to ask is, 'Is this frequency normal for you?'.

In the absence of other symptoms, a high-fibre diet may improve things, as long as sufficient fluid is taken with the fibre. However, constipation may also be due to obstruction (Fig. 8.15).

# ANORECTAL PAIN

Anorectal pain may be caused by spasm of the sphincter, fissures or fistulae *in ano*, haemorrhoids or abscesses (see Chapters 4 and 7).

Fissures *in ano* are cracks in the anal canal. They are intensely painful on defecation, much more so than might be expected from their size. The pain is typically stinging and may last for a while after the bowel motion. Fissures may be caused by trauma from passing a constipated stool. The anal sphincter is usually in spasm.

Fissures, fistulae and other acquired anal abnormalities are a common complication of Crohn's disease (see Chapter 7). Most of them occur in the midline on the posterior margin. They may also occur following childbirth, particularly if a perineal tear occurred.

Patients are understandably reluctant to defecate because of the pain, which leads to a vicious cycle of constipation, the passing of hard constipated stools and further fissuring.

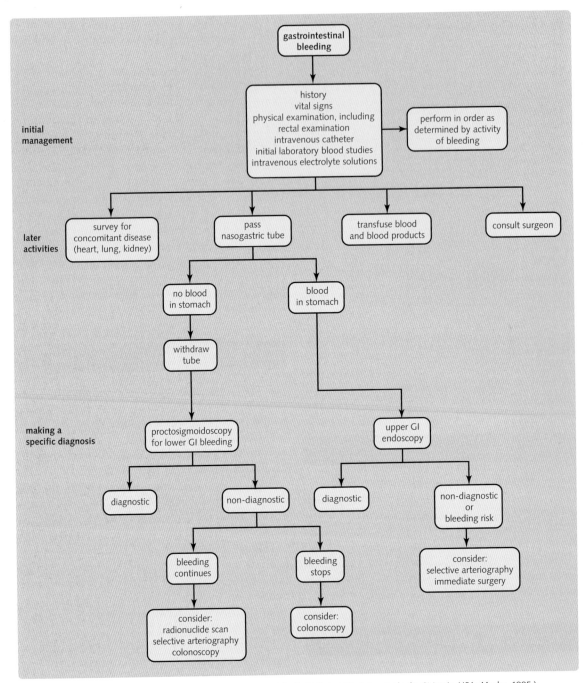

**Fig. 8.12** Management of gastrointestinal bleeding. (From Greene HL et al. Clinical Medicine, 2nd edn. St Louis, USA: Mosby, 1995.)

**Fig. 8.13** Aetiology of diarrhoea. (From Greene HL et al. Clinical Medicine, 2nd edn. St Louis, USA: Mosby, 1995.)

| | |
|---|---|
| Viral | Norwalk agent<br>Rotavirus<br>Enteric adenovirus |
| Bacterial toxin | Staphylococcus<br>*Clostridium perfringens*<br>*Clostridium difficile*<br>*Clostridium botulinum*<br>*Bacillus cereus*<br>Toxigenic *Escherichia coli*<br>*Vibrio cholerae* |
| Bacterial invasion | Shigella<br>Invasive *E. coli*<br>*Salmonella*<br>Gonorrhoea<br>*Yersinia enterocolitica*<br>*Vibrio parahaemolyticus*<br>*Campylobacter fetus* and *jejuni* |
| Parasites | *Giardia lamblia*<br>*Cryptosporidium*<br>*Entamoeba histolytica* |
| After infection | Lactase deficiency<br>Bacterial overgrowth |
| Drugs | Laxatives<br>Antacids with magnesium |
| Food toxins | Ciguatoxin, scombro toxin, pufferfish toxin |
| Metabolic | Hyperthyroidism<br>Adrenal insufficiency<br>Hyperparathyroidism<br>Diabetes mellitus |
| Chronic illness | Inflammatory bowel disease<br>Ischaemic colitis<br>Malabsorption<br>Irritable bowel syndrome |

Treatment is by the application of local anaesthetic cream to the fissure (to prevent the pain of defecation) and laxatives if necessary. Anal stretch, or application of glyceryl trinitrate to relax the sphincter may also be indicated.

# ANAL MASS

The most important thing to exclude is a malignancy. Malignancy is by no means the most common cause of an anal mass, but it is a potentially fatal one.

Patients often complain of tenesmus (an uncomfortable feeling that something is still there after they have defecated).

The most common causes are haemorrhoids (varices), hypertrophied anal papillae, condylomata acuminata (viral warts), rectal prolapse, rectal abscess, faecal impaction and neoplasia (Fig. 8.16).

Anal papillae may hypertrophy in response to chronic irritation or inflammation.

Rectal prolapse occurs where the tone of the sphincter is reduced and the pelvic floor weakened. It may be a late complication of multiple childbirth.

Neoplasms include squamous cell carcinomas, malignant melanoma, Bowen's disease, Paget's disease and basal cell carcinoma.

A rectocoele (the protrusion of the rectum through the weakened posterior wall of the vagina) may also occur in females. The patient may say she can feel 'something drop', especially when straining.

It is essential to perform a rectal examination and proctoscopy at the first opportunity to investigate an anal mass.

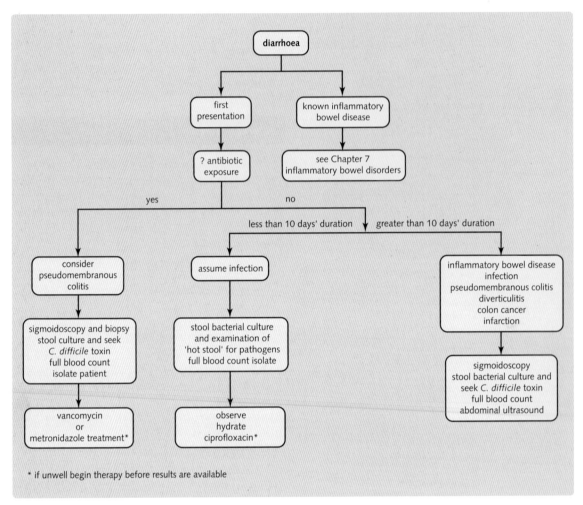

Fig. 8.14 Management of diarrhoea. (Reproduced with permission from Haslett C et al. Davidson's Principles and Practice of Medicine, 18th edn. Edinburgh: Churchill Livingstone, 1999.)

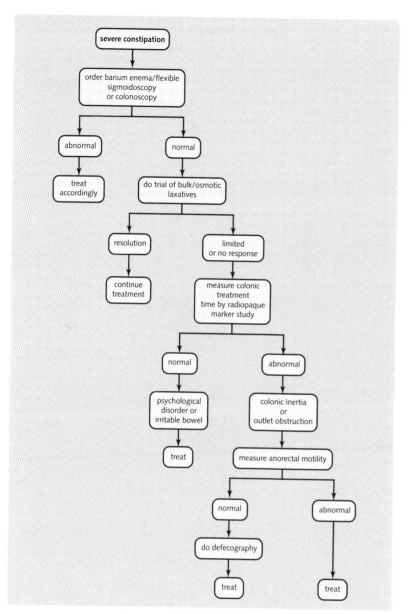

**Fig. 8.15** Management of constipation.
(From Greene HL et al. Clinical Medicine,
2nd edn. St Louis, USA: Mosby, 1995.)

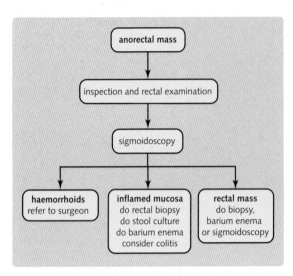

**Fig. 8.16** Investigation and management of an anal mass.

## FAECAL INCONTINENCE

This may be of faeces or of flatus.

The internal sphincter is an involuntary one, relaxing reflexly in response to distension by intestinal contents.

The external sphincter is under voluntary control, allowing us to defer defecation until a convenient moment.

Structural changes such as a loss of the angle of the rectum and anus (which contributes to faecal continence), neuromuscular and neurological lesions may all lead to incontinence.

# History and examination

## Learning objectives

After reading this chapter, you should be able to:

- Describe the process of taking a history with regard to a gastrointestinal system complaint.
- Describe the process of a complete abdominal examination, including rectal and external genital examination.

## INTRODUCTION

These are the core clinical skills you will need as a medical student, so it is well worth taking the time to learn how to do them properly. Use this chapter as a guide, but remember that there is no substitute for practice!

## HISTORY-TAKING

Most diagnoses are made on the history alone—if not, it should allow you to come up with a list of differential diagnoses. In most cases, the examination and investigations should confirm the diagnosis or exclude the differentials.

Remember that when you first meet, the patient has far more information about his or her condition than you do. Introduce yourself, be polite, listen carefully and look interested. Give the patient the time and the opportunity to tell you what you need to know, and put him or her at his or her ease. Many symptoms are embarrassing.

Maintain eye contact, even if the patient doesn't and watch carefully for clues. How ill does the patient look? Is he or she agitated or distressed? Is he or she in pain; can you notice any tremors? Has he or she lost a lot of weight (cachexia)?

Look around the bedside for clues, such as inhalers, oxygen, a walking stick or frame, cards from family and friends, sputum pots, reading material and glasses, special food preparations etc.

## The structure of a history

When recording a history, use the headings below. You are less likely to leave things out if your history is structured. It is also easier for others to find the information they need quickly when looking at your notes.

When writing in the patient's notes, make sure that you include everything, date the entry and sign your name legibly.

### Personal and demographic details of the patient

This should be a brief description giving details of the patient's age, sex, ethnic origins and occupation. It should allow others who have not met the patient to picture him or her in their mind's eye.

### The presenting complaint (PC)

This should be brief—a sentence or two stating the symptoms, not your diagnosis. For example, write 'abdominal pain' or 'chest pain', not 'appendicitis' or 'myocardial infarction'.

If the patient has a number of problems (not uncommon in the elderly) ask them to state the main ones first.

### The history of the presenting complaint (HPC)

Your line of questioning should tie in with the nature of the presenting complaint. Essentially, the

HPC is a complete description of the problem that brought the patient to see you.

It is usually good to start off with:

- How and when the symptoms started.
- The speed of onset: was it rapid, or slow and insidious?
- The pattern of symptoms, their duration and frequency. Are they continuous or intermittent? How often do they appear?

### Gastrointestinal symptoms

If the complaint appears to be gastrointestinal (or if you are asked to take a gastrointestinal history), you should always remember to ask about the following:

- Weight loss or gain and appetite.
- Dysphagia.
- Nausea and vomiting.
- 'Indigestion' or 'heartburn'.
- Abdominal pain (see next section).
- Episodes of jaundice or other liver problems.
- Change in bowel habit—a deviation from what is normal for the patient is the key point, not the absolute number of times they open their bowels.
- Change in the nature of stools: ask about stool colour and consistency, presence of mucus or blood. If blood is present, was it fresh blood and where was it (on the paper, in the toilet bowl, etc.).

### Pain

If pain is present, use the mnemonic SOCRATES as a guide to the questions which need to be asked:

Site: for example, is the pain abdominal or retrosternal?

Onset: you should also ask what the patient was doing at the time and whether the onset was acute or gradual. Ask about its relationship to food.

Character: sharp, dull, shooting, crushing (like a band around the chest), stabbing, colicky, etc.

Radiation.

Associated factors: nausea, vomiting, diarrhoea, migraine, etc.

Timing: duration, episodes.

Exacerbating and relieving factors: lying down, sitting up, food, movement, etc. If movement exacerbates the pain, peritoneum is likely to be involved; if the patient is rolling around, the pain is likely to be visceral colic, e.g. intestinal spasm.

Severity: this should be graded out of 10, with 10 being the most severe.

Additionally, you should ask:

- If the patient has had it before. If yes, is it the same kind of pain?
- What happened last time? Did he or she have any treatment or investigations, or did it go away by itself? If treatment was given, was it effective?
- If the patient did not consult last time, why have they come this time?
- About function. Is there any loss of function, e.g. any movement he or she can't make?
- If there is anything else the patient thinks might be relevant, however trivial?

## Past medical history (PMH)

Has the patient had any medical contact in the past? This question often needs persistence. It is amazing how many people forget operations, spells in hospital, or visits to the GP!

Try to ask for the diagnosis if possible, but if not, ask for symptoms of past complaints. This should allow you to guess what the diagnosis was. It is also good practice to ask whether the patient has or has had any of the following: myocardial infarct, thyroid disease, asthma, tuberculosis, rheumatic fever, diabetes mellitus, epilepsy.

Ask what previous investigations have been carried out and their results. Ask also about past surgery—if they have had any operations, when you examine the abdomen you will know what the scars were for.

## Drug history (DH)

Ask about all drugs, including contraceptive pills and over-the-counter medicines, as well as medicines that have been prescribed. It is a good idea to look at the drug chart at this point, if the patient is an inpatient.

You should always ask about allergies (i.e. type 1 hypersensitivity reactions which might result in anaphylaxis) in this section, as this might affect the drugs you will prescribe or the instruments you will use, e.g. no rubber gloves if the patient is allergic to latex. Lots of people say they are allergic to drugs when what they have actually had is a normal side effect, e.g. diarrhoea after taking penicillin. It is important to establish whether they really are allergic, as you may be denying them the best treatment, but do not give them anything they say they are allergic to unless you are absolutely sure they are not.

Remember to ask if the patient actually took the prescribed medication, if non-compliance is suspected. However, this requires some tact and rapport with the patient.

## Family history (FH)

Ask whether any diseases run in the family. Take note if first-degree relatives (parents and siblings) are affected.

If any first-degree relatives are deceased, ask also about the causes of death. Practise drawing quick sketches of family trees. Make a note on the family tree of any diseases (such as cancer or heart disease) that relatives may have had, to help you notice trends.

## Systems enquiry (SE)

Briefly go through all the systems of the body (Fig. 9.1) and ask specifically whether the patient has experienced any symptoms relating to them.

## Social history (SH)

The purpose of this is to see the patient as a whole and gain some idea of how the illness affects this particular patient, what support he or she has and whether he or she can reduce any health risks.

It should include information about the patient's:

- Marital status.
- Children and other dependants.
- Smoking: is it cigarettes, cigars or a pipe that the patient smokes? How many cigarettes do they smoke per day, and for how long have they been smoking?
- Alcohol: what type of alcoholic beverages do they drink, and how much per week? You should

---

**Fig. 9.1** The systems enquiry.

**Cardiovascular system**
- Chest pain (site, referral, precipitating and relieving factors)
- Palpitations
- Ankle oedema
- Shortness of breath/orthopnoea/ paroxysmal nocturnal dyspnoea

**Respiratory system**
- Chest pain
- Cough
- Sputum production
- Haemoptysis
- Shortness of breath and/or wheeze

**Gastrointestinal system** (also see section on Presenting Complaint above, and Chapter 8)
- Abdominal pain
- Nausea/vomiting
- Diarrhoea/constipation
- Chest pain (non-cardiac)

**Nervous system**
- Headache
- Fits
- Dizziness
- Numbness/tingling/loss of sensation
- Weakness
- Alteration or loss of vision
- Hearing loss
- Weakness

**Endocrine system**
- Polyuria/polydipsia
- Heat/cold intolerance
- Weight loss or gain
- Skin changes
- Mood changes

**Musculoskeletal system and skin**
- Pain
- Swelling
- Stiffness
- Rash

**Genito-urinary system**
- Frequency/oliguria/polyuria/nocturia
- Dysuria
- Haematuria
- Menstrual history in females
- Prostate symptoms in males

calculate weekly consumption using the unit system (Fig. 9.2), but remember that patients often underestimate their drinking.

- Occupational history: this is especially relevant with regard to toxin/chemical exposure and musculoskeletal disorders.
- Accommodation: assess whether the patient will be able to cope at home, e.g. if they have difficulty moving they might have problems with stairs.
- Activities of daily living: can they manage cooking, cleaning, washing themselves and other essential tasks? If not, do they get any help?
- Diet: is it adequate? High cholesterol? Vegetarian?
- Exercise.

## Presenting the history

You may be asked to present your history, for example on a ward round. This should be a concise summary recapping the most important features. For example:

'Reginald Smith, a 69-year-old retired bank manager presented with dysphagia which started about 3 months ago and has become progressively worse, initially only with solids but now with liquids and he has lost 2 kg in weight. Mr Smith had a hernia operation 3 years ago, but there is nothing else of note in his past medical history. His father died of cancer of the stomach at the age of 50. Systems enquiry was unremarkable. He has smoked 30 cigarettes a day since his early 20s, but does not drink. He is managing well at home.'

# GASTROINTESTINAL SYSTEM EXAMINATION

Most clinical examinations comprise inspection, palpation, percussion and auscultation. Of course, not all examinations will require all four components, but you should always remember this sequence and stick to it as much as possible so you do not leave any part undone. Before zooming in on the

**Fig. 9.2** Calculating alcohol consumption using the unit system. (Reproduced with permission from Cameron AD. Crash Course: Psychiatry, 2nd edn. Edinburgh: Mosby, 2004.)

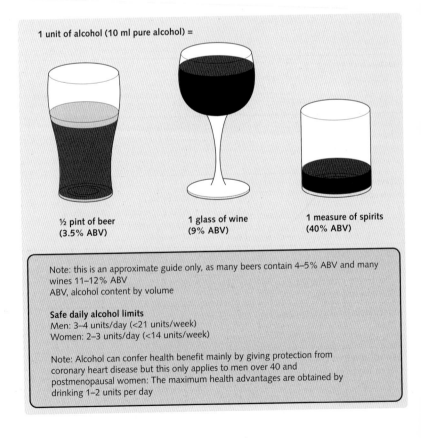

1 unit of alcohol (10 ml pure alcohol) =

½ pint of beer (3.5% ABV)    1 glass of wine (9% ABV)    1 measure of spirits (40% ABV)

Note: this is an approximate guide only, as many beers contain 4–5% ABV and many wines 11–12% ABV
ABV, alcohol content by volume

**Safe daily alcohol limits**
Men: 3–4 units/day (<21 units/week)
Women: 2–3 units/day (<14 units/week)

Note: Alcohol can confer health benefit mainly by giving protection from coronary heart disease but this only applies to men over 40 and postmenopausal women: The maximum health advantages are obtained by drinking 1–2 units per day abdomen, there are a few other steps to the gastro-intestinal system examination.

## General inspection

The main purpose of a general inspection is to determine how ill the patient is (Fig. 9.3). It may also enable you to pick up some clues.

Bear this in mind as you introduce yourself. If the patient is very ill, do not waste valuable time asking questions that can wait until later.

Look at the patient's facial expression. Is he or she comfortable; in obvious distress; looking furtive, receptive, or hostile?

Assess the patient's body posture and mobility as well as his or her weight and size.

Many diseases and conditions do not have a direct effect on the gastrointestinal system. However, always remember that the patient may be receiving medication for a pre-existing condition, which may affect the dose of drug you are intending to give for his or her gut condition, e.g. he or she may already be receiving enzyme-inducing drugs for another condition. Current medication might even be producing his or her gut symptoms, e.g. diarrhoea caused by antibiotic therapy.

Finally, treatment for a pregnant or breastfeeding woman needs to be chosen carefully.

## Inspection of the hands and limbs

Physical examination of the patient should start with an inspection of the hands. This is relatively non-invasive and allows the patient to get used to your touch. It also gives you a lot of information (Fig. 9.4).

Shaking hands at the beginning is commonly done. If the patient takes your hand but cannot release it, you can fairly confidently say that he or

**Fig. 9.3** Possible signs on general inspection.

| Test performed | Sign observed | Diagnostic inference |
|---|---|---|
| Inspection of skin colour | Pallor | Anaemia, shock, myxoedema |
| Inspection | Yellow skin (and sclerae) | Jaundice |
| | Pink nodules and/or areas of baldness on scalp (alopecia neoplastica) | Metastases from internal carcinoma, usually from gastrointestinal tract, breast, kidney, ovary or bronchus |
| | Dark pigmented flexures, especially armpits and under breasts (acanthosis nigricans) | Obesity, endocrine disease, genetic, adenocarcinoma of gastrointestinal tract or other internal malignancy |
| | Vellus hair over face and body (hypertrichosis lanuginosa) | Anorexia, neoplasm |
| | Patient sitting forward on edge of bed using accessory muscles of respiration (respiratory distress) | Airway obstruction, anaemia, heart failure, pulmonary embolism, obesity |
| | Abdominal distension | Fluid, fat, faeces, fetus, flatus |
| | Large masses | Neoplasm, cysts, congenital abnormalities |
| | Telangiectasia (abnormal dilatation of blood vessels) | Cirrhosis, outdoor occupation |
| | Severe muscle wasting and loss of body fat (cachexia) | Severe illness |
| Inspection and questioning | Itchy tissue-paper skin (ichthyosis) | Lymphoma, drugs, malabsorption, malnutrition |
| | Generalized itching | Jaundice, systemic malignancy |
| | Painful tender veins in different sites at different times (thrombophlebitis migrans) | Carcinoma of pancreas |

**Fig. 9.4** Possible signs on examination of the hands.

| Test performed | Sign observed | Diagnostic inference |
|---|---|---|
| Inspection of ends of fingers | Clubbing (an exaggerated longitudinal curvature, loss of the angle between the nail and nail bed and bogginess) | The causes of clubbing may be divided into gastrointestinal, thoracic and cardiac. Gastrointestinal causes include: inflammatory bowel disease (especially Crohn's disease), cirrhosis, gastrointestinal lymphoma and malabsorption (e.g. coeliac disease) |
| Arms straight with wrists fully extended | Hands flap (liver flap or asterixis) | $CO_2$ retention, cirrhosis, portosystemic encephalopathy |
| Inspection of palms of hands | Palmar erythema (redness around the edges of the palms) | Cirrhosis, pregnancy or polycythaemia |
| Inspection of nails | Leuconychia (white nails) | Hypoalbuminaemia |
| | Koilonychia (spoon-shaped nails) | Iron deficiency, syphilis |
| | Terry's lines (white nails with normal pink tips) | Cirrhosis |
| | Mees' lines (paired white parallel bands across the nails) | Hypoalbuminaemia |
| | Beau's lines (horizontal grooves across the nail) | Chemotherapy, previous severe illness |
| Inspection | Purpura (purple lesions which do not blanch on pressure) | Clotting disorder, vasculitis, drugs, infections, amyloidosis |
| Inspection of position of fingers | Dupuytren's contracture (fibrosis and contracture of the palmar fascia) | Ageing, liver disease, trauma (if unilateral) or epilepsy |
| Inspection | Lentigines (small, circumscribed, brown macules) | Peutz–Jeghers syndrome |
| Feel and inspection of skin of palm | Excessive sweating | Alcoholism, anxiety |
| Pinch a fold of skin up on back of hand | Skin fold takes a relatively long time to disappear | Dehydration |
| Inspection | Dark warty palms (tripe palms) | Adenocarcinoma of gastrointestinal tract, other internal malignancy |
| | Calcified nodules | CREST syndrome |
| | Tendon xanthoma | Familial hypercholesterolaemia |
| Inspection of palm | Simian crease | Down syndrome |

she has myotonic dystrophy, an uncommon but chronic condition often cropping up in clinical viva examinations.

When examining a patient, be methodical. Examine the hands and then work your way up the arm to the head and neck. Possible signs on limb examination are listed in Fig. 9.5.

# Examination of the head and neck

## Face, scalp and eyes

You need to pull down the lower eyelid to take a look at the sclerae for pallor (do not say anaemia—this is a haematological finding) or jaundice. This may be uncomfortable, so always warn a patient

**Fig. 9.5** Possible signs on examination of the limbs.

| Test performed | Sign observed | Diagnostic inference |
|---|---|---|
| Palpation | Pulses | Information about cardiovascular system |
| Inspection | Central dilated arteriole with small red vessels radiating out from it, like a spider (spider naevus) | If more than five or six: pregnancy, cirrhosis or other chronic liver disease |
| | Scratches | Pruritus |
| | Muscle wasting | Damage to innervation of muscles, malnutrition, chronic illness |
| | Thinning of skin | Steroid use |

beforehand. You also need to get quite close and ensure that the lighting is good. Remember, however, that jaundice is not clinically detectable unless serum bilirubin levels reach 50 μmol/L (twice the normal value).

Examination of the head and face is covered in Fig. 9.6.

## Mouth

Use a pen torch to inspect the inside of the mouth. Ask the patient to stick their tongue out and then let you look under it. This will tell you if the patient is dehydrated or cyanotic (Fig. 9.7). If necessary, gently depress the tongue with a wooden tongue depressor.

Wear gloves if you need to feel anything in the mouth and ask the patient to remove any false teeth.

Stomatitis simply means ulceration of the mucosal surface of the mouth—it can occur in the mouth or at the edges, where the upper and lower lips meet.

## Neck

Inspect both the front and back of the neck, then stand behind the patient and palpate for enlarged nodes in the back, front and sides of the neck (Fig. 9.8).

Always palpate for the supraclavicular lymph nodes carefully, especially in the left supraclavicular fossa, as this is a common site for gastrointestinal metastases. An enlarged node is indicative of gastric carcinoma (Virchow's node, or Troisier's sign—see Chapter 3).

## Examination of the abdomen

As mentioned earlier, follow the sequence inspection, palpation, percussion and auscultation.

### Inspection

The abdomen should be examined from the nipples to the knees, but not all at once. Respect the patient's dignity and only uncover as much as you need to at any one time.

Ask the patient to remove their clothes and lie flat on the bed or the couch, with the head on one pillow and arms by the sides.

Cover the patient with a folded sheet or blanket. It is easy to move this up or down, exposing or revealing different parts, as you complete your examination.

Briefly expose the patient from the nipples to the pubic bone. Stand at the end of the bed to look at the abdomen as a whole before going nearer and taking a closer look. Look out for the following (Fig. 9.9):

- Asymmetry.
- Distension.
- Dilated veins.
- Caput medusae.
- Purpura.
- Spider naevi – these are found in the distribution of the superior vena cava, i.e. chest and upper back. More than five or six are significant.

**Fig. 9.6** Possible signs on examination of the head and face.

| Test performed | Sign observed | Diagnostic inference |
| --- | --- | --- |
| Inspection of colour of sclera in a good light | Yellow | Jaundice |
| Inspection of colour of conjunctiva of lower lid | Pale | Anaemia |
| Inspection | Red eye from subconjunctival haemorrhage | Bleeding disorder from liver disease or other cause, diabetes, vomiting |
| | Inflamed connective tissue beneath conjunctiva (episcleritis) | Reiter's syndrome (may follow dysentery) |
| | Red eye from conjunctivitis | Stevens–Johnson syndrome |
| | Chronic red eye | Cirrhosis, renal failure, hereditary haemorrhagic telangiectasia (Osler–Weber–Rendu syndrome), iron deficiency anaemia, ataxia telangiectasia |
| | Acute swelling of eyelids | Adverse reaction to penicillin, bee sting or other allergen, infection |
| | Firm, chronic swelling of eyelids | Lymphoma, sarcoidosis |
| | Yellow swelling in periorbital area (xanthelasma) | Hypercholesterolaemia, age |
| | Erythematous, swollen eyelids | Dermatomyositis |
| | Malar flush | Mitral stenosis |
| | White ring around edge of iris (arcus) | Hypercholesterolaemia, ageing |
| | Protruding eye with sclera visible above iris | Graves' disease |
| | Constricted pupils | Ageing, drugs (opiates, glaucoma treatment), damage to sympathetic innervation (e.g.Horner's syndrome if unilateral) |
| | Swollen, purple nose and ears (lupus pernio), prominent scars, orange–brown papules, nodules and plaques | Sarcoidosis |
| | Patches of hair loss on scalp (alopecia neoplastica) | Metastases from internal carcinoma (usually from gastrointestinal tract, kidney, ovary, bronchus or breast) |
| | Flushing | Carcinoid syndrome |
| | Periorbital oedema, erythema of face and neck | Dermatomyositis |
| Inspection of cornea | Brown rings (Kayser–Fleischer rings) at periphery | Wilson's disease |
| Pupil reaction | Pupils constrict to accommodation but not to light (Argyll–Robertson pupil) | Syphilis |

**Fig. 9.7** Possible signs on examination of the mouth.

| Test performed | Sign observed | Diagnostic inference |
|---|---|---|
| Inspection | Puckered mouth | Scleroderma |
| | Swollen gums | Pregnancy, acute leukaemia, puberty, phenytoin, infection |
| | Fissuring at edges of mouth (angular cheilosis or stomatitis) | Iron-deficiency anaemia, malabsorption, candidal or other infection |
| | Vesicles on lips and in perioral area | Herpes simplex infection |
| | Blue spots on mucosa | Hereditary haemorrhagic telangiectasia (Osler–Weber–Rendu syndrome) |
| | Small pigmented areas on lips and on mucosa (lentigines) | Peutz–Jeghers syndrome |
| | Bleeding and necrosis of gums | Acute leukaemia |
| | Bleeding gums | Vitamin C deficiency |
| | Beefy, raw, red tongue | Pernicious anaemia, malabsorption, pellagra |
| | Dry discoloured tongue | Gastrointestinal or other infection |
| | Ulcer | Carcinoma, lymphoma, trauma, infection (tuberculosis, herpes, Vincent's angina, diphtheria, measles), Stevens–Johnson syndrome, Behçet's syndrome, drugs, pemphigus, bullous pemphigoid |
| | Swellings | Cysts, stones in salivary glands, infection |
| | High-arched palate | Marfan's syndrome |
| | Black tongue | Antibiotic treatment |
| | Blue tongue and lips | Cyanosis |
| Inspection and touch with spatula | White patches that cannot be brushed off (leucoplakia) | Trauma, infection (including HIV) |
| | White patches that can be brushed off | Candidal infection (thrush) |
| Smell | Halitosis | Infection, poor hygiene, hepatic coma, uraemia, diabetic coma |

- Bruising.
- Visible peristalsis and/or pulsation.
- Masses.
- Scars.
- Striae.

## Palpation

Make sure your hands are warm and tell the patient that you are about to feel their abdomen.

Before you do so, ask whether the abdomen is tender anywhere. If it is, then start your palpation as far away from the tender area as possible. Start with light palpation before pressing more deeply and

always ask the patient to tell you if he or she feels anything. Most people will understandably tense their abdominal muscles if they think you are about to cause them pain.

Additionally, never take your eyes off the patient's face while you are palpating. You are looking for any signs of pain or discomfort. Do not hurt the patient —you will fail exams if you do!

Light palpation of all four quadrants or nine regions will alert you to any obvious tenderness or peritonism—this is all you want to gain from it.

Patients with tender abdomina are naturally apprehensive about having them palpated. However, when you have been around the quadrants once without

205

**Fig. 9.8** Possible signs on examination of the neck.

| Test performed | Sign observed | Diagnostic inference |
|---|---|---|
| Inspection of JVP (jugular venous pressure) | JVP raised (vertical height of column of blood in internal jugular vein exceeds 3 cm, measured from the sternal angle with the patient lying at 45°) | Superior mediastinal obstruction, e.g. carcinoma of bronchus (if JVP non-pulsatile), right heart failure, fluid overload, tricuspid incompetence, cardiac tamponade (if JVP pulsatile) |
| Palpation | Swellings | Infection, carcinoma, bronchial cyst, thyroglossal or other cyst, goitre (iodine deficiency or thyroid disorder) |
| | Enlarged lymph nodes (lymphadenopathy) | Infection, carcinoma |
| | Enlarged supraclavicular lymph node on the left (Virchow's node) | Carcinoma of stomach |
| Palpation of trachea | Deviation, not central | Superior mediastinal mass, collapse of one lung, fibrosis |
| Palpation of carotid pulse | Character of pulse | Information about cardiovascular system |

**Fig. 9.9** Possible signs on inspection of the abdomen.

| Test performed | Sign observed | Diagnostic inference |
|---|---|---|
| Inspection | Nodule near umbilicus (Sister Joseph's nodule) | Metastasis of gastrointestinal or ovarian carcinoma through the ligamentum teres |
| | Inflamed indurated lesion (carcinoma erysipelatoides) | Lymphatic extension of carcinoma to the skin |
| | Pink nodules on anterior trunk | Cutaneous metastases (usually from gastrointestinal tract, kidney, ovary, breast or bronchus) |
| | Central dilated arteriole with small red vessels radiating out from it, like a spider (spider naevi) | If more than five or six, pregnancy, cirrhosis or other chronic liver disease |
| | Distension | Fat, fetus, fluid, faeces, flatus, obstruction |
| | Firm pressure in the left lower area of distension leaves indentations | Distension caused by faeces (e.g. Hirschsprung's disease or acquired megacolon) |
| | Visible pulsation | Aortic aneurysm |
| | Visible peristalsis from left to right | Pyloric stenosis |
| | Visible peristalsis from right to left | Obstruction in the transverse colon |
| | Visible peristalsis in the middle (like a ladder) | Obstruction in the small bowel |
| | Patient lying rigid, taking very shallow breaths | Peritonitis |
| | Distended stomach but thin limbs | Cushing's syndrome, steroids |
| | Discoloration around umbilicus (Cullen's sign) | Acute pancreatitis, carcinoma of the pancreas |
| | Discoloration in the flanks (Grey Turner's sign) | Acute pancreatitis |
| | Dilated veins (not confined to umbilical region) | Obstruction of inferior vena cava |
| | Purple striae | Cushing's syndrome, steroids |
| | White striae | Obesity, previous pregnancy |
| | Veins radiating out from umbilicus (caput medusae) | Portal hypertension |

hurting them they will often relax the abdominal muscles enough to let you palpate more deeply.

During deep palpation, you should be looking for:

- Tenderness on deep palpation only.
- Guarding (tensing of the abdominal muscles).
- Rovsing's sign (more pain in the right iliac fossa than in the left iliac fossa, when palpated).
- Obvious masses.

To describe any lump in the body, remember the six Ss—site, size, shape, surface, smoothness (as well as consistency and fluctuance) and surroundings, i.e. whether it is tethered or not.

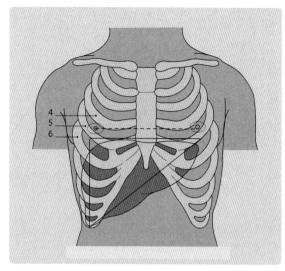

**Fig. 9.10** The position of the normal liver in relation to the nipple line and to the 4th, 5th and 6th ribs.

Following general deep palpation, you will need to palpate for any enlarged abdominal organs (organomegaly). You should attempt to feel the liver, spleen and kidneys.

### Palpating the liver

To examine the liver, start at the right iliac fossa and move your hand up, using the long, flat edge of your index finger to feel for the liver edge. The normal position of the liver is shown in Fig. 9.10.

Its edge can usually be felt just below the edge of the costal margin. You need to palpate quite deeply to feel it. Ask the patient to take deep breaths in and out; the edge should be felt moving against your fingers with respiration.

If you can feel the liver edge, make a note of what it feels like and how many centimetres you can feel. Is it smooth (possible hepatitis) or hard and craggy (tumours)? Remember that cirrhotic livers may not be felt as they often shrink. Some patients may have a palpable extension (Riedel's lobe) to the right lobe which is entirely normal.

### Palpating the spleen

To examine the spleen, start in the right iliac fossa and move up diagonally to the left costal margin. A grossly enlarged spleen can extend into the right iliac fossa. A normal spleen cannot be felt.

A distinguishing feature of the spleen is its notch, which may be palpable in splenomegaly. Additionally, if you can feel an upper margin, you are not feeling the spleen, as you cannot get 'above' it.

### Palpating the kidneys

The kidneys should be 'balloted', using two hands. This is the procedure of bouncing the kidney between the hand at the renal angle and the hand positioned anteriorly to this.

Normally they should not be able to be felt. Enlarged, tender kidneys may indicate infection.

Fig. 9.11 lists the signs elicitable on abdominal palpation.

## Percussion

Percussion is not normally done, unless there is ascites or when confirmation of hepato- or splenomegaly is needed.

The liver and spleen are dull to percussion. You can trace their margins (and confirm organomegaly) by percussing in the directions you palpated when examining them both. Always percuss for the upper border of the liver as well as the lower one. The liver may be pushed down by a hyperinflated chest or other respiratory pathology. Hepatomegaly may be wrongly diagnosed if the upper border has not been located.

If a patient has ascites, there will be shifting dullness (Fig. 9.12). Note that it takes a minute or two for the fluid to drain.

## Auscultation

You should listen for bowel sounds (borborygmi). There should be some and they should not be too

**Fig. 9.11** Possible signs on palpation of the abdomen.

| Test performed | Sign observed | Diagnostic inference |
| --- | --- | --- |
| Palpation | Enlarged liver (hepatomegaly) | Malignancy, infection (especially glandular fever and malaria), hepatitis, sickle-cell disease, porphyria, haemolytic anaemia, connective-tissue disease, portal hypertension, lymphoma, leukaemia, glycogen storage disorders, myelofibrosis |
| | Pulsatile liver | Tricuspid incompetence |
| Palpation of right iliac fossa | The right iliac fossa is more painful than the left (Rovsing's sign) | Acute appendicitis |
| Press on abdomen | Pain occurs when you press in and also when you remove your hand (rebound tenderness) | Peritonitis |
| Place two fingers over right upper quadrant, ask patient to breathe in | Pain on inspiration (Murphy's sign) | Inflamed gall bladder |
| Palpation | Sausage-shaped mass | Pyloric stenosis, intussusception |
| | Mass | Carcinoma, obstruction, hernia, faeces |

**Fig. 9.12** Possible signs on percussion of the abdomen.

| Test performed | Sign observed | Diagnostic inference |
| --- | --- | --- |
| Percuss the abdomen from flank to flank, ask patient to roll onto one side and percuss from flank to flank again | Flanks are dull to percussion, midline is resonant with patient lying on his or her back, upper flank is resonant but lower flank is dull to percussion with patient lying on his or her side (shifting dullness) | Ascites |
| Percussion | Hepatosplenomegaly | Portal hypertension, amyloidosis, leukaemia, sickle-cell anaemia, thalassaemia, glandular fever |
| | Splenomegaly | Lymphoma, leukaemia, portal hypertension, haemolytic anaemia, rheumatoid arthritis, infection |

loud. Listen also for bruits (evidence of disturbed blood flow).

Listen for at least one minute over the ileocaecal valve before declaring that there are absent bowel sounds (Fig. 9.13).

You can also use the stethoscope to confirm the edges of an enlarged liver (the 'scratch test'). Put your stethoscope over the liver and gently scratch the surrounding area with the soft part of the end of your finger (not your nail). The sound will be loud when you are scratching over the liver, but soft as soon as you go over the liver margin. This is not normally done in examination situations however, as it may be uncomfortable for the patient.

You can use the same technique to confirm the edges of an enlarged spleen.

## Examination of the rectum and external genitalia

These are considered part of a complete abdominal examination, although for obvious reasons you will not be asked to do them in examination situations.

**Fig. 9.13** Possible signs on auscultation of the abdomen.

| Test performed | Sign elicited | Diagnostic inference |
|---|---|---|
| Auscultation | Absent bowel sounds | Paralytic ileus |
| | Loud bowel sounds (tinkling) | Intestinal obstruction |
| | Bruit | Disturbed flow (e.g. atherosclerosis) |

## Rectal examination

Always wear gloves and make sure your examining finger is well lubricated.

It is absolutely essential to explain that you are going to perform a rectal or genital examination and why you need to do this.

Make sure you have a chaperone of the same sex as the patient when performing any intimate examination. Many patients find rectal examinations distressing and embarrassing. It is important to establish a rapport with them first and be sensitive to their feelings.

To perform a rectal examination, ask the patient to lie on his or her left side with the knees drawn up. Inspect the anus for redness, bleeding, external haemorrhoids, skin lesions or fistulae. Before you begin, ask the patient if there is any tenderness and ask them to tell you if they feel any pain during the examination.

Gently insert a well-lubricated index finger into the anal canal and rectum. Note the tone of the anal sphincter.

Gently sweep your finger around the walls to check for any masses or abnormalities.

You should be able to feel the prostate in the male and cervix in the female through the anterior wall of the rectum. The prostate has a shallow central groove.

Withdraw your finger: there should be faecal matter on it but no blood or mucus. Take your glove off cuff-first, pulling the glove off inside out, and dispose of it in a clinical waste bag.

Possible abnormal findings are listed in Fig. 9.14.

## Genital examination

You should be looking for any signs of infection, gross abnormality and hernias.

It is best to look for hernias with the patient standing and you kneeling down so that you are at the same level as the area you are examining. Many hernias disappear if the patient lies down. Hernias are common. About 1 in 100 people will have a hernia at some time in their life. About 70% of hernias are inguinal, 20% are femoral and 10% are umbilical.

**Fig. 9.14** Possible signs on rectal examination.

| Test performed | Sign elicited | Diagnostic inference |
|---|---|---|
| Rectal examination and inspection of glove afterwards | Bloody mucus | Chronic inflammatory bowel disease, ulcerating tumour |
| | Watery mucus | Villous adenoma |
| | Pale faecal material | Obstructive jaundice |
| | Bright red blood and slime | Intussusception, colitis |
| Rectal examination | Nodular prostate | Carcinoma, calcification |
| | Tender prostate | Prostatitis |
| | Enlarged, smooth prostate | Age-related benign prostatic hyperplasia |
| | Narrow empty rectum and a gush of faeces and flatus on withdrawing finger | Hirschsprung's disease |

Palpate over the external and internal rings (above and medial to the pubic tubercle) to detect an inguinal hernia and ask the patient to cough. You may feel a lump when he or she does.

Repeat this procedure below and lateral to the pubic tubercle to check for a femoral hernia, and above and below the umbilicus for an umbilical hernia.

Perform the same procedure at other points of weakness, e.g. over scars and at the edges of the rectus muscles.

Try to reduce any swelling. The femoral pulse and lymph nodes in the groin should be palpated.

In the male, inspect the penis and scrotum, carefully palpating the testes, epididymis and spermatic cords. Note any scrotal swelling.

Vaginal examination is not routine and is only performed when indicated.

## Concluding the examination

An examination should also ideally include checking the feet and legs for pitting oedema. This can give clues about respiratory, cardiac or hepatic function.

Urinalysis should also be performed.

# Investigations and imaging

10

## Learning objectives

After reading this chapter, you should be able to outline the following types of investigation with regard to the gastrointestinal tract:

- Tests of organ function.
- Haematological, microbiological and biochemical tests.
- Endoscopic investigations.
- Radiological investigations.

## OVERVIEW

Investigations are part of patient management, and so a good working knowledge of common tests is essential. However, it is worthwhile remembering that 80% of the diagnosis comes from the history and the remainder from the examination and investigations, so investigations cannot replace clinical skill!

Before requesting investigations, a list of differential diagnoses should have been made, from which the most probable diagnosis or diagnoses should have been selected. The tests ordered should be relevant to the possible diagnoses, as unnecessary or inappropriate tests waste time and resources.

## 'ROUTINE' HAEMATOLOGICAL AND BIOCHEMICAL INVESTIGATIONS

A number of simple blood tests are available to confirm (or disprove) diagnoses arrived at from the history and examination.

The results described below are particularly relevant to gastrointestinal disease; other texts in the *Crash Course* series should be consulted for other systems.

Clinical history taking and examination should always take precedence over investigations in the diagnostic process. Remember that although tests have a number of uses, their main function is to confirm or exclude a provisional diagnosis.

## Haematological tests

These, and their results, are described in Fig. 10.1.

## Biochemical tests

Liver function tests (LFTs) are one of the most commonly requested biochemical investigations, and not always because a hepatic cause of disease is suspected—they are also useful when assessing liver function before a certain drug is prescribed, for example. They are discussed below; other biochemical tests concerning the gastrointestinal system are summarized in Fig. 10.2.

### Liver function tests

The functions of the liver are described in Chapter 4 (Fig. 4.11). Liver 'function' can be assessed by measurement of serum levels of albumin, bilirubin, urea, glucose and prothrombin time.

**Fig. 10.1** General haematological tests and possible causes of abnormalities.

| Normal ranges | Raised | Lowered |
|---|---|---|
| Leucocyte count $4-11 \times 10^9$ | Infection—see below for details | Chemotherapy, steroids |
| Erythrocyte count<br>men: $4.5-6.5 \times 10^{12}$<br>women: $3.9-5.6 \times 10^{12}$ | | |
| PCV (packed corpuscular volume)<br>men: 0.4–0.54 L/L<br>women: 0.37–0.54 L/L | Polycythaemia | |
| MCV (mean corpuscular volume)<br>76–96 fL | Excessive alcohol consumption, vitamin $B_{12}$ and folate deficiency, liver disease | Iron-deficiency anaemia, thalassaemia |
| MCH (mean corpuscular haemoglobin)<br>27–32 pg | | |
| Neutrophils<br>$2.0-7.5 \times 10^9$/L<br>40–75% of total white cell count | Bacterial infections, trauma, surgery, haemorrhage, inflammation, infarction, drugs (e.g. steroids), disseminated malignancy, polymyalgia, myeloproliferative disorders, polyarteritis nodosa | Vitamin $B_{12}$ deficiency, folate deficiency, bone marrow failure, tuberculosis, brucellosis, typhoid, kala-azar, septicaemia, hypersplenism, certain autoimmune disease, drugs (e.g. sulfonamides, carbimazole) |
| Lymphocytes<br>$1.3-3.5 \times 10^9$/L<br>20–40% of total white cell count | Viral infection, toxoplasmosis, brucellosis, whooping cough, chronic lymphoid leukaemia | HIV infection, marrow infiltration, drugs (steroids), systemic lupus erythematosus, Legionnaire's disease, uraemia, chemotherapy, radiotherapy |
| Eosinophils<br>$0.04-0.44 \times 10^9$/L<br>1–6% of total white cell count | Atopic conditions, parasitic infections, malignancy, polyarteritis nodosa | |
| Basophils<br>$0-0.1 \times 10^9$/L<br>0–1% of total white cell count | Ulcerative colitis, viral infection, malignancy, polycythaemia rubra, cell-mediated lympholysis, haemolysis, myxoedema | |
| Monocytes<br>$0.2-0.8 \times 10^9$/L<br>2–10% of total white cell count | Acute and chronic infection, malignancy | |
| Platelet count $150-400 \times 10^9$/L | Inflammatory disease, colitis, Crohn's disease | Lymphoma, viral infection, drugs, marrow failure, idiopathic thrombocytopenic purpura, disseminated intravascular coagulation, hypersplenism |
| Reticulocyte count $25-100 \times 10^9$/L | Anaemia, haemorrhage | |
| ESR (erythrocyte sedimentation rate, mm/h) rises with age, upper limit is:<br>men: age ÷ 2<br>women: (age + 10) ÷ 2 | Anaemia, malignancy, infection, sarcoidosis, lymphoma, CT disease, abdominal aneurysm | Heart failure, polycythaemia |
| Prothrombin time 10–14 s (often expressed as INR, by definition 1 is normal) | Liver disease, warfarin | |
| Activated partial thromboplastin time 35–45s | Haemophilia, Christmas disease | |

**Fig. 10.2** General biochemical tests and possible causes of abnormalities. ($\gamma$-GT = $\gamma$-glutamyltransferase; LDH = lactate dehydrogenase.)

| Normal range | Raised | Lowered |
| --- | --- | --- |
| Alanine aminotransferase 5–35 IU/L | Liver disease (hepatocellular damage), shock | |
| Albumin 35–50 g/L | Dehydration | Malabsorption, malnutrition, malignancy, liver disease |
| Alkaline phosphatase 30–300 IU/L | Liver disease (cholestasis) | |
| $\alpha$-fetoprotein <10 kU/L | Hepatocellular carcinoma, hepatitis, chronic liver disease, teratoma | |
| $\alpha$-amylase 0–180 somogyi U/L | Acute pancreatitis | |
| Aspartate transaminase 5–35 IU/L | Liver disease (hepatocellular damage), myocardial infarction, skeletal muscle damage | |
| Bilirubin 3–17 µmol/L | Jaundice | |
| Calcium Ion, 1.00–1.25 mmol/L Total, 2.12–2.65 mmol/L | Malignancy, sarcoidosis, tuberculosis, hyperparathyroidism | Malabsorption, acute pancreatitis, massive blood transfusion, hypoparathyroidism |
| Caeruloplasmin 200–350 mg/L | | Wilson's disease |
| Copper 11.0–22.0 µmol/L | | Wilson's disease |
| Cholesterol 3.9–7.8 mmol/L | Hyperlipidaemia | |
| Creatinine kinase 25–195 IU/L men 25–170 IU/L women | Myocardial infarction | |
| Ferritin 12–200 µg/L | Haemochromatosis | |
| Folate 2.1 µg/L | | Malabsorption, alcoholism, drugs, malignancy, haemolysis |
| $\gamma$-GT 0–0.50 µkat/L | Alcoholic liver disease, biliary obstruction | |
| Iron 14–32 µmol/L men 11–29 µmol/L women | | Iron-deficiency anaemia |
| LDH 70–250 IU/L | Hepatocellular damage, myocardial infarction | |
| Magnesium 0.75–1.05 mmol/L | | Diarrhoea, alcohol, total parenteral nutrition |
| Potassium 3.5–5.0 mmol/L | Trauma (including surgery), catabolic states, renal failure, transfusion of stored blood, haemolysis | Pernicious anaemia treated with $B_{12}$, diarrhoea, laxative abuse, vomiting, villous adenoma |
| Total protein 60–80 g/L | | Malabsorption, Ménétrièr's disease, nephrotic syndrome, malnutrition |
| Sodium 135–145 mmol/L | Dehydration | Vomiting, diarrhoea, fistulae, ileus, intestinal obstruction, cystic, fibrosis |
| Triglyceride 0.55–1.9 mmol/L | Hyperlipidaemia | |
| Urea 2.5–6.7 mmol/L | Dehydration | |
| Urate 210–480 µmol/L men 150–390 µmol/L women | Lymphoma, gout, leukaemia, haemolysis, drugs, alcohol | Coeliac disease, Wilson's disease, pernicious anaemia |
| Vitamin $B_{12}$ 0.13–0.68 µmol/L | | Malabsorption, pernicious anaemia, gastrectomy |

Included in the term LFTs are the liver enzymes, i.e. aminotransferases (AST and ALT), alkaline phosphatase and γ-glutamyltransferase (see later). Although these actually give no information about liver function, raised serum levels reflect some degree of necro-inflammatory change in the liver.

## The prothrombin time

Prothrombin time is a functional test measuring the interaction between a cascade of clotting factors, all of which are made in the liver. Therefore, if any one of these is abnormal or deficient, prothrobin time will be prolonged.

It is a very sensitive test of liver function due to the lability of a number of components, particularly factor V.

Prothrombin time is also increased in vitamin K deficiency as this fat-soluble vitamin is required for activation of factors II, VII, IX and X.

Jaundice due to obstruction will impair absorption of vitamin K so prolonged prothrombin time in obstructive jaundice can be corrected by giving vitamin K but in the presence of hepatocellular damage, where synthesis of other clotting factors is affected, vitamin K administration will have no effect.

## Hepatic enzyme assays

*Aminotransferases* (*transaminases*). These enzymes are present in hepatocytes and leak into the plasma in liver cell damage. Alanine aminotransferase (ALT) is present in the cytoplasm of hepatocytes and its level increases in hepatocellular injury.

Aspartate aminotransferase (AST) is a mitochondrial enzyme present not only in the liver but also in cardiac muscle, the kidneys and the brain. Because of this it is less specific than ALT, as conditions affecting these other organs, e.g. myocardial infarction, muscle injury and congestive heart failure, will also cause it to rise.

*Alkaline phosphatase.* An isoenzyme of this enzyme is present in the canalicular and sinusoidal membranes of the liver. Other isoenzymes are present in bone (it is produced by osteoblasts), intestine and placenta. Bone and liver are the two most important sources.

Levels rise following damage to any of these structures—electrophoresis can be used to determine the particular isoenzyme (and therefore its source) but in practice, a commensurate rise in γ-glutamyltransferase is usually taken to indicate hepatic origin. Hepatic alkaline phosphatase is raised in infiltration of the liver, cirrhosis and cholestasis (from both intrahepatic and extrahepatic causes). The highest levels are seen in hepatic metastases and primary biliary cirrhosis.

*γ-glutamyltransferase* (*γ-GT*). This enzyme is present in the mitochondria of many tissues, including the liver. If γ-GT is raised but alkaline phosphatase levels are normal, the cause of the damage is probably alcohol. If both γ-GT and alkaline phosphatase are high, the cause may be cholestasis or intrahepatic malignancy. If the alkaline phosphatase is raised, but the γ-GT is normal, then one should suspect bone disease, e.g. Paget's disease, or pregnancy.

Note that raised levels of both enzymes are also seen following the administration of phenytoin (an antiepileptic drug and enzyme inducer) and the ingestion of even a moderate amount of alcohol.

When interpreting the results of liver enzyme assays, patterns of abnormality are important in diagnosis:

- Predominantly raised levels of AST and ALT reflect hepatocellular damage.
- Predominantly raised alkaline phosphatase and γ-GT indicate cholestasis or intrahepatic abscess and malignancy.

## Additional tests: the 'liver screen'

As there are many causes of liver failure it is sometimes useful to carry out a number of other tests especially if the standard LFTs are deranged:

- $\alpha_1$-*antitrypsin.* Deficiency of $\alpha_1$-antitrypsin can produce cirrhosis.
- *α-fetoprotein.* This is raised in patients with hepatocellular carcinoma and in pregnant women. Less elevated levels are found in hepatitis, teratoma and chronic liver disease.
- *Ferritin.* In haemachromatosis, the serum ferritin will be raised due to the increased serum iron, as will transferrin saturation levels.
- *Caeruloplasmin.* This is relevant if Wilson's disease is suspected. Patients will have low levels of the protein, although occasionally there is no apparent abnormality. Note that any cause of advanced liver failure may cause low caeruloplasmin.
- *24-hour urinary copper.* As with caeruloplasmin, this aids in the diagnosis of Wilson's disease. The urinary excretion rate of copper will be raised.

- *Viral hepatitis serology* for hepatitis A, B and C viruses. This is useful to screen for an infective cause. The presence of anti-viral IgM suggests an acute infection, while the presence of IgG suggests immunity due to past infection or vaccination.
- *Autoantibody screen.* Certain diseases are associated with particular autoantibodies, for example autoimmune hepatitis (anti-smooth muscle and anti-nuclear in type I; anti-liver-kidney-microsomal in type II), primary biliary sclerosis (anti-mitochondrial) and primary sclerosing cholangitis (perinuclear anti-neutrophil cytoplasmic antibodies, p-ANCA).
- *Glucose, lipids and HbA$_{1c}$.* To screen for metabolic diseases, e.g. diabetes mellitus which may have symptoms common to liver disease. For instance, acute liver failure can cause hypoglycaemia.

The pattern of deviation from normal levels is more important than individual rises or falls: do not rely too heavily on a single abnormal result. If all the tests were conducted on a healthy person, the chances are that at least one of them would be abnormal!

## Histology and cytology

Histology is the study of tissue samples taken on biopsy or following surgical removal. The sample may be examined using light microscopy or electron microscopy. Histological examination is useful in cases of malignancy, or in diseases where there are structural changes, e.g. Crohn's disease.

Cytology is the study of cell samples taken by means of swabs or fine-needle aspiration. The cells are stained and examined under a microscope to detect the presence of abnormal, e.g. neoplastic, and inflammatory cells.

## Microbiology

Medical microbiology is the study of microorganisms and their effects on humans. Bacteria, viruses, fungi and parasites can cause disease. A typical request to the microbiology laboratory would be for microscopy, culture and (antibiotic) sensitivity.

Many bacteria, fungi and parasites can be identified using light microscopy, but viruses are too small and other methods, e.g. electron microscopy or serological testing must be employed for their detection.

In gastrointestinal disease, samples for microbiological investigation include raw stools and swabs.

Gram staining of microscopic samples is particularly useful, as it classifies bacteria as being either Gram-positive or Gram-negative, allowing provisional identification.

Culture is a slower method of identification—some bacteria require certain types of culture medium to grow. It is also useful in deciding which antibiotic is most effective against a particular organism.

A simple sensitivity test involves smearing samples on an agar plate, placing antibiotic discs onto the plate and then incubating it. Small patches of agar on which no bacteria have grown can be seen around those antibiotics that are most effective against the bacteria in question. Other, more sophisticated sensitivity tests are available but are not within the scope of this book.

## Breath tests

The general principle of a breath test is that if an enzyme which catalyses a reaction causing the production of gases such as hydrogen or $CO_2$ is present in the gut lumen, then giving the patient the relevant substrate will cause the gas to be detectable in the patient's breath (Fig. 10.3). This is because the gas is absorbed by diffusion and then exhaled via the lungs.

An example of this is the hydrogen breath test, which can be performed after giving the patient a lactulose solution to drink. This can detect an overgrowth of bacteria if there are more than 20 parts per million of hydrogen gas in less than 2 hours. Normally, breath hydrogen is undetectable, hence raised levels suggest bacterial hydrolysis. In a similar way, lactase deficiency can be detected by giving a lactose drink.

A urea breath test can be performed to confirm the presence of *Helicobacter pylori* in the stomach. This uses $^{14}C$-urea or $^{13}C$-urea isotopes. The *H. pylori* urease enzyme converts the urea to ammonia and radiolabelled $CO_2$, which is collected in a breath sample. It is a good non-invasive investigation.

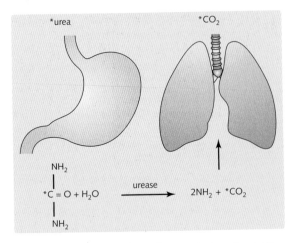

**Fig. 10.3** The basis of a breath test. The example shown here is the urea breath test for detection of *H. pylori*, where the bacterial urease splits radiolabelled urea into ammonia and $CO_2$, the latter of which is detected in the exhaled breath. (Reproduced with permission from Fox C, Lombard M. Crash Course: Gastroenterology, 2nd edn. Edinburgh: Mosby, 2004.)

## Oesophageal manometry

Oesophageal manometry measures pressure changes in different parts of the oesophagus and is used to investigate suspected motility disorders.

A fluid-filled continuously perfused catheter is passed through the nose into the oesophagus, in much the same way as a nasogastric tube. Contraction of the oesophagus causes a pressure change that is transmitted up the fluid column and recorded as a trace.

In normal individuals, a pressure wave should pass down the oesophagus to the lower oesophageal sphincter, which then relaxes to allow the oesophageal contents to pass into the stomach. Abnormal traces are seen in motility disorders, e.g. achalasia.

## Investigation of gastric function

Refluxed acid may overwhelm the normal protective lining of the oesophagus, leading to ulceration. Suspected reflux may be investigated by measuring the pH in the lower oesophagus over the course of 24 hours with a pH-sensitive probe.

A normal trace shows a pH above 4 for most of the time—if the pH is below 4 for more than 4% of the time significant reflux is said to have occurred.

Disorders of gastric acid secretion may be investigated using the pentagastrin test. The patient fasts overnight and the resting juice in the stomach is aspirated using a nasogastric tube. Pentagastrin, a synthetic analogue of gastrin, is then given (6 mg/kg body weight) to stimulate acid secretion, and gastric contents are again aspirated for 1 hour and analysed.

Generally, a large volume of resting juice suggests gastric stasis, a high acid secretion suggests Zollinger–Ellison syndrome and a failure to stimulate acid secretion with pentagastrin indicates achlorhydria.

Plasma levels of gastrin (a hormone which stimulates gastric acid secretion and growth of the gastric mucosa) may also be measured.

The levels of gastrin will be high in the Zollinger–Ellison syndrome as G cells in the pancreas, duodenum or, more rarely, the stomach, secrete large amounts of gastrin in this disorder and cause hyperacidity, leading to ulceration.

Levels will also be high if the patient is taking drugs that inhibit gastric acid secretion and such drugs should be stopped before gastrin levels are measured.

## ENDOSCOPIC EXAMINATIONS

Endoscopy gives very valuable information about a number of gastrointestinal tract disorders. It is less invasive than surgery and allows visualization of the interior of the alimentary tract on a monitor.

Endoscopy can also be used therapeutically for the following:

- Removal of submucosal lesions or polyps (polypectomy, sub-mucosal resection).
- Control of bleeding, e.g. variceal banding or diathermy.
- Relief of strictures, e.g. with stents.
- Treatment of tumours, e.g. with lasers.
- Gallstones in the bile duct (retrieval or sphincterotomy).

## Gastroscopy (oesophagogastroduodenoscopy)

In this procedure, the patient is laid on the left side and the endoscope is passed down the oesophagus.

Patients must fast overnight beforehand and the endoscopy is performed as a day-case procedure.

Some patients are given mild sedation (which can cause slight amnesia), but many manage with just an oral local anaesthetic spray.

Gastroscopy is commonly used to investigate upper gastrointestinal disorders. Forceps for taking biopsies can be passed through the biopsy channel of the endoscope.

> Gastroscopy should not be performed in patients with upper gastrointestinal bleeding until the haemorrhage is controlled, as the procedure can increase the severity of the haemorrhage.

## Colonoscopy, sigmoidoscopy and proctoscopy

These procedures give information about the lower gastrointestinal tract.

Proctoscopy is commonly performed in out-patients and involves the use of a proctoscope, a rigid tube with a detachable, disposable end that is used for one patient only and then removed and thrown away. Before the proctoscope is used, an obturator is inserted into its lumen to avoid the discomfort of inserting a hollow tube into the patient's anal canal and the end of the instrument is well lubricated.

The patient is then asked to lie on the left side with knees drawn up to the chest; the proctoscope is gently inserted; the obturator is removed; and air is pumped in through the proctoscope to inflate the rectum. It is kinder to explain to the patient that any associated noise is caused by the air being pumped in, otherwise they may think it is caused by flatulence and become very embarrassed!

Proctoscopy gives valuable information about the anal canal and rectum but, because the instrument is rigid, it cannot be used to visualize structures above the flexure.

The fibre sigmoidoscope and colonoscope are both flexible instruments, with the former being shorter. The colonoscope will allow inspection of the entire large bowel, but the sigmoidoscope gives information only on the anal canal, rectum and sigmoid colon.

The procedure in sigmoidoscopy and colonoscopy is similar to proctoscopy. However, bowel preparation, e.g. with sodium picosulphate to clear out the bowel, is required for 2 days before colonoscopy. Patients are given analgesia and may be sedated for the procedure.

> Always perform a digital rectal examination before proctosigmoidoscopy or colonoscopy. The patient may have a large tumour in the anal canal or rectum and damage may be caused if a scope is inserted without checking first.

## Endoscopic ultrasound

Endoscopic ultrasound (EUS) is a procedure in which an ultrasound image is obtained while performing an endoscopy. The ultrasound transducer is incorporated into the end of the endoscope to produce images alongside the camera image (Fig. 10.4).

## Endoscopic retrograde cholangiopancreatography

Endoscopic retrograde cholangiopancreatography (ERCP) involves injection of contrast material into the biliary and pancreatic systems, via endoscopy, followed by radiological screening (Fig. 10.5).

Two different contrasts are used: low iodine for the common bile duct (so as not to obscure gallstones) and a higher iodine contrast for the pancreatic duct.

Diathermy instruments and grasping forceps can be passed through the endoscope and used to remove stones in the common bile duct after the sphincter of Oddi has been incised (sphincterotomy). Obstructions in the biliary tree can also be relieved using a stent.

ERCP may introduce infection leading to cholangitis and prophylactic antibiotics are usually given. Pancreatitis may also occur.

Nowadays, EUS or magnetic resonance cholangiopancreatography (MRCP—see later) is replacing ERCP for diagnostic purposes.

## IMAGING OF THE GASTROINTESTINAL SYSTEM

## Plain radiography and contrast technique

Substances absorb X-rays to different extents, depending on their atomic number. Those that absorb most appear white, e.g. bone, while those that absorb least, e.g. air, appear black.

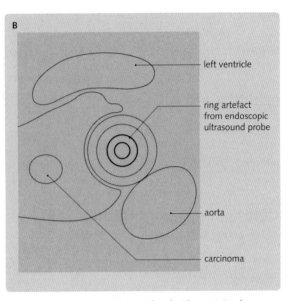

**Fig. 10.4** Endoscopic ultrasound image of oesophageal carcinoma (A) and explanatory diagram (B). ([A] Reproduced with permission from Haslett C et al. Davidson's Principles and Practice of Medicine, 19th edn. Edinburgh: Churchill Livingstone, 2002.)

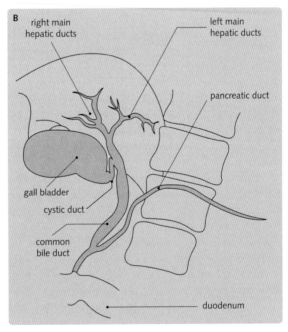

**Fig. 10.5** Endoscopic retrograde cholangiopancreatography (ERCP) image showing a normal biliary and pancreatic duct system (A) and explanatory diagram (B). ([A] Reproduced with permission from Haslett C et al. Davidson's Principles and Practice of Medicine, 18th edn. Edinburgh: Churchill Livingstone, 1999.)

Borders are seen only at the interfaces between different densities, e.g. the interface between the wall of the stomach and the gastric air bubble, but may be enhanced by the introduction of contrast media, for example, barium.

When commenting on any X-ray, always follow the same order. Do not come straight out with a diagnosis, evident though it may be!

1. Check that the film has been taken properly and the information recorded on it:
   - Look at the name and the date. Is it the correct patient and the X-ray you want to examine?
   - Is it an AP (anteroposterior) or PA (posteroanterior) film?
   - Check the alignment of the spine (or the clavicles on a chest X-ray). Was the patient straight when it was taken? If not, organs may be displaced and look abnormal even if they are not.
2. Check the outlines of all the structures you would expect to see on a normal X-ray. Are they all visible? Can you see anything you would not normally expect? Is any area more (or less) opaque than normal?
3. Describe the gross pathology that might have caused these abnormalities, e.g. stricture in the oesophagus, rose-thorn ulcers in the ileum.
4. Suggest the most probable diagnosis and some differential diagnoses.

## Abdominal radiographs

Abdominal films may be taken with the patient supine (best for seeing the distribution of gas) or erect (better for spotting air under the diaphragm and for seeing fluid levels).

The intestines are lower down in erect X-rays than in the supine position. Before X-rays became available doctors had seen intestines only in supine bodies at dissections and operations and a number of unfortunate people had completely unnecessary operations to hitch up their guts when erect abdominal X-rays were first taken! Look at the pattern of gas (central in ascites, displaced to the left lower quadrant in splenomegaly). Extraluminal gas in the liver or biliary system suggests a gas-forming infection or the passing of a stone. In the colonic wall it suggests infective colitis.

Important causes of air under the diaphragm are:

- Perforation of the bowel—this is an emergency and should not be missed.
- A section of intestine lying between the liver and the diaphragm.
- A gas-forming infection.
- A pleuro-peritoneal fistula (tuberculosis, trauma or carcinoma), following surgery or laparoscopy.

Look for opaque areas of calcification, commonly caused by stones (although only 10% of gallstones are radio-opaque), pancreatitis or atherosclerosis.

A loop of intestinal gas (sentinel loop) can be caused by local peritoneal inflammation resulting in a localized ileus.

Fig. 10.6 shows the structures normally visible on plain abdominal X-ray.

## Contrast radiographs

These may be single (barium only) or double contrast (e.g. air and barium). Double-contrast films give a better picture of surface mucosa.

Barium may be administered orally and different parts of the gastrointestinal tract can be visualized using this technique depending on the delay before taking the X-ray.

A barium enema is often used to visualize the lower gastrointestinal tract (Fig. 10.7).

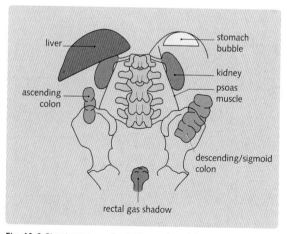

**Fig. 10.6** Structures normally visible on plain abdominal X-ray. (Reproduced with permission from Hope RA et al. Oxford Handbook of Clinical Medicine, 3rd edn. Oxford: Oxford University Press, 1993.)

Fig. 10.7 A small bowel barium study in Crohn's disease showing narrowing and distortion of the terminal ileum. (Courtesy of Dr A Grundy, St George's Hospital, London.)

## Angiography

Angiography is a form of contrast imaging used to visualize blood vessels.

It may show the site of gastrointestinal bleeding (although endoscopy is often the investigation of choice) and the blood supply to specific organs such as the liver (showing architectural abnormalities).

## Computerized tomography

Computerized tomography (CT) scanners produce computerized images of the body in a series of slices, based on the amount of X-rays absorbed by different tissues at different angles (Fig. 10.8). They are more effective for imaging soft tissues (including tumours) than radiography, and the level of radiation is generally lower. CT scans may be plain or contrast—contrast is often used to delineate the bowel.

## Magnetic resonance imaging

Magnetic resonance imaging (MRI) scanners are large electrical coils that align the nuclei of hydrogen atoms in the body so that they lie parallel to each other (normally they lie in random directions).

Fig. 10.8 Computerized tomography (CT) scan of a renal cyst. The cyst (C) is displacing the pelvicalyceal system (compare with right kidney, K). (L = liver.) (Courtesy of Dr A Grundy, St George's Hospital, London.)

The nuclei are then temporarily knocked out of alignment by radio pulses and they emit radio signals as they fall back into alignment. These signals are analysed to produce sliced images of the body, similar to CT scans.

Most scanners will be set so that fatty tissue, containing a high density of hydrogen atoms, produces a bright image. Conversely, bone tissue produces dark images. However, techniques used may vary according to the requirements of the scan.

MRI scans are often preferred in pregnancy as they do not use radiation, but they can interfere with pacemakers, hearing aids and other electrical devices.

As its name suggests, MRCP (magnetic resonance cholangio-pancreatography) uses a large magnet surrounding the body to detect differences in the electromagnetic characteristics of different body components or fluids. The signals obtained are compiled by computer graphics into very detailed anatomical images which can be used to visualize the common bile duct and pancreatic duct. However, because it is not invasive it cannot be used for therapeutic purposes.

Another related, but also not endoscopic, investigation is percutaneous transhepatic cholangiography, which is an interventional radiological technique. While it can be used for therapeutic interventions, it does not allow the visualization of the ampulla of Vater or pancreatic duct.

> In many cases, CT is preferred over MRI, as it is faster, exposes the patient to lower levels of radiation and costs less.

## Radioisotope scanning

Radioisotope scanning is used to study the uptake of isotopes by various organs.

Different isotopes are taken up by different organs and structures. 'Hot' lesions are those which take up

**Fig. 10.9** Ultrasound image of a cirrhotic liver showing its classical coarse, grainy appearance. (Courtesy of Dr J Pilcher, St George's Hospital, London.)

more isotope than the surrounding tissue, while 'cold' ones take up less.

An example of radioisotope scanning is the use of technetium ($^{99m}$Tc) colloid to scan the liver and assess gastric emptying. Another is $^{99m}$Tc HIDA (hepatic iminodiacetic acid) which is used to scan the biliary tree, as it is taken up by the liver, cleared to the gall bladder and excreted in the bile. Liver lesions greater than 2 cm in diameter show up as cold spots in scanning with $^{99m}$Tc colloid.

## Ultrasonography

Ultrasonography has been used since the 1970s and is often the investigation of choice for abdominal masses (Fig. 10.9).

Ultrasonographic machines emit very-high-frequency sound waves, which pass readily through fluids, but are reflected back from acoustic interfaces such as soft tissue, bone or gas—the reflected echoes are analysed to produce images.

Ultrasonographic scans are non-invasive and safe in pregnancy.

# SELF-ASSESSMENT

Indicate whether each statement is true or false.

## Chapter 1—Introduction to the gastrointestinal system

1.  **Regarding the different food groups:**
    (a) Pellagra is a manifestation of protein deficiency.
    (b) Carbohydrates with β-glycosidic linkages are easily absorbed.
    (c) Fat-soluble vitamins are stored mostly in the liver.
    (d) Water is needed in the digestive process.
    (e) Protein provides much more energy than carbohydrate.

2.  **The following statements on the embryology of the alimentary tract are true:**
    (a) The branchial arches contribute to the development of the oesophagus.
    (b) The superior mesenteric artery supplies those parts derived from the foregut.
    (c) The part of the colon derived from the midgut ends at approximately the first third of its length.
    (d) The vitelline duct persists in about 2% of the population.
    (e) The nerve supply of the hindgut derivatives comes from the vagus nerve.

3.  **Concerning the gastrointestinal tract:**
    (a) Malformation may result from absence of the fifth branchial arch.
    (b) Lymphoid tissue is found in the submucosa.
    (c) Vitamins are digested in the small intestine.
    (d) Meissner's plexus is located between the longitudinal and smooth muscle layers.
    (e) It is longer in a cadaver than it is in a living person.

4.  **Regarding the alimentary system:**
    (a) Hormones play an important role in its function.
    (b) It is sterile due to its internal location.
    (c) The muscles of mastication are supplied by the trigeminal nerve.
    (d) The gut herniates between weeks 9–13 of embryological development.
    (e) It maintains the same basic structure throughout its length.

## Chapter 2—The upper gastrointestinal tract

5.  **Regarding appetite and food intake:**
    (a) High temperatures decrease appetite.
    (b) Leptin acts on receptors in the thalamus to inhibit appetite.
    (c) Carbohydrates are the main energy source during the day while fats are the main energy source at night.
    (d) Diabetics have a higher satiety threshold than normal.
    (e) Damage to the paraventricular nucleus of the hypothalamus results in aphagia.

6.  **The oesophagus:**
    (a) Joins the stomach just behind the 7th costal cartilage.
    (b) Is constricted by the aortic arch.
    (c) Has two anatomical sphincters, one at each end.
    (d) Develops in association with the descent of the heart and lungs.
    (e) Inclines to the right before it contacts the arch of the aorta.

7.  **Concerning the salivary glands:**
    (a) There are six large glands in the normal person.
    (b) The sublingual glands comprise predominantly serous secretory cells.
    (c) Intercalated ducts are lined with columnar secretory cells.
    (d) Surgery to the parotid gland runs the risk of damaging the facial nerve.
    (e) The secretory unit is called an acinus.

8.  **The following are risk factors for gastro-oesophageal reflux disease (GORD):**
    (a) Age.
    (b) Obesity.
    (c) Female sex.
    (d) Hiatus hernia.
    (e) Cigarette smoking.

9.  **Regarding swallowing:**
    (a) It is controlled by the medulla oblongata.
    (b) The epiglottis protects against food entering the trachea.
    (c) Tertiary peristaltic waves are caused by distension of the oesophagus.
    (d) In the absence of peristalsis, food does not enter the stomach.
    (e) It inhibits respiration.

10. **Concerning the mouth and oropharynx:**
    (a) Cleft palate is more common than cleft lip.
    (b) Cleft lip is more common in females.
    (c) Leukoplakia is a malignant condition.

225

(d) Cold sores are a sign of recurrent herpes simplex virus infection.
(e) Oral candidiasis is a common condition.

11. **The following are true statements regarding saliva and salivation:**
    (a) Muscarinic blockers inhibit salivation.
    (b) A normal person produces half a litre of saliva daily.
    (c) In saliva, potassium is present in hypotonic concentrations at high flow rates.
    (d) Sympathetic stimulation produces thick saliva.
    (e) Immunoglobulin A is present in saliva.

12. **The following statements are true of the oesophagus:**
    (a) The upper third is made up of smooth muscle.
    (b) The upper oesophageal sphincter is part of the cricopharyngeus muscle.
    (c) Seromucous glands are most prominent in the middle third.
    (d) Oesophageal varices are harmless.
    (e) Oesophageal atresia and fistulae usually occur together.

13. **Regarding the tongue:**
    (a) Circumvallate papillae are found anterior to the sulcus terminalis.
    (b) The extrinsic muscles of the tongue, except the palatoglossus, are supplied by the IXth cranial nerve.
    (c) The lingual artery is a branch of the external carotid artery.
    (d) Fungiform papillae appear red.
    (e) A lesion of the IXth cranial nerve will cause the tongue to deviate to the normal side when the tongue is protruded.

14. **Oesophageal carcinoma:**
    (a) Is a common malignant tumour.
    (b) Is commonly found in the upper and lower thirds.
    (c) Has an association with Barrett's oesophagus.
    (d) Is usually squamous cell carcinoma or adenocarcinoma.
    (e) Has a good prognosis.

15. **Concerning diseases of the oesophagus:**
    (a) Proton pump inhibitors are indicated in gastro-oesophageal reflux disease.
    (b) Chagas' disease may lead to a beak deformity seen on barium swallow.
    (c) Oesophageal diverticula may be treated with banding.
    (d) Sliding hiatus hernias are less common than rolling hiatus hernias.
    (e) In Barrett's oesophagus, the normal columnar epithelium is replaced by squamous epithelium in response to gastric acid reflux.

16. **Concerning vomiting:**
    (a) The chemoreceptor trigger zone (CTZ) is situated in the fourth ventricle.
    (b) The CTZ is part of the vomiting centre.
    (c) A side effect of metoclopramide (a dopamine-receptor antagonist) is increased intestinal motility.
    (d) $H_1$-receptor antagonists are effective against vomiting produced by substances acting directly on the CTZ.
    (e) The blood–brain barrier is relatively permeable in the region of the CTZ.

17. **Concerning anti-emetic drugs:**
    (a) Ondansetron (a $5\text{-}HT_3$ antagonist) is effective against motion sickness.
    (b) Metoclopramide is a muscarinic receptor antagonist.
    (c) Cannabinoids prevent vomiting caused by substances acting on the vomiting centre.
    (d) $5\text{-}HT_3$ antagonists are effective against emetic stimuli originating from the stomach.
    (e) Dry mouth is a side-effect of hyoscine.

# Chapter 3—The stomach

18. **In the stomach:**
    (a) Stem cells are found mainly at the bases of the gastric glands.
    (b) Peptic (chief) cells secrete intrinsic factor.
    (c) Gastric juice has a pH of 3–4.
    (d) Gastrin-secreting cells are found in the pylorus.
    (e) Peptic (chief) cells have abundant mitochondria and ribosomes.

19. **Regarding the stomach:**
    (a) The greater omentum is a reflection of peritoneum at the greater curvature.
    (b) The pylorus is usually on the right.
    (c) The gastroduodenal vein drains into the hepatic portal system.
    (d) It has both sympathetic and parasympathetic innervation.
    (e) The fundus may herniate through the diaphragm giving rise to a sliding hiatus hernia.

20. **Concerning tumours of the stomach:**
    (a) They may be caused by a hereditary disorder.
    (b) Malignancy may present as dysphagia.
    (c) Squamous cell carcinoma is the most common malignant neoplasm.
    (d) A swollen lymph node in the right supraclavicular fossa is suggestive of gastric carcinoma.
    (e) Lack of gastric acid secretion is a risk factor for gastric carcinoma.

21. **The following are true statements on vomiting:**
    (a) The vagus nerve plays a role in vomiting.
    (b) The chemoreceptor trigger zones are part of the vomiting centres.
    (c) It may be caused by excessive stimulation of the vestibular system.
    (d) The epiglottis is closed during vomiting.
    (e) There is increased production of saliva prior to vomiting.

22. **Concerning the stomach:**
    (a) During its embryological development, the anterior wall grows faster than the posterior wall.
    (b) The left and right gastroepiploic arteries anastomose.
    (c) It rotates 90° on its vertical axis during its embryological development.
    (d) Its lymphatic drainage is towards the curvatures.
    (e) Gastric varices can be safely biopsied.

23. **The following statements on gastric emptying are true:**
    (a) It depends on the myogenic properties of gastric smooth muscle.
    (b) It can be increased by domperidone.
    (c) The rate is decreased if the vagus nerve is damaged.
    (d) Fats are emptied most quickly.
    (e) It is inhibited by cholecystokinin.

24. **The gastric parietal cell:**
    (a) Has a pump which actively transports chloride.
    (b) Is essential for the absorption of vitamin $B_{12}$.
    (c) Is most numerous in the pyloric part of the stomach.
    (d) Stains red with haematoxylin and eosin.
    (e) Has a 'fried-egg' appearance.

25. **The following are true statements on peptic ulcers:**
    (a) They are an example of a chronic inflammatory process.
    (b) Most peptic ulcers are associated with *Helicobacter pylori*.
    (c) Misoprostol protects the gastric mucosa from ulceration.
    (d) Use of non-steroidal anti-inflammatory drugs is a risk factor for developing peptic ulcers.
    (e) A perforated peptic ulcer is life-threatening.

26. **Regarding gastric secretion:**
    (a) The intestinal phase is the longest of the three phases.
    (b) It occurs before food intake.
    (c) It is decreased by products of fat digestion.
    (d) Gastric lipase plays a major part in fat digestion.
    (e) Gastric hydrochloric acid is essential for life.

27. **The bacterium *Helicobacter pylori*:**
    (a) Is a Gram-positive organism.
    (b) Causes type B chronic gastritis.
    (c) Produces vacuolating toxin (VacA).
    (d) Can be detected by the hydrogen breath test.
    (e) Can be eradicated with a combination of three antibiotics.

28. **Concerning gastric motility:**
    (a) Most of the mixing of food with gastric secretions takes place in the fundus.
    (b) The lag phase occurs when the stomach is full.
    (c) The pacemaker cells for gastric peristalsis are found in the antrum.
    (d) Vagotomy greatly diminishes gastric motility.
    (e) The pressure in the antrum between contractions is slightly higher than the intra-abdominal pressure.

29. **Concerning drugs affecting gastric acid secretion:**
    (a) Omeprazole (a proton-pump inhibitor) is a weak base.
    (b) $H_2$-receptor antagonists decrease acetylcholine-stimulated acid secretion.
    (c) Misoprostol is prescribed in the chronic use of non-steroidal anti-inflammatory drugs (NSAIDs).
    (d) Proton-pump inhibitors competitively inhibit $H^+/K^+$-ATPase.
    (e) Ranitidine (a $H_2$-receptor antagonist) may be used as part of triple therapy to eradicate *Helicobacter pylori*.

30. **The following statements on gastric acid secretion are true:**
    (a) A pH of 1–2 will inhibit secretion.
    (b) Cimetidine (a $H_2$-receptor antagonist) increases cyclic AMP production in the parietal cell.
    (c) Calcium salts may be used as antacids.
    (d) Proglumide acts by blocking gastrin receptors.
    (e) Histamine acts as a neurotransmitter on the parietal cell causing increased gastric acid secretion.

31. **The following are true statements regarding disorders of the stomach:**
    (a) Diaphragmatic hernias are treated surgically.
    (b) Untreated type A chronic gastritis will result in a low mean corpuscular volume (MCV) on a full blood count.
    (c) Pyloric stenosis is more common in female infants.
    (d) The Zollinger–Ellison syndrome is a cause of peptic ulcer disease.
    (e) Gastroparesis can be treated with ranitidine (a $H_2$-receptor antagonist).

32. **Concerning the stomach:**
    (a) Pepsin is secreted as a proenzyme.
    (b) The mucus layer inhibits the activity of pepsin.
    (c) Acetylcholine stimulates hydrochloric acid secretion via activation of cyclic AMP.
    (d) Resting gastric juice is acidic.
    (e) The bacterium *Helicobacter pylori* is protected from the acidity of the stomach by its ability to produce urease.

33. **Concerning gastric pharmacology:**
    (a) Bismuth has a similar mechanism of action as sucralfate.
    (b) Proton-pump inhibitors act on the terminal step of the acid secretory pathway.
    (c) Aluminium salts cause diarrhoea.

(d) Relapses of ulceration are unlikely when treatment with $H_2$-receptor antagonists is stopped.

(e) Prostaglandin analogues protect against ulceration by decreasing mucosal blood supply.

**34. Based on data in the table:**

In a trial of a new gastrin analogue on volunteer subjects conducted by a drug company, the following results were obtained. The experiment was based on collection of gastric juice samples and involved an intravenous infusion of the gastrin analogue before and after each subject was given a certain type of drug.

| | | Subject A | Subject B | Subject C |
|---|---|---|---|---|
| Baseline | Sample volume (mL) | 41 | 37 | 43 |
| | Collection time (min) | 46 | 40 | 52 |
| | Proton concentration (mmol/mL) | 124 | 129 | 105 |
| After infusion of gastrin analogue | Sample volume (mL) | 31 | 30 | 25 |
| | Collection time (min) | 14 | 15 | 15 |
| | Proton concentration (mmol/mL) | 140 | 163 | 112 |
| After infusion of gastrin analogue following drug administration | Sample volume (mL) | 29 | 44 | 33 |
| | Collection time (min) | 12 | 10 | 13 |
| | Proton concentration (mmol/mL) | 120 | 158 | 109 |

(a) The number of protons in subject C's baseline sample was 3205.

(b) After infusion of the gastrin analogue, the rate of proton output for subject B was 326 mmol/min.

(c) Subject A may have received a proton-pump inhibitor.

(d) Subject B may have received a selective $H_1$-receptor antagonist.

(e) Subject C may be achlorhydric.

# Chapter 4—The liver;
# Chapter 5—The pancreas and biliary tract

**35. Regarding jaundice:**

(a) In hepatic jaundice, both conjugated and unconjugated bilirubin accumulate in the blood.

(b) Incompatible blood transfusion may cause jaundice.

(c) Jaundice due to obstruction of the common bile duct presents with dark stools and light-coloured urine.

(d) Serum transaminase levels may be helpful in determining the type of jaundice.

(e) A high level of urobilinogen in the urine is a sign of post-hepatic jaundice.

**36. The liver:**

(a) Is entirely covered by peritoneum.

(b) Weighs about 1.5 kg normally.

(c) Is separated from the diaphragm by the suprahepatic recess.

(d) Receives most of its blood supply from the hepatic artery.

(e) Is most easily palpated when it is cirrhotic.

**37. Concerning the liver:**

(a) It has a wide range of pathological responses to injury.

(b) Zone 3 of the acinus is most susceptible to toxin-mediated damage.

(c) Councilman bodies may be found in patients with hepatitis B.

(d) Chronic active hepatitis causes piecemeal necrosis.

(e) A nutmeg liver results from occlusion of the portal venous system.

**38. Bile:**

(a) Is produced by the epithelial cells of the gall bladder wall.

(b) Has an emulsifying function mainly carried out by phospholipids.

(c) Is expelled into the duodenum in response to the presence of lipids.

(d) Is needed for pancreatic lipase to be most effective.

(e) Has a role in the absorption of fats.

**39. The following statements on tumours of the liver and biliary tract are true:**

(a) Haemangiomas of the liver are common.

(b) Hepatocellular carcinoma is the most common liver malignancy.

(c) Cholangiocarcinomas may have jaundice as a presenting feature.

(d) Infection with hepatitis A virus predisposes to hepatocellular carcinoma.

(e) Gallstones are a risk factor for carcinoma of the gallbladder.

**40. Regarding the anatomy of the liver:**

(a) The layers of the coronary ligaments form the right triangular ligament.

(b) The right lobe is the larger lobe and so includes the caudate lobe and most of the quadrate lobe.

(c) The hepatorenal recess is located between the right lobe and the right kidney.

(d) Its draining lymphatics converge at the bare area.

(e) The hepatogastric ligament is part of the greater omentum.

**41. Concerning the hepatitis viruses:**

(a) Hepatitis B virus is a picornavirus.

(b) Hepatitis A and hepatitis E viruses are transmitted in a similar way.

(c) Infection with hepatitis D virus carries a moderate risk of hepatocellular carcinoma.

(d) The presence of hepatitis B e antigen (HBeAg) is associated with chronic liver disease.

(e) Hepatitis A virus causes a self-limiting infection.

**42. The liver:**

(a) Like the pancreas, is a foregut derivative.

(b) Begins to develop from the fourth week of the embryonic period.

(c) Begins its haematopoietic function from the 6th week of embryonic life.

(d) Is sympathetically innervated by nerves arising from the coeliac plexus.

(e) Is not a common site for metastatic tumours.

**43. The following are true statements on the liver:**

(a) Hepatic damage may affect blood clotting.

(b) It is the main store of vitamins A, B, E and K.

(c) Wilson's disease predisposes to liver cirrhosis.

(d) Hepatocytes in each of the three zones of the acinus are functionally dissimilar.

(e) It has a protective function.

**44. Regarding the histology of the liver:**

(a) The hepatic lobule is divided into three zones.

(b) The space of Disse separates the sinusoids from the hepatocytes.

(c) The intrahepatic bile ducts are lined by squamous epithelium.

(d) Kupffer cells are found in the sinusoids.

(e) A portal triad consists of the hepatic artery, a lymphatic and the portal vein.

**45. The following are symptoms and signs of chronic liver failure:**

(a) A flapping tremor.

(b) Spider naevi.

(c) A decreased prothrombin time.

(d) An enlarged spleen.

(e) Raised serum albumin levels.

**46. The gallbladder:**

(a) Is made up of three parts called the fundus, neck and antrum.

(b) Is lined with columnar epithelium.

(c) Is adherent to the liver.

(d) Is supplied by an artery arising from the left hepatic artery.

(e) Causes referred pain to the pelvic region when inflamed.

**47. The following statements concerning gallstones are true:**

(a) Being a fair, fat middle-aged female increases the risk of gallstones.

(b) Most are made up of bile pigments.

(c) They usually cause biliary colic.

(d) Cholesterol stones are large and irregular in shape.

(e) The presence of stones in the gallbladder thins its wall due to erosion.

**48. Concerning the gallbladder and biliary tract:**

(a) The ampulla of Vater is formed by the convergence of the cystic duct and the pancreatic duct.

(b) The gallbladder wall has a folded pattern when empty.

(c) The sphincter of Oddi includes the choledochal and pancreatic sphincter.

(d) Mucous glands are found in the extrahepatic biliary tree.

(e) The biliary tract may be obstructed by pancreatic neoplasms.

**49. The following are true statements on drugs and the liver:**

(a) Mallory's hyaline is a sign of alcoholic hepatitis.

(b) Fatty change due to alcohol abuse is irreversible.

(c) Serum levels of liver transaminases and alkaline phosphatase are elevated in alcoholic hepatitis.

(d) Paracetamol overdose may cause acute liver necrosis.

(e) Alcoholic cirrhosis results in a smooth, shrunken liver.

**50. Concerning disorders of the liver and biliary tract:**

(a) $\alpha_1$-antitrypsin deficiency causes cirrhosis in homozygotes for the M allele.

(b) Gilbert's syndrome is harmless in the majority of sufferers.

(c) Infection with hepatitis D virus can only occur in the presence of hepatitis B virus.

(d) High levels of anti-mitochondrial antibodies are found in primary sclerosing cholangitis.

(e) A Zahn infarct occurs when a branch of the hepatic artery is occluded.

**51. Regarding infections of the liver and biliary tract:**

(a) Hepatitis E is particularly dangerous in pregnant women.

(b) Acute hepatitis B infection is self-limiting in most patients.

(c) Chronic biliary bacterial infection predisposes to gallstones.

(d) Hepatitis C virus is a DNA virus.

(e) Liver abscesses usually resolve untreated.

**52. Regarding bile and its constituents:**

(a) Bile acids are reabsorbed in the terminal ileum.

(b) Bile is concentrated by the active transport of potassium from the gallbladder epithelium.

(c) Bilirubin is a green-coloured pigment.
(d) Cholecystokinin increases bile acid secretion.
(e) Cholesterol is important in the production of bile acids.

53. **The following are true statements on the liver:**
    (a) The coronary ligament attaches it to the anterior abdominal wall.
    (b) It moves with respiration.
    (c) Synthesis of chylomicrons takes place within it.
    (d) It stores carbohydrates mainly in the form of starch.
    (e) It bleeds relatively little when traumatized.

54. **The following statements on portal hypertension are true:**
    (a) A palpable spleen may be a sign.
    (b) Cirrhosis due to alcohol abuse is the most common cause worldwide.
    (c) It may cause haemorrhoids.
    (d) It may cause transudation of fluid into the peritoneal cavity.
    (e) Caput medusae on the thorax may be a manifestation.

55. **Concerning secretions of the pancreas:**
    (a) Trypsinogen has proteolytic activity.
    (b) The brush border is the site of action of enterokinase.
    (c) Vagotomy enhances pancreatic secretion.
    (d) The presence of chyme in the duodenum increases pancreatic secretion.
    (e) Pancreatic amylase is first secreted as a zymogen.

56. **Regarding the pancreas:**
    (a) It is a retroperitoneal organ.
    (b) Blood supply to the head is from branches of the splenic artery.
    (c) It contacts the hilum of the left kidney.
    (d) It is innervated by the pelvic splanchnic nerves and the vagus nerve.
    (e) The pancreatic duct opens into the second part of the duodenum.

57. **Concerning the exocrine pancreas:**
    (a) Its secretions are alkaline.
    (b) The proportion of enzyme types in its secretions varies according to the composition of ingested food.
    (c) Chloride is actively exchanged for bicarbonate in the main collecting ducts.
    (d) Insufficiency results in steatorrhoea.
    (e) The secretory unit is called the pancreon.

58. **The following are true statements on the histology of the pancreas:**
    (a) The δ cells secrete digestive enzymes.
    (b) The intercalated ducts drain into interlobular ducts.

(c) The secretory cells have prominent nucleoli and rough endoplasmic reticulum.
(d) Insulin is produced by the β cells.
(e) The intercalated ducts are lined with squamous epithelium.

59. **Regarding tumours of the pancreas:**
    (a) Most carcinomas occur in the body.
    (b) Pancreatic carcinoma has a poor prognosis.
    (c) The gallbladder may be palpable in carcinomas of the head of the pancreas.
    (d) The incidence of carcinoma of the pancreas in the West is increasing.
    (e) A tumour in the pancreas may cause the Zollinger–Ellison syndrome.

60. **The pancreas:**
    (a) Develops from endoderm.
    (b) Develops from three buds which go on to form its three parts.
    (c) Has lymphatic drainage to nodes located along the splenic artery.
    (d) Has the common bile duct in a groove in the body.
    (e) Has a neck adjacent to the gastric pylorus.

61. **The following are true statements on pancreatitis:**
    (a) Most cases are caused by gallstones or alcohol.
    (b) Grey Turner's sign is pathognomonic for acute pancreatitis.
    (c) It may cause hypercalcaemia.
    (d) A pseudocyst may result from acute pancreatitis.
    (e) Pancreatic enzymes play a minor part in the overall picture.

62. **Concerning disorders of the pancreas:**
    (a) Acute pancreatitis may have an iatrogenic cause.
    (b) Pseudocysts are lined with squamous epithelium.
    (c) Non-fusion of the pancreatic buds results in an annular pancreas.
    (d) The 'sweat test' is useful in testing for cystic fibrosis.
    (e) Elevated serum amylase is highly sensitive for acute pancreatitis.

# Chapter 6—The small intestine

63. **Regarding the small intestine:**
    (a) The entire length of the duodenum lies behind the peritoneum.
    (b) When the ligament of Treitz contracts, it facilitates movement of duodenal contents.
    (c) Loss of the terminal ileum may lead to a microcytic anaemia.
    (d) The jejunum and ileum are supplied by the superior mesenteric artery.
    (e) Venous drainage of the small intestine is mostly to the systemic venous system.

64. The following are true statements on the small intestine:
    (a) The average enterocyte has a lifespan of about 12–13 days.
    (b) Migratory motility complexes occur in the fed state.
    (c) The ileocaecal valve is a one-way valve.
    (d) The juices of the small intestine contain trypsin and lipase secreted by the enterocytes.
    (e) Coeliac disease may result in protein malabsorption.

65. The following statements regarding disorders of the small bowel are true:
    (a) Lactase deficiency causes an osmotic diarrhoea.
    (b) Hirschprung's disease typically occurs in the small intestine.
    (c) Meckel's diverticulum typically occurs 2 inches from the caecum.
    (d) Crohn's disease may cause malabsorption.
    (e) Peutz–Jeghers polyps are pre-malignant.

66. Concerning carcinoid tumours of the small intestine:
    (a) Their cells originate from the neural crest.
    (b) They are fast-growing.
    (c) They may present with diarrhoea.
    (d) Symptom control is with octreotide (a somatostatin analogue).
    (e) They are malignant in 90% of cases.

67. The small bowel:
    (a) Has lymphatics in the villi of the jejunum and ileum.
    (b) Is not easily distinguished from the large bowel on abdominal radiographs.
    (c) Has a distal section derived from the embryonic hindgut.
    (d) Has a mesentery in its proximal 2 cm only.
    (e) Has lymphoid nodules in its mucosal layer.

68. Regarding the small intestine:
    (a) The cores of the villi are extensions of the muscularis mucosae.
    (b) Paneth cells have a defensive function.
    (c) The intraepithelial lymphocytes are mostly of the B cell type.
    (d) Goblet cells produce an alkaline mucus.
    (e) The villi are lined with simple columnar epithelium.

69. The following statements on Crohn's disease are true:
    (a) It is most common in the West.
    (b) Granulomas similar to those of tuberculosis may be found in affected parts of the bowel.
    (c) It is most common over the age of 40.
    (d) Lesions affect the entire thickness of the intestine.
    (e) A cobblestone appearance of the mucous membrane is pathognomonic.

70. Concerning the small intestine:
    (a) Secretin is produced by S cells in the proximal small bowel.
    (b) The migrating motility complex is under hormonal control.
    (c) The gastroileal reflex is mediated by the hormone gastrin.
    (d) Glucose and galactose are transported into the enterocyte together with sodium.
    (e) The water-soluble vitamins require water or carrier proteins alone for absorption.

71. Regarding absorption in the small bowel:
    (a) Lipids are absorbed directly into the blood.
    (b) Absorbed iron may be stored in the enterocytes.
    (c) Vitamin D stimulates the passive absorption of calcium.
    (d) Amino acids are absorbed by a secondary active transport mechanism.
    (e) Infection with the bacterium *Tropheryma whipplei* may cause malabsorption.

72. Regarding the small intestine:
    (a) The brush border is formed by villi.
    (b) Migrating motility complexes originate in the stomach and travel down the small bowel.
    (c) Peristalsis is the main factor responsible for the mixing of chyme.
    (d) Its inner surface is thrown into folds.
    (e) Brunner's glands are found throughout its length.

# Chapter 7—The large intestine

73. Regarding the large intestine:
    (a) The transverse colon has a variable position.
    (b) The ascending colon is immobile.
    (c) The splenic flexure is attached to the diaphragm.
    (d) The transverse colon is the part most prone to volvulus.
    (e) The external anal sphincter is made up of smooth muscle.

74. The appendix:
    (a) Has its base one-third of the way along the line joining the right anterior superior iliac spine and the umbilicus.
    (b) Is a common site for malignancy.
    (c) May be obstructed, usually by faecal material.
    (d) Has a mesentery.
    (e) Is supplied by a branch of the superior mesenteric artery.

75. In the colon:
    (a) Mass movements happen about three or four times a day.
    (b) The gastrocolic reflex is usually strongest after the first meal of the day.
    (c) Haustra extend throughout its entire circumference.

(d) Peristalsis occurs at the same rate as in the small intestine.
(e) Minimal digestion takes place.

76. **Concerning the histology of the large intestine:**
    (a) There are two muscle coats, an outer circular layer and an inner longitudinal layer.
    (b) The luminal surface of the glands is lined with goblet cells.
    (c) The absorptive cells are columnar.
    (d) The muscularis mucosae are not as prominent as in the small intestine.
    (e) Stem cells are found at the bases of the glands.

77. **Regarding defecation:**
    (a) If circumstances are unfavourable, the internal anal sphincter can be voluntarily tightened.
    (b) Both the intrathoracic and intra-abdominal pressures are raised when a person defecates.
    (c) Impulses in the defecation reflex are transmitted by acetylcholine.
    (d) There is contraction of the pelvic floor muscles during defecation.
    (e) Hirschprung's disease causes excessive defecation.

78. **Concerning bowel obstruction:**
    (a) Vomiting is usually a sign of proximal bowel obstruction.
    (b) Previous surgery may predispose to obstruction.
    (c) The most common form of intussusception is ileo-ileal.
    (d) Hernias only obstruct the bowel when they become strangulated.
    (e) A 'bent inner-tube' sign on radiography is characteristic of obstruction due to diverticula.

79. **Concerning the colon:**
    (a) The caecum is located in the right lower quadrant of the abdomen.
    (b) The transversus abdominis muscle lies anterior to the descending colon.
    (c) The arterial 'watershed area' lies halfway along the transverse colon.
    (d) The appendix develops from the caecal diverticulum of the primitive gut tube.
    (e) Perforation of the anal membrane occurs in the 6th week of development.

80. **Irritable bowel disease:**
    (a) Has two forms, Crohn's disease and ulcerative colitis.
    (b) Is common in the Western world.
    (c) Has a relapsing and remitting course in most patients.
    (d) Has weight loss as a prominent feature.
    (e) Can be treated with mesalazine.

81. **The following statements on tumours of the colon are true:**
    (a) Familial adenomatous polyposis is inherited in a dominant manner.

(b) Carcinomas occurring on the left side cause obstruction late.
(c) A Duke's Stage B carcinoma implies spread to pericolic lymph nodes.
(d) A diet low in fibre is a risk factor for adenocarcinomas of the colon.
(e) Familial adenomatous polyposis-associated cancer is more common than hereditary non-polyposis colorectal cancer.

82. **Regarding large intestine pathology:**
    (a) Pseudomembranous colitis is a complication of taking broad-spectrum antibiotics.
    (b) Colonic diverticula are common in the developing world.
    (c) Colonic diverticula are commonly found in the ascending colon.
    (d) Colonoscopy should be performed as a confirmatory measure if ischaemia is suspected.
    (e) Bacterial overgrowth causes malabsorption of vitamin $B_{12}$.

83. **Concerning laxatives:**
    (a) Senna has a direct effect on the myenteric plexus.
    (b) Lactulose is a stimulant purgative.
    (c) Bulk laxatives take several hours to work.
    (d) Osmotic laxatives may cause abdominal cramps and vomiting.
    (e) Prolonged use of magnesium sulphate may lead to atonic colon.

84. **The following are true statements on anti-diarrhoeal agents and drugs affecting gut motility:**
    (a) Domperidone acts on $D_2$-receptors.
    (b) Morphine may cause diarrhoea as it increases the rhythmic contractions of the intestine.
    (c) Muscarinic antagonists are often used in the treatment of diarrhoea.
    (d) Cisapride promotes acetylcholine release in the myenteric plexus.
    (e) Loperamide is relatively selective for the gastrointestinal tract.

85. **In the large bowel:**
    (a) Haustrations are the chief propulsive movements.
    (b) The defecation reflex is triggered by the gastrocolic reflex.
    (c) Sodium and chloride are actively absorbed, which causes water to follow osmotically.
    (d) Most of the bowel gas is derived from bacterial fermentation.
    (e) Mucus protects against trauma to the bowel wall.

86. **The following are true statements on ulcerative colitis and Crohn's disease:**
    (a) Toxic megacolon is a complication of Crohn's disease.
    (b) Lesions in ulcerative colitis are continuous.

(c) 5-aminosalicylates are used more often in the treatment of Crohn's disease than in ulcerative colitis.

(d) Crypt abscesses are seen in Crohn's disease.

(e) Smoking appears to be protective against ulcerative colitis.

# Chapter 8—Common presentations of gastrointestinal disease

### 87. The following statements concerning dysphagia are true:

(a) There is pain with swallowing.

(b) It may be caused by carcinoma.

(c) Dysphagia due to the Plummer–Vinson syndrome is responsive to treatment with vitamin $B_{12}$.

(d) Patients with dysphagia due to achalasia are young with a long history.

(e) A gurgling sound on swallowing is suggestive of a pharyngeal pouch.

### 88. Regarding gastrointestinal (GI) bleeding:

(a) The most common cause of an acute upper GI haemorrhage is bleeding from a peptic ulcer.

(b) Anaemia occurs after a severe acute GI haemorrhage.

(c) The diagnosis is an important prognostic factor in an acute upper GI haemorrhage.

(d) The most common cause of a chronic lower GI haemorrhage is diverticular disease.

(e) Haemorrhoidal bleeding is usually easily noticed.

### 89. Concerning anal pathology:

(a) Internal haemorrhoids usually present with severe anal pain.

(b) Anal fissures may present with long-lasting pain after defecation.

(c) Constipation is a complication of anal fissures.

(d) Tenesmus is a common feature of an anal mass.

(e) Unusually strong pelvic floor muscles may cause rectal prolapse.

### 90. Regarding abdominal pain:

(a) Colicky pain is suggestive of obstruction.

(b) An erect chest X-ray is essential if a perforated viscus is suspected.

(c) Involvement of the parietal peritoneum produces poorly localized pain.

(d) Pain in midgut organs is referred to the umbilical region.

(e) Pain due to inflammation develops gradually.

### 91. The following are true statements on dyspepsia:

(a) It is well defined.

(b) It is common in the general population.

(c) Associated dysphagia must always be promptly investigated.

(d) Investigations are often normal.

(e) The bacterium *Helicobacter pylori* may be a cause.

# Chapter 9—History and examination

### 92. Concerning signs and symptoms:

(a) Palmar erythema is a sign of cirrhosis.

(b) Hypoalbuminaemia is a cause of koilonychia.

(c) Aphthous ulcers may be seen in chronic liver disease.

(d) Pain in the right iliac fossa on palpation exceeding that in the left iliac fossa is called Murphy's sign.

(e) Mechanical intestinal obstruction causes absent bowel sounds.

### 93. The following are causes of finger clubbing:

(a) Carcinoma of the pancreatic head.

(b) Malabsorption.

(c) Lymphoma of the alimentary tract.

(d) Type A gastritis.

(e) Cirrhosis.

### 94. Regarding the full abdominal examination:

(a) A normal spleen cannot be felt.

(b) Veins radiating out from the umbilicus may be due to cirrhosis.

(c) A liver edge felt below the costal margin implies hepatomegaly.

(d) A complete examination includes examination of the external genitalia.

(e) The sigmoid colon may be able to be palpated.

### 95. Regarding signs and symptoms:

(a) The presence of three or four spider naevi is highly suggestive of chronic liver disease.

(b) Brown rings at the corneal peripheries are a sign of Wilson's disease.

(c) A pulsatile liver may be caused by mitral regurgitation.

(d) Jaundice with an enlarged gallbladder is likely to be found in association with gallstones.

(e) An enlarged lymph node in the left supraclavicular fossa is suggestive of gastric carcinoma.

### 96. Concerning signs and symptoms:

(a) Shifting dullness to percussion implies peritonitis.

(b) A mass that is pulsatile but not expansile is suggestive of an aortic aneurysm.

(c) Patients are best examined for hernias in the lying position.

(d) Peri-umbilical nodules are very likely to be benign in adults.

(e) A patient with peritonitis will be shocked, in severe pain and taking frequent deep breaths.

# Chapter 10—Investigations and imaging

### 97. Concerning liver function tests:

(a) Viral hepatitis causes a rise in serum transaminases.

(b) γ-glutamyltransferase levels are increased in $\alpha_1$-antitypsin deficiency.

(c) Alkaline phosphatase levels are a sensitive marker of liver damage.

(d) The prothrombin time will be increased in fat malabsorption.

(e) Alanine aminotransferase is more specific than aspartate aminotransferase as a marker of hepatic damage.

98. **Concerning radiological investigations:**

(a) The majority of gallstones can be seen on plain radiography.

(b) A supine abdominal X-ray is best for showing fluid levels in the intestine.

(c) Rose-thorn ulcers on a plain abdominal radiograph are a sign of inflammatory bowel disease.

(d) Fat appears bright on a $T_2$-weighted magnetic resonance imaging scan.

(e) Both anatomical lesions and abnormalities of motility in the oesophagus are well-demonstrated on a barium swallow.

99. **Regarding investigations in gastrointestinal disease:**

(a) Intestinal function tests are commonly performed.

(b) Iron deficiency causes a low mean corpuscular volume.

(c) High neutrophil counts are seen in viral hepatitis.

(d) Wilson's disease causes a high serum copper level.

(e) High-powered light microscopy is the best method for detecting viruses in a stool sample.

100. **Concerning endoscopic investigations:**

(a) They need to be performed under general anaesthetic.

(b) Sigmoidoscopy can be performed in the outpatient clinic.

(c) They may be used to remove gallstones.

(d) Upper gastrointestinal endoscopy is both diagnostic and therapeutic.

(e) Bleeding is a significant risk.

# Short-answer questions (SAQs)

1. State the intrinsic and extrinsic muscles of the tongue, and their attachments. What is the nerve supply of the lingual muscles?

2. Briefly outline the phases of gallbladder contraction.

3. Describe the mechanism of action of (a) proton-pump inhibitors and (b) antacids. Give two examples of each class of drug.

4. List the sites of porto-systemic anastomoses. What pathological processes might cause these to dilate?

5. Draw a diagram of a salivon. How does the electrolyte concentration of saliva vary with flow rate?

6. Briefly describe the various types of gallstones. How may a patient with gallstones present?

7. Define 'intestinal atresia'. What are the causes and consequences of intestinal atresia?

8. Compare and contrast the gastric chief cell and the gastric parietal cell.

9. What are the functions of bile acids?

10. What congenital disorders might affect the pancreas?

11. State the substances assayed in liver function tests. Why is the prothrombin time described as a 'true' liver function test as opposed to measurement of hepatic enzymes?

12. List the causes of acute pancreatitis, and state how it is diagnosed. Why may Grey Turner's sign occur in acute pancreatitis?

13. Write short notes on achalasia.

14. Give a concise account of the urea breath test. What is the purpose of carrying out this investigation?

15. Briefly describe how carbohydrates are digested. Why are humans not able to digest cellulose?

16. A 43-year-old man presents complaining of lethargy and of having lost 6 kg of weight over the last 2 months. He also says that his urine is unusually dark, while his stools are unusually pale. He denies being in pain. On examination, his sclerae are yellow.
    (a) What is the likely diagnosis?
    (b) Briefly justify your diagnosis in (a).
    (c) What investigations might you request to confirm your diagnosis?

17. A 22-year-old woman goes to see her GP because she has been passing stools significantly more than normal over the last 3 weeks. The stools are bloody and watery, and each time she finishes defecating she feels like she 'still has some left'. She also says she is feeling tired and has lost her appetite. She does not smoke, but eats a diet high in saturated fats.
    (a) What is the most likely diagnosis?
    (b) Outline the available treatment options.

18. You are a GP. A 26-year-old man comes to see you with a complaint of flu-like symptoms, malaise and loss of appetite. He is a bank clerk who has previously been fit and well. However, his girlfriend, with whom he maintains sexual relations, is a final-year medical student who returned from her elective to southern Thailand 3 months ago. She has admitted to him that she injected heroin on one of her weekends off.
    (a) What investigations might you request?
    (b) What advice might you give?

19. A middle-aged man consults his GP because he has noticed his skin getting more 'tanned' even though it is winter. He also says his libido has been decreased over the past few weeks. On examination, the GP notes that the man has hepatomegaly.
    (a) What is the diagnosis? Explain the aetiology.
    (b) What results might be expected on investigation?
    (c) How is the condition treated?

20. You are on your elective in Bangladesh. During your last week in the country, an outbreak of cholera occurs.
    (a) Name the causative organism, and state how it is spread.
    (b) How does the organism cause the symptoms of the disease?
    (c) What is the most effective treatment?

# Extended-matching questions (EMQs)

For each scenario described below, choose the most likely corresponding option from the list given. Each option may be used once, more than once or not at all.

## 1. Abdominal pain.

A. Crohn's disease.
B. Pancreatitis.
C. Gallstones.
D. Appendicitis.
E. Viral gastroenteritis.
F. Diverticulitis.
G. Irritable bowel syndrome.
H. Obstruction.
I. Sigmoid volvulus.
J. Acute bowel ischaemia.

1. A 63-year-old lady presented complaining of colicky pain in her abdomen and associated vomiting for the past four days. She has a history of gastro-oesophageal reflux disease. On examination, she appeared dehydrated. The abdomen was slightly distended and tender. Tinkling bowel sounds were heard on auscultation. ☐

2. A 22-year-old man is referred from his GP with pain in the right iliac fossa. He says that previously the pain was central but in the last few hours it has shifted to its current location. He also described vomiting. On examination, he had a fever of 38°C and there was tenderness and guarding over the right iliac fossa. ☐

3. A 75-year-old man presented with colicky abdominal pain which he says is 'killing him'. He says he is also suffering from constipation due to some new medication he is taking. On examination, the abdomen is distended but not particularly tender. An abdominal radiograph was taken which showed a shadow on the left side which looked like a bent inner tube. ☐

4. A previously fit and well 34-year-old woman comes into Accident and Emergency complaining of very severe abdominal pain which came on suddenly. On examination, the abdomen was tender and bowel sounds were absent. After being examined, she stands up and then collapses. ☐

5. A 25-year-old medical student is brought into hospital after a night out to celebrate passing his finals, complaining of a sudden pain in his abdomen which radiates into the back and associated vomiting. He grades the severity of the pain as 10/10. According to his friends, he had drunk 12 pints of lager and eight shots of whisky. Examination revealed a tender abdomen with guarding, worst in the epigastrium. ☐

## 2. Pharmacology of the gastrointestinal system.

A. Oral rehydration solution.
B. Lactulose.
C. Sodium picosulphate.
D. Metoclopramide.
E. Pantoprazole.
F. Ondansetron.
G. Loperamide.
H. Misoprostol.
I. Hyoscine.
J. Ranitidine.

1. A mother goes to see her GP with her 6-year-old son. They are going on a long car trip to Scotland to visit relatives, but the boy has motion sickness and his mother would like the GP to prescribe a prophylactic drug. ☐

2. A 65-year-old man with a history of peptic ulcer disease diagnosed 20 years ago consults his GP. He has been taking the medication prescribed on diagnosis but is dissatisfied because each time he feels well and stops taking it his symptoms come on again. ☐

3. You are a newly appointed Senior House Officer in colorectal surgery. On your first day, you are told by the consultant to consent the patients for surgery the next day, as well as ensure that their bowels are prepared for the operation. ☐

4. A 45-year-old woman develops severe rheumatoid arthritis and is prescribed indometacin (a non-steroidal anti-inflammatory drug) by her rheumatologist. She has a longstanding history of peptic ulcer disease. ☐

5. A 16-year-old boy has diarrhoea. His GP gives him medication, which he takes as advised. Unfortunately, he develops abdominal cramps and drowsiness, and within a few days becomes constipated. ☐

## 3. Neoplasms of the gastrointestinal tract.

A. Carcinoid tumour.

B. Cholangiocarcinoma.

C. Pancreatic carcinoma.

D. Peutz–Jeghers syndrome.

E. Gastric carcinoma.

F. Oesophageal carcinoma.

G. Leiomyoma of the small intestine.

H. Intestinal T cell lymphoma.

I. Familial adenomatous polyposis.

J. Hepatocellular carcinoma.

1. A 55-year-old man presented with pain in the epigastrium. He says he has lost a lot of weight in the past few months and his appetite is not as good as it used to be. He also suffers from autoimmune gastritis. On examination, he is cachectic. A palpable lymph node is found in the left supraclavicular fossa. ☐

2. A 60-year-old man consulted his GP complaining of having lost two stone in 3 months. On taking a detailed history, the GP finds out that he is an infectious carrier of the hepatitis B virus. The patient was jaundiced on examination. ☐

3. A 45-year-old man presented with difficulty swallowing. He is now able to eat only liquid foods, but with difficulty. Apart from that, he also says he has been losing weight and has lost his appetite. His voice appears hoarse. ☐

4. A 30-year-old woman presented complaining of tiredness and rectal bleeding. On examination, there was abnormal skin pigmentation, but nothing else of note. Colonoscopy revealed multiple polyps in the colon. ☐

5. A 51-year-old man presented with severe weight loss and anorexia. On examination, the patient was jaundiced and a mass was felt in the right upper quadrant. There was no tenderness, and neither did the patient complain of pain. ☐

## 4. Malabsorption syndromes.

A. Coeliac disease.

B. Disaccharide deficiency.

C. Rapid transit.

D. Bacterial overgrowth.

E. Whipple's disease.

F. Giardiasis.

G. Tropical sprue.

H. Abetalipoproteinaemia.

I. Resection of the small intestine.

1. A 52-year-old man presented with tiredness and weight loss. He was previously fit and well with no history of foreign travel. A full diagnostic work-up, including biopsy of the jejunum was requested. The biopsy showed the presence of macrophages staining positive with periodic acid–Schiff (PAS). ☐

2. A 26-year-old woman who has just returned from travelling in South Asia presented complaining of weight loss, tiredness and the passage of greasy stools. Examination was unremarkable, but stool microscopy showed the presence of kite-shaped organisms. ☐

3. An 80-year-old lady presented with diarrhoea and steatorrhoea. The rest of the history and examination were unremarkable. Investigations revealed an increased plasma vitamin K level and an elevated hydrogen level on a breath test. ☐

4. A 3-year-old girl is brought to see the GP by her parents, who are concerned that she is not growing as quickly as she should and that she is not as active as other children her age. The GP advises the parents to change her diet, in particular to stop giving foods containing wheat. On the next visit, the child appears much healthier. ☐

5. A 32-year-old Jamaican man who has recently migrated to the UK presents with weight loss, tiredness and diarrhoea. He says that most of his family in Jamaica suffer from similar symptoms. The rest of the history and examination yielded nothing suspicious. ☐

## 5. Dysphagia.

A. Achalasia.

B. Pharyngeal pouch.

C. Congenital oesophageal atresia.

D. Inflammatory stricture.

E. Presence of a foreign body.

F. Oesophageal tumour.

G. Oesophageal web.

H. Crohn's stricture.

1. A 79-year-old lady presents with a recurrent chest infection. She says she has been accidentally inhaling food particles as she is having trouble swallowing. Her breath was foetid and a gurgling lump was found on her neck. ☐

2. A 66-year-old woman presents with tiredness and difficulty swallowing. The rest of the history was unremarkable. A full blood count revealed a low haemoglobin, together with microcytic erythrocytes. ☐

3. A 35-year-old woman presents with a chest infection. She also says she is having difficulty swallowing, which has got worse over the past few months, and has lost about 3 kg. Tapering of the oesophagus towards the lower end was evident on barium swallow. ☐

4. A week-old baby is brought in by his mother, who says he has been having trouble swallowing his milk. On examination, he appears lethargic but otherwise normal. The mother says her obstetrician told her she had polyhydramnios when she was pregnant with her baby. ☐

5. A 43-year-old man with a longstanding history of gastro-oesophageal reflux disease presents with difficulty swallowing. The rest of the history and examination were unremarkable. ☐

## 6. Diarrhoea.

A. Bacterial overgrowth.
B. Amoebic dysentery.
C. Ulcerative colitis.
D. Rapid transit.
E. Pseudomembranous colitis.
F. Disaccharidase deficiency.
G. Viral gastroenteritis.
H. Cholera.
I. Giardiasis.

1. This condition has a relapsing and remitting course. The diarrhoea is bloody, and tenesmus may be a feature. Histology shows a haemorrhagic, granular colonic mucosa, with other tissue layers being normal. It is the commonest cause of prolonged bloody diarrhoea in the Western world. ☐

2. This disease is endemic in parts of the developing world. The major symptom is a profuse, 'rice-water' diarrhoea. In affected people, there is a rise in intracellular adenylate cyclase and cyclic AMP. ☐

3. A day after a sumptuous dinner at a scientific conference, which included oysters on the half-shell, a large group of eminent microbiologists fall ill. Their symptoms include profuse vomiting, diarrhoea and abdominal pain. ☐

4. An 89-year-old woman is admitted to hospital with a fractured neck of femur. While on the ward, she is given ceftriaxone (a cephalosporin). Some days later, she develops a fever and painful bloody diarrhoea. ☐

5. This disorder is more likely to be acquired than congenital. Symptoms include diarrhoea, bloating and flatulence. It is more likely to be seen in those with a high-milk diet. ☐

## 7. Intestinal obstruction.

A. Stricture.
B. Congenital atresia.
C. Inguinal hernia.
D. Hirschsprung's disease.
E. Adhesions.
F. Volvulus.
G. Intussusception.
H. Malignancy.
I. Faecal impaction.
J. Diverticulitis.

1. A 33-year-old woman presents with colicky abdominal pain. She suffers from endometriosis, and has had intestinal surgery a year ago. Examination showed a distended abdomen. ☐

2. A 25-year-old man presented with continuous pain in the abdomen. A day ago, he had been doing some heavy lifting. On examination, he was pyrexial, tachycardic and there was a mass in his groin. ☐

3. A 33-year-old woman with longstanding Crohn's disease presented with colicky abdominal pain. She also complained of constipation. On examination, the abdomen was distended. ☐

4. A 1-year-old girl is taken to see her GP by her father. The GP was told that a day ago she started crying and vomiting a lot. Her father also said she had been passing stools which resembled redcurrant jelly. ☐

5. A 60-year-old man presents complaining of tiredness and loss of appetite. He says he has lost quite a lot of weight over the past few months. ☐

## 8. Liver pathology.

A. Haemochromatosis.
B. Hepatitis B infection.
C. Hepatitis A infection.
D. Hepatitis C infection.
E. Portal hypertension.
F. Hepatocellular carcinoma.
G. Gilbert's syndrome.
H. Alcoholic hepatitis.
I. Budd–Chiari syndrome.
J. $\alpha_1$-antitrypsin deficiency.

1. A 45-year-old man presented because he has noticed that his skin is becoming unusually brown. He also complained of tiredness and loss of libido. Investigations revealed a raised ferritin level. ☐

2. A 16-year-old boy presented to his GP because he has noticed a slight yellowish discoloration of his skin and eyes. He has no other symptoms. Liver function tests showed a slightly raised bilirubin level. The GP tells him not to worry, because the condition he has is not serious and is asymptomatic. ☐

3. A 34-year-old woman presents with flu-like symptoms. On questioning, she reluctantly reveals that she is an intravenous drug user.

A 2 cm liver edge was felt on inspiration, and liver function tests showed raised transaminase levels. ☐

4. A 38-year-old woman presented as an emergency with haematemesis and was successfully resuscitated. Further examination showed dilated vessels around the umbilicus and an enlarged spleen. ☐

5. A 28-year-old traveller presented shortly after returning from India with jaundice and gastroenteritic-type symptoms. He admitted to having eaten from roadside stalls on his travels. Investigations were performed, but the doctor said that the illness was likely to be self-limiting. ☐

## 9. Gastro-oesophageal disorders.

A. Hypertrophic pyloric stenosis.
B. Type B gastritis.
C. Type A gastritis.
D. Peptic ulcer disease.
E. Gastric carcinoma.
F. Hiatus hernia.
G. Oesophageal carcinoma.
H. Oesophageal diverticula.
I. Mallory–Weiss tear.
J. Gastro-oesophageal reflux disease.

1. In this disorder, an acute inflammatory response is present. This causes protease release, which destroys gastric glands. Infection with the bacterium *Helicobacter pylori* is seen in approximately 90% of cases. The stomach may become fibrotic. ☐

2. This condition usually manifests about 4–6 weeks after birth. Projectile vomiting is the most typical symptom. It has a male preponderance, occurring in 1/150 male births compared to 1/750 female births. ☐

3. This condition is typified by massive haematemesis. Patients have usually been vomiting or coughing for a prolonged period before the bleeding occurs. It is most common in alcoholics. ☐

4. This disease is most common in patients with blood group O. The majority of cases are associated with *H. pylori* infection, but severe stress or burns may also cause it. Non-steroidal anti-inflammatory drugs are a risk factor for this condition. ☐

5. In this condition, the squamo-columnar junction of the oesophagus is abnormally high. It is the commonest cause of oesophagitis. A decreased lower oesophageal sphincter tone may be one of the causes. ☐

## 10. Intestinal disorders.

A. Crohn's disease.
B. Ulcerative colitis.
C. Irritable bowel syndrome.
D. Hirschsprung's disease.
E. Meckel's diverticulum.
F. Infectious enterocolitis.
G. Appendicitis.
H. Diverticulitis.
I. Colorectal carcinoma.

1. A 20-year-old woman presented with longstanding abdominal pain, bloatedness and 'slimy stools'. Examination showed abdominal tenderness on palpation, but nothing else. Investigations yielded no abnormal results. ☐

2. A 1-week-old boy is brought to the GP by his parents, who are worried that he has not defecated at all. On examination, the abdomen was distended and the rectum empty. ☐

3. A 17-year-old boy presented with diarrhoea, cramping abdominal pain and weight loss. On examination, there was abdominal tenderness and mouth ulcers. Intestinal biopsy showed fissuring lesions extending throughout the full thickness of the bowel wall. ☐

4. A 22-year-old university student presents with severe diarrhoea, projectile vomiting and cramping abdominal pain. The night before, he had eaten a Chinese take-away meal. ☐

5. A 60-year-old pensioner who lives alone presented complaining of localized pain in the left iliac fossa. On examination, she was pyrexial and tachycardic, and the left iliac fossa was tender to palpation. ☐

# Chapter 1 – Introduction to the Gastrointestinal System

1. (a) False – it is a manifestation of vitamin $B_3$ deficiency.
   (b) False – they can only be absorbed as monosaccharides; β-glycosidic linkages are found in oligosaccharides and polysaccharides.
   (c) True – as the liver has a high fat content.
   (d) True – the digestive process is accomplished by hydrolytic enzymes.
   (e) False – carbohydrate and protein provide roughly the same amount of energy.

2. (a) True – the caudal arches contribute to its superior third.
   (b) False – the foregut is supplied by the coeliac artery.
   (c) False – it ends at approximately half to two-thirds along its length.
   (d) True – this is the Meckel's diverticulum.
   (e) False – the hindgut derivatives are supplied by the pelvic splanchnic nerves.

3. (a) False – the fifth arch is often absent.
   (b) False – it is found in the lamina propria of the mucosa, hence the name mucosa-associated lymphoid tissue (MALT).
   (c) False – vitamins are not digested!
   (d) False – it is located in the submucosa; the Auerbach's or myenteric plexus is situated between the two muscle coats.
   (e) True – ongoing contraction during life shortens the alimentary tract.

4. (a) True – they control digestion and motility, among other functions.
   (b) True – as it is open to the external environment.
   (c) True – more precisely, its motor branch.
   (d) False – it herniates between weeks 7 and 11.
   (e) True – the basic structure comprises the mucosa, submucosa, muscularis mucosae and serosa.

# Chapter 2—The upper gastrointestinal tract

5. (a) True – low temperatures do the opposite.
   (b) False – leptin receptors are found in the hypothalamus.
   (c) True – the hypothalamus is responsible for the diurnal variation in substrates.
   (d) True – increased insulin secretion in response to increased blood glucose levels, such as during a meal, is a signal for satiety.
   (e) False – lesions in the ventromedial wall and paraventricular nucleus of the hypothalamus (the satiety centre) will cause hyperphagia.

6. (a) True – this is the cardiac orifice of the stomach.
   (b) True – the other sites of constriction are where it crosses the left main bronchus and where it passes through the diaphragm.
   (c) False – the lower sphincter is a physiological sphincter.
   (d) True – the descent of the heart and lungs causes it to lengthen rapidly.
   (e) False – it lies to the left before the aortic arch pushes it to the median plane.

7. (a) True – there are three pairs of large salivary glands in the normal person.
   (b) False – the cells of the sublingual gland are primarily mucus-secreting.
   (c) False – they are lined with cuboidal epithelium.
   (d) True – the facial nerve and its branches run through the parotid gland superficially.
   (e) False – the basic secretory unit is called the salivon, which comprises an acinus and a duct.

8. (a) False – GORD has no association with age.
   (b) True – it increases intra-abdominal pressure.
   (c) False – GORD is not associated with either sex.
   (d) True – hiatus hernias impair the function of the lower oesophageal sphincter.
   (e) True – smoking is a risk factor for almost anything!

9. (a) True – it is a programmed sequential motor activity generated in the medullary centres.
   (b) True – the food bolus pushes it down over the closed glottis as a further protective measure.
   (c) False – secondary peristaltic waves are initiated by oesophageal distension.

(d) True – as in the case of achalasia where food collects at the bottom of the oesophagus.

(e) True – the swallowing centre briefly inhibits the respiratory centre during swallowing.

10. (a) False – the incidence of cleft palate is 1/2500 births compared with 1/1000 births in cleft lip.

(b) False – it is more common in males.

(c) False – they are either benign or pre-malignant.

(d) True – the virus is latent in the trigeminal ganglion and may be reactivated by a number of stimuli.

(e) False – *Candida albicans* is a common oral commensal but oral candidiasis is rare.

11. (a) True – this is why atropine is used before surgery to reduce the aspiration risk.

(b) False – the average rate of production is about 1–2 litres per day.

(c) False – it is present in hypertonic concentrations; electrolyte concentration is mediated by the duct cells.

(d) True – this causes the dry-mouth sensation during fight-or-flight situations.

(e) True – it serves a defensive function against invasion of microorganisms.

12. (a) False – it comprises striated muscle as the first phase of swallowing is voluntary.

(b) True – it is an anatomical sphincter and normally constricted.

(c) False – they are most numerous in the upper and lower thirds.

(d) False – they may burst causing fatal haematemesis.

(e) True – they occur together in 90% of cases.

13. (a) True – they form a row immediately anterior to the sulcus terminalis.

(b) False – all muscles of the tongue except the palatoglossus are supplied by the XII$^{th}$ cranial nerve.

(c) True – it arises from the external carotid and its branches supply the tongue.

(d) True – this is because they have a highly vascular core.

(e) False – the action of the unaffected genioglossus muscle on the normal side causes the tongue to deviate to the paralysed side.

14. (a) True – it is the eighth most common malignancy in the world.

(b) False – carcinoma of the upper third is very rare.

(c) True – the risk of adenocarcinoma is 30–40 times higher with Barrett's oesophagus.

(d) True – these account for 95% of oesophageal carcinomas.

(e) False – it has a very poor prognosis; 5-year survival is only about 5%.

15. (a) True – they are effective in reducing gastric acid secretion.

(b) True – as invading trypanosomes destroy the intrinsic nerve plexuses causing achalasia.

(c) False – treatment for oesophageal diverticula is surgical.

(d) False – sliding hiatus herniae account for 80% of all cases.

(e) False – metaplastic change causes the normal squamous epithelium to change to a columnar type.

16. (a) True – it is located in the area postrema on the floor of the fourth ventricle.

(b) False – they are two separate units in the medulla.

(c) True – this adds to its anti-emetic effect.

(d) False – they are effective against vomiting due to motion sickness and substances acting in the stomach.

(e) True – this allows circulating mediators to act on it directly.

17. (a) False – the vestibular nuclei do not have 5-HT$_3$ receptors.

(b) False – it is a dopamine-receptor antagonist.

(c) False – it prevents vomiting caused by substances acting on the chemoreceptor trigger zone.

(d) True – they block receptors on the visceral afferent nerves.

(e) True – as it is a muscarinic receptor antagonist.

# Chapter 3—The stomach

18. (a) False – they are found at the necks of the glands where they divide continuously to replace worn-out cells.

(b) False – intrinsic factor is secreted by the parietal cells.

(c) False – it is much more acidic, with a pH of 0.9–1.5.

(d) True – these are the neuroendocrine G cells.

(e) True – this is because they produce pepsinogen.

19. (a) True – it descends and folds back to attach to the transverse colon.

(b) True   –   the location varies in the erect position from L2 to L4 vertebrae but it is normally on the right.

(c) False   –   there is no such thing as the gastroduodenal vein!

(d) True   –   the sympathetic supply is from T6 to T9 segments of the spinal cord while the parasympathetic supply is from the vagus nerve.

(e) False   –   this is a rolling hiatus hernia.

**20.** (a) True   –   as in the case of hamartomas in Peutz–Jeghers syndrome.

(b) True   –   this is a presentation of diffuse infiltrative carcinoma (linitis plastica).

(c) False   –   adenocarcinomas make up 90% of all gastric malignancies.

(d) False   –   it is a swollen lymph node in the left supraclavicular fossa (Troisier's sign).

(e) True   –   this causes an increase in bacterial flora, particularly *Helicobacter pylori*.

**21.** (a) True   –   vagal afferent nerves from the gut may be stimulated by mucosal irritation.

(b) False   –   they stimulate the vomiting centres in response to stimuli such as drugs but are not part of the centres proper.

(c) True   –   this is what happens in motion sickness.

(d) True   –   this protects the airways and prevents aspiration.

(e) True   –   this helps to protect the oral mucosa from the acidity of gastric contents.

**22.** (a) False   –   the posterior wall grows faster and forms the curvatures.

(b) True   –   they anastomose at the lesser curvature.

(c) True   –   this is why the left vagus nerve innervates the left surface and vice-versa.

(d) True   –   the lymphatic vessels accompany the gastric arteries on the curvatures.

(e) False   –   varices must never be biopsied as a fatal bleed may result.

**23.** (a) False   –   it is gastric motility, not emptying, in which this is a factor.

(b) True   –   the mechanism by which it does this is unknown.

(c) True   –   parasympathetic stimulation via the vagus nerve quickens gastric emptying.

(d) False   –   they are emptied most slowly as they increase the contractility of the pyloric sphincter.

(e) True   –   cholecystokinin is released in the duodenum in the presence of fatty chyme and slows gastric emptying.

**24.** (a) False   –   the proton pump actively transports $H^+$; chloride follows passively.

(b) True   –   it produces intrinsic factor which is needed for vitamin $B_{12}$ absorption.

(c) False   –   it is most abundant in the body of the stomach.

(d) True   –   hence its alternative name, the oxyntic cell.

(e) True   –   it has a central nucleus.

**25.** (a) True   –   continuing necrosis, organization and repair occur simultaneously in a peptic ulcer.

(b) True   –   they are associated with 80% of gastric ulcers and 95% of duodenal ulcers.

(c) True   –   it increases the mucosal blood supply, thus increasing the production of mucus.

(d) True   –   they decrease prostaglandin synthesis.

(e) True   –   if untreated, it will cause generalized peritonitis and ultimately oligaemic shock.

**26.** (a) False   –   the gastric phase, lasting up to $2\frac{1}{2}$ hours, is the longest.

(b) True   –   the cephalic phase is initiated by the sight, smell and taste of food.

(c) True   –   these release cholecystokinin which inhibits gastric secretion.

(d) False   –   it only plays a significant role in pancreatic insufficiency.

(e) False   –   however it does have a defensive function against ingested microorganisms.

**27.** (a) False   –   it is Gram-negative.

(b) True   –   remember 'B' for 'bacterial'!

(c) True   –   VacA alters intracellular vesicular trafficking in gastric cells, causing large vacuoles to form.

(d) False   –   the hydrogen breath test detects bacterial overgrowth in the intestine; the urea breath test is used to detect *H. pylori*.

(e) False   –   triple therapy usually takes the form of two antibiotics plus a proton pump inhibitor.

**28.** (a) False   –   it is in the antrum and the distal end of the fundus that mixing of food with gastric juices occurs.

(b) True   –   this is when gastric secretions are chemically digesting the food to form chyme.

(c) False   –   they are found in the distal fundus.

(d) True   –   cholinergic stimulation from the vagus nerve upregulates gastric motility.

(e) False   –   it only nearly approximates to the intra-abdominal pressure.

**29.** (a) False – thus it is active in the acidic environment of the stimulated parietal cell canaliculi.

(b) True – along with histamine- and gastrin-stimulated acid secretion.

(c) True – it is a prostaglandin E1 analogue and so prevents NSAID-induced gastric damage.

(d) False – they are non-competitive inhibitors of the proton-pump.

(e) False – it does not feature in any triple-therapy regimen.

**30.** (a) True – secretion is inhibited if the pH falls to below 2.5.

(b) False – it acts to decrease cyclic AMP production.

(c) False – calcium salts are effective stimulants of gastric acid production.

(d) True – but proglumide is only used experimentally.

(e) False – it acts as a local hormone.

**31.** (a) True – this allows the breach in the diaphragm to be repaired.

(b) False – it will result in a macrocytic anaemia due to lack of vitamin $B_{12}$.

(c) False – it is more common in male infants (incidence 1/150 versus 1/750).

(d) True – the adenomas produce gastrin resulting in hyperacidity which predisposes to ulceration.

(e) False – the medical treatment for gastroparesis is prokinetic drugs such as metoclopramide.

**32.** (a) True – it is secreted as pepsinogen, which is then hydrolysed to pepsin by gastric hydrochloric acid.

(b) True – as it is alkaline.

(c) False – it acts directly on the parietal cells.

(d) False – it is alkaline, with a pH of about 7.7.

(e) True – the urease converts urea to carbon dioxide and ammonia, which is basic.

**33.** (a) True – they act as mucosal strengtheners by coating the bases of ulcers and neutralizing acid.

(b) True – they irreversibly inhibit the $H^+/K^+$-ATPase of parietal cells.

(c) False – they cause constipation, whereas magnesium salts cause diarrhoea.

(d) False – relapses are likely on stopping these drugs.

(e) False – they protect against ulceration by increasing the blood supply, so increasing mucus production.

**34.** (a) False – it is 4515; the answer is derived from [concentration × volume].

(b) True – the answer is derived from [(concentration × volume)/time].

(c) True – the rate of secretion is reduced after administration of the drug.

(d) False – these do not affect gastric acid secretion.

(e) True – the rate of secretion in subject C is much lower than the other two subjects.

## Chapter 4—The liver;
## Chapter 5—The pancreas and biliary tract

**35.** (a) True – as the liver is unable to conjugate bilirubin effectively, and also less is excreted into the bile canaliculi.

(b) True – as it will cause haemolysis.

(c) False – as common bile duct obstruction prevents bilirubin excretion.

(d) True – they are an indication of liver damage, and therefore may be raised in hepatic jaundice.

(e) False – in post-hepatic jaundice urobilinogen is absent from the urine.

**36.** (a) False – it has a bare area posteriorly, demarcated by the layers of the coronary ligament.

(b) True – it is the largest gland in the body.

(c) False – it is the subphrenic recess that does this – the suprahepatic recess does not exist!

(d) False – 70% of its blood supply is from the portal vein.

(e) False – cirrhosis results in a shrunken liver.

**37.** (a) False – the range of responses of the liver to injury is limited.

(b) False – it is the furthest zone from the portal triad and so is least susceptible to toxins in the bloodstream.

(c) True – they are apoptotic, shrunken cells.

(d) True – this is death of liver cells in a scattered manner next to portal triad connective tissue.

(e) False – it is caused by right-sided heart failure.

**38.** (a) False – it is produced in the liver.

(b) False – fat emulsification is carried out by bile acids.

(c) True – this is mediated by cholecystokinin which stimulates gallbladder contraction.

(d) True – it emulsifies fats so facilitating their hydrolysis by pancreatic lipase.

(e) True – bile acids form micelles with the products of fat digestion and facilitate transport to the brush border.

**39.** (a) True – it is made up of abnormal vascular channels in a collagenous stroma.
(b) False – metastases are the most common type of malignant neoplasm in the liver.
(c) True – if they cause sufficient obstruction of the bile ducts.
(d) False – it does not cause chronic hepatitis and so is not a risk factor for hepatocellular carcinoma.
(e) True – gallstones and chronic cholecystitis are the main risk factors.

**40.** (a) True – the layers meet at the right of the liver to form the right triangular ligament.
(b) False – it is the left lobe which contains the caudate and most of the quadrate lobes.
(c) True – it separates the visceral surface of the liver from the right kidney.
(d) False – they converge at the porta hepatis.
(e) False – it is part of the lesser omentum which extends between the liver and the stomach.

**41.** (a) False – it is a hepadnavirus.
(b) True – they are both transmitted via the faecal–oral route.
(c) False – this is because it seldom resolves.
(d) True – most patients with HbeAg will develop chronic hepatitis and have a high risk of cirrhosis.
(e) True – symptomatic hepatitis A typically lasts for a few weeks.

**42.** (a) True – it arises from the hepatic diverticulum, which is an outgrowth of the primitive foregut.
(b) True – this is when the hepatic diverticulum appears.
(c) True – this gives it its reddish appearance in embryonic life.
(d) True – the sympathetic fibres in the hepatic plexus are derived from the coeliac plexus.
(e) False – it is a very common site for metastases, mainly from the alimentary tract, breast and lungs.

**43.** (a) True – one of the functions of the liver is to synthesize clotting factors.
(b) False – it is the main store of vitamins A, D, E and K; vitamin B is not fat-soluble.
(c) True – the excess copper causes a chronic hepatitis which progresses to cirrhosis.

(d) True – this is due to their relative locations.
(e) True – toxins and microorganisms in the portal blood supply are filtered out in the liver.

**44.** (a) False – it is the liver acinus which is divided into three zones.
(b) True – the space of Disse drains into the portal lymphatics.
(c) False – they are lined by columnar or cuboidal epithelium.
(d) True – they serve a phagocytic function.
(e) False – it is made up of the hepatic artery, portal vein and bile duct.

**45.** (a) True – this is a sign of hepatic encephalopathy.
(b) True – more than five is a clinically significant sign.
(c) False – it would be raised as the production of clotting factors is impaired.
(d) True – this is due to portal hypertension.
(e) False – as the liver's synthetic function is decreased.

**46.** (a) False – it comprises the fundus, neck and body.
(b) True – the lining is made up of tall simple columnar epithelial cells.
(c) True – it adheres to the liver at its anterior surface.
(d) False – it is supplied by the cystic artery which comes from the right hepatic artery.
(e) False – inflammation causes pain in the right hypochrondriac and epigastric regions.

**47.** (a) False – they have the same risk of gallstones as everyone else.
(b) False – most gallstones are of the cholesterol type.
(c) False – over 70% are asymptomatic.
(d) False – they are large but regular; typically they are round and faceted.
(e) False – they cause muscle hypertrophy and thickening of the wall.

**48.** (a) False – it is formed by the convergence of the common bile duct and the pancreatic duct.
(b) True – this allows it to distend with stored bile.
(c) True – this allows the flow of bile and pancreatic juice into the duodenum to be controlled.
(d) True – the mucus may serve a protective function for the biliary tract.
(e) True – carcinoma of the head of the pancreas presents early with obstructive jaundice.

**49.** (a) True – they are made up, among others, of intermediate filament aggregates.

(b) False – it is reversible if the patient abstains from alcohol.

(c) True – they are intrahepatic enzymes and so are markers of liver damage.

(d) True – this mainly happens in the centrilobular areas.

(e) False – cirrhosis causes a nodular appearance.

**50.** (a) False – it causes cirrhosis in ZZ homozygotes.

(b) True – most will require no treatment.

(c) True – it is a defective virus and requires hepatitis B virus for assembly.

(d) False – they are found in primary biliary sclerosis.

(e) False – it occurs in occlusion of a branch of the portal vein.

**51.** (a) True – as it may result in acute fulminant hepatitis and death.

(b) True – more than 90% recover, while 10% develop chronic infection.

(c) True – the bacteria act as a nidus for gallstone formation.

(d) False – it is an RNA virus.

(e) False – untreated liver abscesses have a high mortality rate.

**52.** (a) True – this happens as part of enterohepatic recirculation.

(b) False – it is active transport of sodium which causes water to follow passively, thus concentrating the bile.

(c) False – it is yellow, hence the yellowness of jaundice.

(d) True – this occurs during the intestinal phase of digestion in response to the presence of lipids.

(e) True – bile acids are synthesized from cholesterol in the hepatocytes.

**53.** (a) False – it is the falciform ligament which does this.

(b) True – as it is attached to the diaphragm.

(c) True – the liver makes all lipoproteins.

(d) False – carbohydrate is stored in the liver as glycogen.

(e) False – as it is a highly vascular organ.

**54.** (a) True – back-pressure in the portal vascular bed leads to splenomegaly.

(b) False – cirrhosis due to viral infection is the most common cause.

(c) True – as collateral channels open up between the superior, middle and inferior rectal veins.

(d) True – this is ascites.

(e) False – caput medusae are found around the umbilicus.

**55.** (a) False – it is a proenzyme and so is inactive.

(b) True – enterokinase converts trypsinogen to trypsin.

(c) False – it will result in a loss of parasympathetic stimulation and so a reduction in secretion.

(d) True – this is mediated by cholecystokinin.

(e) False – as it does not have the ability to digest pancreatic tissue.

**56.** (a) True – it lies transversely across the posterior abdominal wall behind the peritoneum.

(b) False – the head is supplied by the superior and inferior pancreaticoduodenal arteries.

(c) False – the tail contacts the hilum of the spleen.

(d) True – the nerve fibres reach the pancreas by running along arteries from the coeliac and superior mesenteric plexuses.

(e) True – it drains into the ampulla of Vater.

**57.** (a) True – to neutralize gastric acid in the duodenum.

(b) False – the enzyme proportions do not vary with ingested food composition.

(c) True – this results in the concentrations of chloride and bicarbonate being reciprocal.

(d) True – as fats will not be able to be digested.

(e) False – it is called the acinus.

**58.** (a) False – they are endocrine cells which secrete somatostatin.

(b) False – they open into intralobular ducts.

(c) True – this reflects their protein-secreting function.

(d) True – these are situated in the islets of Langerhans.

(e) True – whereas the intralobular ducts are lined with cuboidal or columnar epithelium.

**59.** (a) False – about 60% occur in the head.

(b) True – 90% of patients are dead within 6 months of diagnosis.

(c) True – as the tumour may obstruct the common bile duct.

(d) True – however, no definite risk factors except smoking have been identified.

(e) True – this occurs in a gastrinoma where excess gastric acid is secreted.

60. (a) True – the pancreatic buds arise from the foregut endoderm.
    (b) False – they arise from two buds, the dorsal and the ventral.
    (c) True – these are the pancreaticosplenic nodes.
    (d) False – the common bile duct lies in a groove on the posterosuperior surface of the head.
    (e) True – it also overlies the superior mesenteric vessels and the portal vein.

61. (a) True – gallstones are present in half the cases, and alcohol causes most of the rest.
    (b) True – it is a bluish discoloration in the loins occurring a few days after a severe attack.
    (c) False – it may cause hypocalcaemia partly due to fat saponification.
    (d) True – this results from collection of necrotic material and inflammatory exudates in the lesser sac.
    (e) False – they are the main factors involved in the autodigestive process.

62. (a) True – it may occur, for example, after ERCP.
    (b) False – they are not true cysts and so do not have an epithelial lining.
    (c) False – this results in pancreas divisum.
    (d) True – the sweat will have an increased level of sodium chloride in cystic fibrosis.
    (e) False – other causes include perforated peptic ulcers and severe diabetic ketoacidosis.

# Chapter 6—The small intestine

63. (a) False – only those parts distal to the duodenal cap are retroperitoneal.
    (b) True – as it then widens the angle of the duodenojejunal flexure.
    (c) False – it will cause a macrocytic anaemia as vitamin $B_{12}$ cannot be absorbed.
    (d) True – as they are midgut derivatives.
    (e) False – drainage is mainly to the portal system.

64. (a) False – its lifespan is about 2–3 days.
    (b) False – they occur in the fasting state.
    (c) True – this prevents reflux into the small intestine.
    (d) False – the digestive enzymes in the small intestine come from the pancreas.
    (e) True – it will cause malabsorption of all nutrients due to the villous atrophy.

65. (a) True – as lactose will not be able to be absorbed.
    (b) False – it usually affects the rectum and distal large intestine.

(c) False – it is typically 2 feet from the caecum.
(d) True – due to mucosal damage.
(e) False – they are hamartomas, and hence benign.

66. (a) False – this is a common misconception.
    (b) False – they grow very slowly.
    (c) True – due to the production of 5-hydroxytryptamine (5-HT) by the tumour cells.
    (d) True – octreotide inhibits 5-HT release.
    (e) False – they are potentially malignant, but relatively benign.

67. (a) True – these are the lacteals.
    (b) False – its central location and the presence of valvulae conniventes distinguish it from the colon.
    (c) False – the small intestine is a midgut structure distal to the entry of the common bile duct.
    (d) False – most of the small intestine has a mesentery.
    (e) True – they are called Peyer's patches.

68. (a) False – they are formed by extensions of the lamina propria.
    (b) True – they are phagocytic besides containing various antimicrobial peptides.
    (c) False – they are mainly T cells.
    (d) False – they produce an acidic mucus, unlike the Brunner's glands.
    (e) True – the epithelium is continuous with that of the crypts of Lieberkühn.

69. (a) True – it is in fact increasing.
    (b) False – Crohn's disease granulomas are non-caseating, unlike tuberculous granulomas.
    (c) False – it most commonly affects those between 20 and 40 years of age.
    (d) True – typically, there is fibrosis, lymphoedema and a chronic inflammatory infiltrate.
    (e) True – this is due to mucosal ulceration and intervening oedema.

70. (a) True – among other functions, it augments the function of cholecystokinin.
    (b) True – it is regulated by the hormone motilin.
    (c) True – the reflex causes segmentation in the ileum.
    (d) True – this is known as secondary active transport.
    (e) False – vitamin $B_{12}$ requires intrinsic factor to be absorbed.

247

71. (a) False – the capillary basement membrane prevents the entry of chylomicrons.
    (b) True – when stored in the enterocyte, it is bound to ferritin.
    (c) False – it stimulates the active transport of calcium.
    (d) True – similar to the mechanism of absorption of glucose and galactose.
    (e) True – it causes Whipple's disease.

72. (a) False – it is formed by microvilli.
    (b) True – they take 100–150 minutes to reach the end of the small bowel.
    (c) False – it is segmentation which primarily mixes chyme.
    (d) True – these serve to increase its absorptive capacity.
    (e) False – they are found in the duodenum only.

## Chapter 7—The large intestine

73. (a) True – this is due to the transverse mesocolon.
    (b) True – as it is retroperitoneal and fixed to the posterior abdominal wall.
    (c) True – it is attached via the phrenicocolic ligament.
    (d) False – most cases of volvulus affect the sigmoid colon.
    (e) False – it is a voluntary sphincter, and so is made up of striated muscle.

74. (a) True – this is McBurney's point.
    (b) False – malignancies of the appendix are rare.
    (c) True – this may result in appendicitis.
    (d) True – it is called the mesoappendix.
    (e) False – the appendicular artery, which supplies the appendix, is a branch of the ileocolic artery.

75. (a) True – they occur usually after meals.
    (b) True – this causes mass movements and the urge to defecate.
    (c) False – this makes it easy to distinguish the colon from the small bowel on radiographs.
    (d) False – peristalsis occurs at a higher rate in the small intestine.
    (e) False – no digestion happens in the large intestine!

76. (a) False – the outer coat is longitudinal and the inner circular.
    (b) False – it is lined with absorptive cells.
    (c) True – they have oval basal nuclei.
    (d) False – it is a prominent feature of the colonic mucosa.
    (e) True – they continually replace the epithelium.

77. (a) False – the internal sphincter is made up of smooth muscle and so is not under voluntary control.
    (b) True – as the respiratory muscles contract on full lungs.
    (c) True – they are conveyed by the cholinergic pelvic parasympathetic nerves.
    (d) False – the pelvic floor muscles relax during defecation.
    (e) False – as the internal anal sphincter does not relax, thus causing difficulty in defecating.

78. (a) True – as opposed to distal bowel obstruction which usually causes distension.
    (b) True – as it may cause adhesions.
    (c) False – the most common type is ileo-colic, occurring in 75% of cases.
    (d) True – the strangulation will also cause gangrene if untreated.
    (e) False – this is pathognomonic of a volvulus.

79. (a) True – it lies in the right iliac fossa.
    (b) False – it lies behind the descending colon, together with the quadratus lumborum and the lateral border of the left kidney.
    (c) False – it is located at the splenic flexure.
    (d) True – this happens in the 6th week of development.
    (e) False – this occurs in the 9th week of development.

80. (a) False – these are the forms of inflammatory bowel disease.
    (b) True – it afflicts about 20% of the general population.
    (c) True – exacerbations may be brought on by stress.
    (d) False – patients are constitutionally well in spite of their symptoms.
    (e) False – management is mainly reassurance and/or symptomatic treatment; mesalazine is used in the treatment of ulcerative colitis.

81. (a) True – it is an autosomal dominant condition.
    (b) False – they cause early obstruction as the faeces are more solid.
    (c) False – it is Dukes' Stage B carcinoma which affects the lymph nodes.
    (d) True – however, the mechanism is yet to be fully explained.
    (e) False – hereditary non-polyposis colorectal cancer is much more common.

**82.** (a) True – it is caused by the bacterium *Clostridium difficile*.

(b) False – they are very rare in developing countries but common in the West.

(c) False – in the colon they decrease in incidence from left to right.

(d) False – this should never be done due to the risk of perforation.

(e) True – as the bacteria bind vitamin $B_{12}$ preventing its absorption.

**83.** (a) True – it is the anthracene derivatives in senna which do this.

(b) False – it is an osmotic laxative.

(c) False – they take several days to have an effect.

(d) True – this is due to an increased volume of fluid in the gut lumen.

(e) False – it is the stimulant purgatives which have this side-effect.

**84.** (a) True – hence it is also used as an anti-emetic.

(b) False – it has an overall constipating effect.

(c) False – this is because they have effects on other systems.

(d) True – this results in an increase in gut motility.

(e) True – but it also has side-effects such as drowsiness and dizziness.

**85.** (a) False – while they are the main method of motility, haustrations are not propulsive.

(b) True – as the contents of the colon are pushed into the rectum, distending it.

(c) False – sodium is actively absorbed but chloride follows passively down the electrical gradient.

(d) False – most bowel gas comes from swallowed air.

(e) True – it acts as a lubricant.

**86.** (a) False – it is a rare complication of ulcerative colitis.

(b) True – they are also superficial.

(c) False – they are used more often in the treatment of ulcerative colitis.

(d) False – they are found in ulcerative colitis.

(e) True – the incidence is decreased in smokers; it is the other way around in Crohn's disease.

# Chapter 8—Common presentations of gastrointestinal disease

**87.** (a) False – dysphagia is difficulty swallowing; pain with swallowing is odynophagia.

(b) True – these may cause malignant strictures.

(c) False – it responds to iron-replacement therapy.

(d) True – usually there is no weight loss as well.

(e) True – other symptoms are a lump in the neck and regurgitation of collected. food

**88.** (a) True – it accounts for 35–50% of cases.

(b) False – it takes time for haemodilution to occur; in the intervening period the haemoglobin level is normal.

(c) True – varices and cancer have the worst prognosis.

(d) False – haemorrhoids are the most common cause.

(e) True – patients usually report 'seeing blood on the toilet paper'.

**89.** (a) False – unless they undergo thrombosis.

(b) True – the pain may last up to 2 hours.

(c) True – as the pain discourages patients from defecating.

(d) True – be sure to note other symptoms which may indicate the nature of the mass as well.

(e) False – it is weak pelvic floor muscles which predispose to this.

**90.** (a) True – as the gut goes into spasm.

(b) True – if perforation is present there will be air under the diaphragm.

(c) False – it causes well-localized pain as the parietal peritoneum is supplied by somatic nerves.

(d) True – due to the embryological development of the alimentary system.

(e) True – usually over several hours.

**91.** (a) False – it is an ill-defined collective term for upper gastrointestinal tract symptoms.

(b) True – it affects up to 80% of the population at some time.

(c) True – it may be a feature of serious gastrointestinal disease.

(d) True – especially in younger patients.

(e) True – as it causes peptic ulcer disease, which is a cause of dyspepsia.

# Chapter 9 – History and examination

**92.** (a) True – along with a host of other signs.

(b) False – iron deficiency causes koilonychia.

(c) False – they have many causes, among them Crohn's disease and coeliac disease, but not chronic liver disease.

(d) False – this is Rovsing's sign.

(e) False – obstruction causes tinkling bowel sounds.

93. (a) False – apart from the general signs and symptoms of malignancy, the commonest feature is painless jaundice.
    (b) True – for example, in coeliac disease.
    (c) True – other malignancies may also cause clubbing.
    (d) False – this does not cause clubbing.
    (e) True – cirrhotic liver disease is an important cause of clubbing.

94. (a) True – it is covered by the ribcage.
    (b) True – they are called caput medusae and are due to the resulting portal hypertension.
    (c) False – it is not possible to be sure until the location of the upper border of the liver is determined.
    (d) True – although not usually done in practice!
    (e) True – it may sometimes be felt in thin patients.

95. (a) False – they are only significantly suggestive of liver disease if more than 5–6 are present.
    (b) True – they are called Kayser–Fleischer rings.
    (c) False – this is caused by tricuspid regurgitation.
    (d) False – as the gallbladder is likely to be fibrotic and so unable to expand; this is Courvoisier's law.
    (e) True – this is Virchow's node, or Troisier's sign.

96. (a) False – it is a sign of ascites.
    (b) False – aortic aneurysms are both pulsatile and expansile.
    (c) False – as many hernias regress when the patient is lying.
    (d) False – benign umbilical lesions are rare in adults; they may be a sign of metastasis from a gastrointestinal or ovarian carcinoma.
    (e) False – the patient will be taking shallow breaths as movement irritates the peritoneum causing pain.

# Chapter 10—Investigations and imaging

97. (a) True – as the infection causes hepatocellular damage causing the enzyme to leak out into the blood.
    (b) False – alcohol or cholestasis may cause this, but not $\alpha_1$-antitrypsin deficiency.
    (c) False – they are not sensitive, as alkaline phosphatase is also found in bone, intestine and placenta.
    (d) True – as it is dependent on vitamin K, which is a fat-soluble vitamin.
    (e) False – alanine aminotransferase is the more specific of the two.

98. (a) False – only about 10% are seen on plain X-rays.
    (b) False – an erect abdominal film will show fluid levels best.
    (c) True – more specifically, Crohn's disease.
    (d) True – as it has a high density of hydrogen atoms.
    (e) True – however the level of mucosal detail is poor.

99. (a) False – they are not common investigations.
    (b) True – as it causes a microcytic anaemia.
    (c) False – they are seen in bacterial infections.
    (d) False – it causes low serum copper and caeruloplasmin levels.
    (e) False – viruses are too small to be seen using light microscopy.

100. (a) False – usually only sedation is necessary.
     (b) True – for rigid sigmoidoscopy.
     (c) True – as in ERCP.
     (d) True – for example, biopsies can be taken and varices banded.
     (e) True – due to trauma during the procedure.

1. There are four pairs of intrinsic tongue muscles: transverse, vertical and superior and inferior longitudinal. The intrinsic muscles do not have attachments outside the tongue.

    The extrinsic muscles and their attachments are:

    (a) Genioglossus—mandible.
    (b) Hyoglossus—hyoid bone.
    (c) Styloglossus—styloid process.
    (d) Palatoglossus—soft palate.

    All the tongue muscles are innervated by the XIIth cranial nerve except for palatoglossus, which is innervated by fibres from the cranial root of the XIth nerve which pass through the pharyngeal branch of the vagus nerve.

---

2. The function of the gallbladder is to store and concentrate bile. Soon after the ingestion of food, the gallbladder contracts to release its contents. This happens in three stages:

    (a) In the cephalic phase, vagal stimulation to increase gallbladder emptying occurs by means of the smell and taste of food, as well as the presence of food in the mouth and pharynx.
    (b) The second phase is the gastric phase, where gastric distension stimulates similar vagal impulses.
    (c) Cholecystokinin released from the duodenum in the intestinal phase in response to products of fat digestion results in the highest rate of emptying.

---

3. The mechanisms of action, with examples, are:

    (a) Proton-pump inhibitors (PPIs) act by irreversible inhibition of the $H^+/K^+$-ATPase of gastric parietal cells (the proton pump). The proton pump is the final step in the acid secretory pathway. PPIs therefore drastically inhibit gastric acid secretion. Two examples of PPIs are omeprazole (the first PPI) and lansoprazole.
    (b) Antacids neutralize gastric acid, and therefore raise the gastric pH. They thus inhibit peptic activity. Two common antacids are magnesium hydroxide and aluminium hydroxide. Because magnesium salts cause diarrhoea and aluminium salts cause constipation, mixtures of both are usually used to ensure normal bowel function.

---

4. Porto-systemic anastomoses occur at four places:

    (a) Between oesophageal veins which drain into the left gastric vein (portal) or the azygos vein (systemic).
    (b) Between para-umbilical veins (portal) and the small epigastric veins of the anterior abdominal wall (systemic).
    (c) Between the superior rectal vein (portal) and the middle and inferior rectal veins (systemic).
    (d) Between colic veins (portal) and retroperitoneal veins (systemic).

    The anastomoses may dilate if the flow of venous blood through the liver is obstructed by cirrhosis, or if the portal vein is obstructed, e.g. by a thrombus.

---

5. See Fig. 2.13 for a diagram of a salivon.

    The main electrolytes in saliva are $Na^+$, $K^+$, $Cl^-$ and $HCO_3^-$. While the concentrations of $Na^+$ and $Cl^-$ are hypotonic with respect to plasma, they increase with flow rate. $K^+$ and $HCO_3^-$ concentrations are hypertonic with respect to plasma. However, the concentration of $K^+$ is more or less constant, while that of $HCO_3^-$ increases, plateauing at a salivary flow rate of around 2 mL/min. Refer to Fig. 2.3 for a diagrammatic representation of the above.

---

6. Generally, there are three types of gallstones:

    (a) Cholesterol stones (20%), which have greasy yellow surfaces. They may occur as a single stone, two stones joined together, or a cluster.
    (b) Bile pigment stones (5%), which are small, black and multiple. They are amorphous and fragile.
    (c) Mixed stones (75%), which comprise both cholesterol and pigment. They are multiple and faceted, the cut surface showing alternating dark and light concentric rings of pigment and cholesterol respectively.

    Some 80% of gallstones are asymptomatic, but if they impact in the common bile duct then biliary pain, jaundice and cholangitis may manifest. Impaction in the cystic duct will cause biliary pain without jaundice.

---

7. 'Intestinal atresia' refers to the failure of the intestine to canalize. It is most common in the duodenum, although it can occur anywhere in the gastrointestinal tract. There are a number of causes for this phenomenon, for instance gastroschisis and malrotation may occur in the distal duodenum, or the proximal duodenum may fail to recanalize.

    Atresia causes total obstruction. If, as occurs in malrotation and gastroschisis, the blood supply to a section of intestine is cut off, that part will undergo necrosis. Patients with intestinal atresia may have imperforate anuses.

---

8. Both parietal and chief cells are found in the gastric glands. However, chief cells are located deeper than parietal cells in the glands. They secrete pepsinogen, which is the inactive precursor of the enzyme pepsin, while the parietal cells secrete hydrochloric acid and intrinsic factor, which is needed for vitamin $B_{12}$ absorption.

In terms of ultrastructure, chief cells have many mitochondria, rough endoplasmic reticula and Golgi bodies, which reflect their protein-secreting role. Parietal cells have fewer Golgi bodies and rough endoplasmic reticula, but are also rich in mitochondria as acid production requires much energy. They have a 'fried egg' appearance due to their central nuclei.

9. Bile acids have five main roles:
   (a) Transport of lipids—by forming micelles with the products of fat digestion and facilitating transport to the brush border.
   (b) Induction of bile flow—because they attract water and electrolytes by osmosis as they are secreted.
   (c) Triglyceride assimilation—bile acids emulsify lipids, providing a larger surface area for the action of lipases. This is done with the help of lecithin.
   (d) Regulation of bile acid synthesis—when they are absorbed from the bowel, the synthesis of more bile acids in the liver is inhibited.
   (e) Water and electrolyte secretion—this occurs when they are present in the large intestine.

10. A number of congenital abnormalities may affect the pancreas. An annular pancreas results when migration of the ventral pancreatic bud around the back of the duodenum is incomplete, or when migration occurs in the wrong direction. This may cause constriction or obstruction of the duodenum. If fusion of the buds does not occur, the condition is called pancreas divisum.

Occasionally, ectopic pancreatic tissue is found, for instance in gastric mucosa. It may produce normal pancreatic secretions. In addition to the conditions above, the pancreas may be incompletely developed (hypoplasia), or there may be agenesis.

11. Liver function tests (LFTs) assay the serum levels of the following: aminotransferases (alanine aminotransferase and aspartate aminotransferase), γ-glutamyltransferase, alkaline phosphatase, albumin and bilirubin.

The prothrombin time is said to be a 'true' LFT because it indicates how well the liver is synthesizing clotting factors (a measure of the synthetic function of the liver) and therefore a prolonged prothrombin time indicates liver dysfunction. Note, however, that the prothrombin time may be increased by vitamin K

deficiency, in which case vitamin K should be given to the patient and the test repeated after at least 18 hours. In contrast to the prothrombin time, assays for hepatic enzymes will show liver damage but not the actual functioning of the liver.

12. The main causes of acute pancreatitis are gallstones, alcohol, trauma, steroids, mumps, autoimmunity, scorpion bites, hyperlipidaemia, hypercalcaemia, hypothermia, post-ERCP, post-operation and drugs, for example azathioprine. Other causes are carcinoma of the pancreas, malignant hypertension, cholesterol emboli and polyarteritis nodosa.

It is diagnosed by means of serum amylase levels. A marked increase (five times or more) is indicative. However, some other conditions also cause a drastic increase in sereum amylase levels, for example renal failure and severe diabetic ketoacidosis so it is unwise to rely on serum amylase levels alone.

Grey Turner's sign may occur in acute pancreatitis because the released pancreatic enzymes digest blood vessel walls causing extravasation of blood and hence the discoloration of the flanks.

13. Achalasia is a rare neuromuscular condition where the lower end of the oesophagus fails to relax. There is spasm of the lower oesophageal sphincter and uncoordinated peristalsis. As a result, the oesophagus progressively dilates, and the upper region often undergoes hypertrophy. The patient will have progressive dysphagia, and regurgitation of oesophageal contents may cause an aspiration pneumonia.

The disorder is most common in the third decade, although it may occur at any age. It is more common in females, with a female-to-male ratio of 3:2. Chagas' disease, in which the trypanosomes destroy the intrinsic plexuses of the oesophagus, is a cause, although its other causes are unknown.

Diagnostic investigations include barium swallow, which shows a beak deformity, oesophagoscopy and oesophageal manometry. Treatment is with Heller's cardiomyotomy.

14. A urea breath test is used for the non-invasive diagnosis of gastric infection with the bacterium *Helicobacter pylori*. The test is simple to perform. Because *H. pylori* produces urease, it is able to convert urea into carbon dioxide and ammonia, which allows it to neutralize gastric acid. The test therefore involves patients being given radioactively labelled urea ($^{13}C$ or $^{14}C$). If *H. pylori* is present, the resulting carbon dioxide will be radioactive, and this is detected in the breath sample.

15. Most of the carbohydrate ingested is in the form of starch, which is a polymer of glucose. The glucose residues in starch are linked by α-1,4 and α-1,6

glycosidic linkages. Digestion of carbohydrates begins in the mouth, where salivary amylase (ptyalin) breaks some of the $\alpha$-1,4 bonds, resulting in a mixture of malto-oligosaccharides and $\alpha$-limit dextrans. In the stomach, carbohydrate digestion stops temporarily as gastric acid inactivates ptyalin.

In the duodenum, bicarbonate secreted by the pancreas neutralizes the acidity of the stomach contents, and pancreatic amylase continues carbohydrate digestion. Maltase and isomaltase found at the duodenal brush border complete the digestion of starch into its constituent glucose units. Other saccharides like lactose and sucrose are also digested here. The end-products of carbohydrate digestion are the monosaccharides glucose, galactose and fructose, which are then absorbed.

Cellulose, like starch, is a polymer of glucose. We are not able to digest cellulose because the glucose residues are linked by $\beta$-1,4 glycosidic bonds, for which we do not have the necessary enzymes to hydrolyse.

---

16. With regard to this patient:
    (a) The likely diagnosis is carcinoma of the head of the pancreas.
    (b) The diagnosis may be justified as follows. The tumour is obstructing the common bile duct. This causes leakage of conjugated bilirubin into the blood, resulting in dark urine. The faeces are pale because of the lack of stercobilinogen. His lethargy and severe weight loss are suggestive of carcinoma, as does the fact that the jaundice is painless, which makes it very unlikely to have been caused by gallstones.
    (c) Ultrasound and CT are usually sufficient to confirm the diagnosis of pancreatic carcinoma in a patient presenting with obstructive jaundice, such as this man. Biopsy is another option, as is ERCP.

---

17. With regard to this patient:
    (a) Ulcerative colitis is the most likely diagnosis.
    (b) Pharmacological treatment for ulcerative colitis consists of 5-aminosalicylates or sulfasalazine. Additionally, some patients may need corticosteroids such as prednisolone, or immunosuppressants such as azathioprine. Surgery is curative for this condition.

---

18. With regard to this patient:
    (a) I would request serological testing for hepatitis B surface antigen and e antigen for hepatitis B infection, as well as for anti-hepatitis C virus.

The polymerase chain reaction may also be used to test for infection with the hepatitis C virus.
    (b) I would advise them of the way the viruses spread (sexual contact, infected blood and vertical transmission from mother to baby), and, based on that, advise them against activities that might pose a risk to others. Additionally I would advise them of the need for contact tracing so that appropriate measures, e.g. vaccination of contacts, can be carried out.

---

19. With regard to this patient:
    (a) The patient has haemochromatosis. The disease is caused by a defective gene on chromosome 6 which causes excessive absorption of iron from the small intestine. This occurs even when transferrin, which binds iron, is saturated. The iron is deposited in the liver, pancreas, heart and also in other organs to a much lesser extent.
    (b) Biochemical testing on blood samples will show a raised ferritin level. If a liver biopsy is performed, the hepatocytes will be rich in haemosiderin, reflecting the excessive accumulation of iron. Liver function tests may be deranged.
    (c) Haemochromatosis is treated by venesection once or twice weekly to get the iron levels down to normal, after which it is done three or four times a year. If venesection cannot be done, for instance in an anaemic patient, chelation therapy, e.g. with desferrioxamine, is a viable alternative.

---

20. Concerning the features of cholera:
    (a) The organism which causes cholera is *Vibrio cholerae*. It is spread via the faecal–oral route.
    (b) Once the small intestine is successfully colonized by *V. cholerae*, the bacteria produce cholera toxin. This is an enterotoxin which binds to receptors on the immature cells of the crypts of Lieberkühn and causes an increase in intracellular adenylate cyclase levels, which in turn increases cyclic AMP. Consequently, there is an increase in the secretion of sodium, chloride and water into the gut lumen, which manifests itself as secretory diarrhoea.
    (c) Oral rehydration therapy to replace water and electrolytes is curative.

## 1. Abdominal pain.

1. H  Obstruction. The tinkling bowel sounds are diagnostic. The obstruction is likely to be higher up in the alimentary tract as there was vomiting (which caused the dehydration) and the abdomen was only slightly distended. Her past history of gastro-oesophageal reflux disease is a red herring!

2. D  Appendicitis. The location of the pain, as well as the fact that it changed from being central to localized in the right iliac fossa (as the peritoneum surrounding the appendix becomes inflamed) is characteristic of acute appendicitis. The examination findings are also typical.

3. I  Sigmoid volvulus. The patient fits the demographic stereotype for sigmoid volvulus— he is old, male and constipated. The constipation is the most likely cause, as it results in overloading of the sigmoid colon causing it to twist.

4. J  Acute bowel ischaemia. The onset and severity of the pain are indicative, among others, of acute intestinal ischaemia. The absent bowel sounds, as well as the collapse (due to hypovolaemic shock) are diagnostic.

5. B  Acute pancreatitis. This is a classical description of acute pancreatitis caused by overconsumption of alcohol. The severe epigastric pain radiating to the back and guarding are typical features.

## 2. Pharmacology of the gastrointestinal system.

1. I  Hyoscine. Hyoscine, a muscarinic-receptor blocker, is the first-choice drug for motion sickness and acts on the vomiting centre and nucleus tractus solitarius. The other anti-emetic in the list, ondansetron, acts on the chemoreceptor trigger zone and is not effective against motion sickness but is used to treat vomiting caused by cytotoxic drugs.

2. J  Ranitidine. This is an $H_2$-receptor antagonist, and is older than the proton-pump inhibitors, which are the first-line drugs in peptic ulcer disease now. The relapse of symptoms after stopping the drug is characteristic.

3. C  Sodium picosulphate. Sodium picosulphate (Picolax) is a stimulant laxative. It increases secretion of mucus and water by stimulating enteric nerves, thus encouraging evacuation of bowel contents. It is commonly used to prepare the bowel for surgery.

4. H  Misoprostol. This is a prostaglandin analogue, and thus has mucosa-protective properties. It is therefore necessary for this patient, as she is at increased risk for gastrointestinal ulceration given her history of peptic ulcer disease and the fact that she needs to be on indometacin (non-steroidal anti-inflammatory drugs are a risk factor for peptic ulceration).

5. G  Loperamide. The side-effects described are characteristic of those for loperamide. They are due to the opioid action of the drug. Loperamide also has anti-secretory effects. It should not be used in young children.

## 3. Neoplasms of the gastrointestinal tract.

1. E  Gastric carcinoma. The palpable node in the left supraclavicular fossa (Virchow's node) is characteristic of gastric carcinoma. The location of the abdominal pain is suggestive of a gastric lesion, while the non-specific weight loss is an indication that the patient may have cancer.

2. J  Hepatocellular carcinoma. The most likely cause is progression of the patient's hepatitis B. The jaundice should make you think of a hepatobiliary cause.

3. F  Oesophageal carcinoma. Dysphagia is indicative of an oesophageal or upper gastric lesion. Hoarseness of the voice suggests that the tumour has invaded the left recurrent laryngeal nerve.

4. D  Peutz–Jeghers syndrome. This is an autosomal dominant condition where numerous polyps are found in the alimentary tract. These may bleed, as in this case. The skin pigmentation is characteristic; it may also be found around the mouth.

5. C  Pancreatic carcinoma. Painless progressive jaundice is a sign of carcinoma of the head of the pancreas. The mass felt in the right upper quadrant is not the tumour, but rather the swollen gallbladder, as the tumour compresses the common bile duct, obstructing it.

## 4. Malabsorption syndromes.

1. E  Whipple's disease. This is caused by the bacterium *Tropheryma whipplei* and usually occurs in men over 50. The appearance on jejunal biopsy is diagnostic. The man should be treated with tetracycline.

2. F  Giardiasis. The protozoon *Giardia lamblia* is endemic in the tropics and is a cause of traveller's diarrhoea, although some carriers may show no symptoms. The kite-shaped forms are the trophozoites.

3. D  Bacterial overgrowth. This usually occurs if a structural abnormality is present in the intestine, but may also occur in the elderly. Vitamin K levels may be high as the bacteria produce it. The hydrogen breath test is diagnostic.

4. A  Coeliac disease. This is caused by an abnormal reaction to gluten in wheat, and in children may present as failure to thrive. Small intestine biopsy shows short, stumpy villi (villous atrophy).

5. G  Tropical sprue. Tropical sprue is an infectious condition, although the exact organism is unknown. Endemic areas include parts of Asia and the Carribean. Treatment is with broad-spectrum antibiotics, e.g. tetracycline.

## 5. Dysphagia.

1. B  Pharyngeal pouch. This is an oesophageal diverticulum, occurring most commonly in Killian's dehiscence, the weak area between the thyropharyngeus and cricopharyngeus muscles. The recurrent pneumonia and the gurgling swelling in her neck are characteristic.

2. G  Oesophageal web. This is associated with the Plummer–Vinson syndrome, which comprises dysphagia and iron-deficiency anaemia. The fact that the lady has iron-deficiency anaemia is evident from the results of her full blood count.

3. A  Achalasia. The cause of this condition is unknown. It is a neuromuscular failure of the lower part of the oesophagus. Chest infection may be caused by regurgitation of food and fluid from the dilated upper part. The tapering deformity seen on barium swallow is characteristic.

4. C  Congenital oesophageal atresia. This is common, occurring in 1 in 200 births. It is easily diagnosed as the infant has difficulty swallowing. Polyhydramnios may be a sign that the fetus has congenital atresia, as it cannot swallow amniotic fluid.

5. D  Inflammatory stricture. This is a complication of gastro-oesophageal reflux disease, due to gastric acid damaging the oesophageal mucosa. Treatment is surgical.

## 6. Diarrhoea.

1. C  Ulcerative colitis. The symptoms mentioned are typical, and the histological findings characteristic. Females are affected more than males.

2. H  Cholera. This is caused by the bacterium *Vibrio cholerae*. The 'rice-water' diarrhoea is characteristic. The bacterium produces a toxin, which binds to cellular receptors in the crypts of Lieberkühn, causing a rise in adenylate cyclase and cyclic AMP, which in turn causes increased secretion into the gut lumen.

3. G  Viral gastroenteritis. A number of viruses can cause this, e.g. astroviruses, noroviruses, caliciviruses, rotaviruses and adenoviruses. Raw shellfish is one of the modes of transmission for the first three.

4. E  Pseudomembranous colitis. This occurs when the normal intestinal flora is suppressed, e.g. on administration of broad-spectrum antibiotics, hence the caution against giving elderly people cephalosporins. The causative organism is *Clostridium difficile*. The surface of the colon is coated with a whitish pseudomembrane, hence the name.

5. F  Disaccharidase deficiency. The symptoms are typical of lactase deficiency, which is commoner in Oriental, African and Mediterranean populations than in Caucasian ones. The undigested lactose causes an osmotic diarrhoea.

## 7. Intestinal obstruction.

1. E  Adhesions. These are connections between two parts of the bowel which are normally separate. Most adhesions are a complication of abdominal surgery, but other inflammatory conditions such as peritonitis and endometriosis may also cause them. The obstruction is due to external constriction.

2. C  Inguinal hernia. The groin lump and the history of heavy lifting are suggestive of a hernia. Confirmation is obtained if the lump moves when the patient coughs. The pyrexia, tachycardia and continuous pain indicate that the hernia is strangulated.

3. A  Stricture. This is a recognized complication of Crohn's disease, and may obstruct the bowel.

4. G  Intussusception. This occurs when a segment of intestine prolapses into an adjacent segment, usually precipitated by a mass projecting into the lumen being pushed along the intestine. It is most common in early childhood. The passage of 'redcurrant jelly' stools is suggestive.

5. H  Malignancy. Tiredness, weight loss, cachexia and loss of appetite are symptoms suggestive of malignancy and should always be investigated thoroughly. Colonoscopy should be requested for this patient.

## 8. Liver pathology.

1. A   Haemochromatosis. This is an autosomal recessive disorder. Signs and symptoms are caused by the absorption of excess iron. It usually occurs in men over the age of 40, who often complain of loss of libido.

2. G   Gilbert's syndrome. This is a congenital disorder caused by insufficient UDP-glucuronyltransferase. Serum unconjugated bilirubin levels are mildly increased and hepatic jaundice occurs as a result.

3. B   Hepatitis B infection. Infection with the hepatitis B virus in the developed world is usually due to high-risk activities like intravenous drug use or unprotected homosexual sex. The symptoms are non-specific, but the examination findings and investigation results are suggestive. Serology should be performed.

4. E   Portal hypertension. The haematemesis is probably due to ruptured oesophageal varices, which are a site of a porto-systemic anastomosis, as are the veins around the umbilicus (caput medusae). Splenomegaly is another sign of portal hypertension.

5. C   Hepatitis A infection. This is spread via the faecal–oral route from consuming contaminated food or water. The incubation period is 2–3 weeks, and the illness does not become chronic or result in a carrier state.

## 9. Gastro-oesophageal disorders.

1. B   Type B gastritis. This usually begins in the antrum, but may spread to other parts of the stomach. Besides fibrosis, atrophy and metaplasia may ensue.

2. A   Hypertrophic pyloric stenosis. The disorder is caused by hypertrophy of the pyloric circular smooth muscle, which obstructs the flow of gastric contents into the duodenum, thus causing vomiting. Peristaltic waves may be visible, and a sausage-shaped mass felt in the right upper quadrant.

3. I   Mallory–Weiss tear. This is a tear at the gastro-oesophageal junction, and may be fatal if the patient is not resuscitated adequately. Prolonged vomiting and coughing lead to sustained increases in intra-abdominal pressure, causing the tear.

4. D   Peptic ulcer disease. Peptic ulcers are lesions occurring where gastric acid and pepsin are present, i.e. the stomach and duodenum. *Helicobacter pylori* infection is seen in 95% of duodenal ulcers and 80% of gastric ulcers. Gastric hyperacidity, acid reflux and smoking are other risk factors.

5. J   Gastro-oesophageal reflux disease. Besides poor lower oesophageal sphincter tone, increased intra-abdominal pressure, hiatus hernia and delayed gastric emptying are other risk factors for this condition. Prolonged reflux may cause metaplasia of the cells of the lower oesophagus and lead to malignant change.

## 10. Intestinal disorders.

1. C   Irritable bowel syndrome. This is a common disorder which affects more women than men. Diagnosis is obtained by exclusion of other conditions. Other symptoms include tenesmus, changes in bowel habit and urgency.

2. D   Hirschsprung's disease. Absence of ganglion cells in Meissner's and Auerbach's plexus is the cause of this disease. It is seen more often in males. Severely obstructed cases will be apparent soon after birth, with less severe cases presenting with chronic constipation.

3. A   Crohn's disease. This is a common disease in the West, particularly in white people. It may affect anywhere in the gastrointestinal tract, and the distribution of ulcers is patchy ('skip lesions'). The aphthous ulcers are suggestive.

4. F   Infective enterocolitis. The cause may be bacterial or viral. Treatment is symptomatic, with fluid replacement essential to prevent dehydration. If a bacterial cause is suspected, antibiotics should be given.

5. H   Diverticulitis. This is inflammation of diverticula. The presentation may be similar to that of appendicitis, except that the pain is localized in the left iliac fossa instead of the right. Radiographs should be taken to exclude perforation, which is an emergency.

**achalasia** A condition in which the lower oesophageal sphincter goes into spasm and there is loss of coordinated peristalsis in the lower oesophagus.

**achlorhydria** Absence of gastric hydrochloric acid.

**acinus** A general definition is a sac or cavity surrounded by secretory cells of a gland. See individual chapters for more specialized definitions.

**ascites** accumulation of fluid in the peritoneal cavity.

**asterixis** A flapping tremor seen in liver disease or carbon dioxide retention when the hands are outstretched.

**atresia** Congenital absence of a duct or opening.

**borborygmi** Bowel sounds.

**cachexia** Abnormally low weight with a wasted appearance and weakness, usually seen in chronic disease, e.g. malignancy.

**cholangiocarcinoma** Carcinoma of the bile ducts.

**cholangitis** Inflammation of the bile ducts.

**cholelithiasis** Gallstone disease.

**cirrhosis** A condition in which the liver undergoes nodular fibrosis in response to injury and/or cell death. A number of complications may ensue, including liver failure and portal hypertension.

**dysentery** An infection of the gut causing severe bloody, mucoid diarrhoea.

**endoscopy** Any investigation using an instrument (an endoscope) to view the inside of a body cavity, e.g. the gut. Examples include gastroscopy, proctoscopy and colonoscopy.

**ERCP** Endoscopic retrograde cholangiopancreatography, a radiological diagnostic or therapeutic technique in which the pancreatic duct and bile ducts are visualized by passing a catheter through a duodenoscope into the ampulla of Vater and injecting a radio-opaque dye into the biliary tract. See also MRCP.

**faecaliths** Small, hard masses of faeces which may cause obstruction, e.g. of the appendix.

**fistula** An abnormal connection between two epithelium-lined surfaces, e.g. the gut and the bladder.

**glossitis** Inflammation of the tongue.

**haustra** The pouches on the external surface of the colon.

**melaena** Faeces which are black and tarry due to the presence of partly digested blood originating from higher up the alimentary tract.

**mesentery** A double layer of peritoneum which attaches an organ, or part of an organ, to the posterior abdominal wall and confers motility. Not all abdominal organs have mesenteries.

**MRCP** Magnetic resonance cholangiopancreatography, a radiological diagnostic technique using magnetic resonance imaging to visualize the pancreatic duct and bile ducts. Unlike ERCP, it is not invasive and cannot be used for therapeutic purposes. See also ERCP.

**omentum** A double layer of peritoneum attaching the stomach to other abdominal organs, e.g. the liver and large intestine. There are two omenta, the greater omentum and the lesser omentum.

**plicae circulares** Circular folds in the small intestine which extend across its entire width and are visible on radiographs. Also known as valvulae conniventes or Kerckring's valves.

**porta hepatis** The opening on the visceral surface of the liver through which its associated nerves and vessels (hepatic artery, portal vein, hepatic ducts and lymphatics) pass.

**portosystemic anastomosis** A connection between the hepatic portal and systemic venous systems. They are not significant except in portal hypertension, in which they may distend and possibly bleed.

**pseudocyst** A fluid-filled sac which is not covered by epithelium, e.g. a pancreatic pseudocyst (cf. a true cyst, which has an epithelial lining).

**salivon** The basic unit of a salivary gland.

**stenosis** An abnormal narrowing of a tube or opening.

**stomatitis** Ulceration of the oral mucosal surface.

**tenesmus** The sensation of incomplete evacuation of the bowels, especially after defecation.

**volvulus** Twisting of part of the intestine, which may lead to infarction or obstruction.

Page numbers in *italics* refer to figures and tables.

# A

abdomen
    acute, 185–6, *189*
    auscultation, 207–8, *209*
    distension, 184, *185*
    examination, 203–8, *206*
    imaging, 219
    pain, 184–6, *186*
    palpation, 205–7, *208*
    percussion, 207, *208*
abetalipoproteinaemia, 143, 150
abscesses
    crypt, 169
    liver, 98–9
    rectal, 174
absorption
    large intestine, 158
    small intestine, 6
accessory pancreatic duct of Santorini, 110
acetaldehyde dehydrogenase, 60
acetylcholine
    gastric secretion, 51, 53
    motility
        large intestine, 159
        small intestine, 137
    salivation, 15
*N*-acetylcysteine, 77
achalasia, 37, 181
achlorhydria, 47, 216
aciclovir, 30
acini
    liver, 70, 74
    pancreas, 110, *110,* 111
    salivary glands, 25, *27*
acquired megacolon, 163
'acquired pedicle,' 17
acute abdomen, 185–6, *189*
adenoids (pharyngeal tonsils), 28
adenoma
    bowel, 177
    hepatocellular, 94
    pancreatic, 61
    salivary glands, 31
    stomach, 62
    Zollinger–Ellison syndrome, 57, 61, 142, 216
adenosine triphosphate (ATP), 7
adhesions, post-inflammatory scarring, 172

adrenocorticotrophic hormone (ACTH), 178
AIDS, 30, 35
alcohol, 51, 77
    caution, metronidazole, 60
    gastritis, 59
    intake, history-taking, 199–200, *200*
    metabolism, 60, *101*
    pancreatitis, 117–18
alcoholic cirrhosis, 102, 105
alcoholic hepatitis, 100–2
alcoholic liver disease, *100,* 100–2
alginic acid, 53
alkaline phosphatase, 214
allergies, history-taking, 198–9
alpha$_1$-antitrypsin, 93, 214
alpha-fetoprotein, 214
alpha-interferon, 98
amino acids
    appetite regulation, 13
    protein synthesis, 7–8
    transamination, 76
amino precursor uptake and decarboxylation cells,
    48, 132, 178
5-aminosalicylic acid (5-ASA), 169
aminotransferases, 76, 214
ammonia, 76, 90
amoebic dysentery, 164–5
amphotericin, 30
ampulla of Vater, 108, 109, 110, 119, 120, 125–6
amylase
    pancreatic, *113,* 114, 117, 139
    salivary, 16, 139
anaemia, 148
    haemolytic, 88, 123
    macrocytic, 59, 144
    megaloblastic, 148
    pernicious, 50, 59, 76, 99, 144
anal canal, *154,* 156
    defaecation control, 160
    mucosa, 157
anal columns, 156
anal cushions, 176
anal fissure, 187, 189
anal mass, 191, *194*
anal papillae, 191
anal sphincter, *5, 154,* 156, 162, 194
    innervation, 156–7
angiodysplasia, 62, 176
angiography, 220

# M